WENNER-GREN CENTER
INTERNATIONAL SYMPOSIUM SERIES

VOLUME 32

CENTRAL NERVOUS
CONTROL MECHANISMS
IN BREATHING

Already published in this series:

CENTRAL NERVOUS CONTROL MECHANISMS IN BREATHING

Physiological and Clinical Aspects of Regular, Periodic and Irregular Breathing in Adults and in the Perinatal Period

Proceedings of the International Symposium
held at
The Wenner-Gren Center, Stockholm
September 4-6, 1978

Edited by

Curt von Euler

Nobel Institute for Neurophysiology, Karolinska Institute, Stockholm, Sweden

and

Hugo Lagercrantz

Department of Physiology, Karolinska Institute and Department of Pediatrics, Karolinska Hospital, Stockholm, Sweden

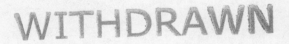

PERGAMON PRESS

OXFORD · NEW YORK · TORONTO · SYDNEY · PARIS · FRANKFURT

U.K.	Pergamon Press Ltd., Headington Hill Hall, Oxford OX3 0BW, England
U.S.A.	Pergamon Press Inc., Maxwell House, Fairview Park, Elmsford, New York 10523, U.S.A.
CANADA	Pergamon of Canada, Suite 104, 150 Consumers Road, Willowdale, Ontario M2J 1P9, Canada
AUSTRALIA	Pergamon Press (Aust.) Pty. Ltd., P.O. Box 544, Potts Point, N.S.W. 2011, Australia
FRANCE	Pergamon Press SARL, 24 rue des Ecoles, 75240 Paris, Cedex 05, France
FEDERAL REPUBLIC OF GERMANY	Pergamon Press GmbH, 6242 Kronberg-Taunus, Pferdstrasse 1, Federal Republic of Germany

First edition 1979

British Library Cataloguing in Publication Data

Central nervous control mechanisms in breathing.
(Wenner-Gren Center. International symposium series; 32).
1. Respiration - Regulation - Congresses
I. Euler, Curt von II. Lagercrantz, Hugo
III. Series
612'.21   QP123   79-40862
ISBN 0-08-024942-6

In order to make this volume available as economically and as rapidly as possible the authors' typescripts have been reproduced in their original forms. This method unfortunately has its typographical limitations but it is hoped that they in no way distract the reader.

*Printed and bound in Great Britain by
William Clowes (Beccles) Limited, Beccles and London*

CONTENTS

B. DRIVE MECHANISMS IN FETUSES AND NEONATES

SESSION II
GENERATION AND REGULATION OF PATTERN OF BREATHING
A. BASIC MECHANISMS IN THE ADULT ORGANISM

CONTRIBUTORS AND INVITED PARTICIPANTS

P.O.Åstrand
Department of Physiology III
Karolinska Institutet
Stockholm, Sweden

A.L.Bianchi
Département de Physiologie
Université de Droit, d'Economie
et des Sciences d'Aix-Marseille
Marseille, France

H.Bjurstedt
Department of Environmental
Medicine
Karolinska Institutet
Stockholm, Sweden

E.N.Bruce
Nobel Institute for Neuro-
physiology
Karolinska Institutet
Stockholm, Sweden

A.C.Bryan
Department of Respiratory
Physiology
Hospital for Sick Children
Toronto, Ontario, Canada

M.H.Bryan
Department of Respiratory
Physiology
Hospital for Sick Children
Toronto, Ontario, Canada

N.S.Cherniack
Pulmonary Division
Veterans Administration Hospital
Cleveland, Ohio, USA

M.I.Cohen
Department of Physiology
Albert Einstein College of
Medicine of Yeshiva University
Bronx, N.Y., USA

D.J.C.Cunningham
University Laboratory of
Physiology
Oxford, England

G.S.Dawes
Nuffield Institute for Medical
Research
Oxford, England

J.A.Dempsey
Department of Preventive Medicine
University of Wisconsin
Madison, Wisconsin, USA

M.Denavit-Saubié
Département de Neurophysiologie
Appliquée
C.N.R.S.-L.P.N. 1
Gif-sur-Yvette, France

B.Duron
Laboratoire de Neurophysiologie
Université de Picardie à Amiens
Amiens, France

F.L.Eldridge
Department of Physiology
University of North Carolina
Chapel Hill, N.C., USA

C. von Euler
Nobel Institute for Neuro-
physiology
Karolinska Institutet
Stockholm, Sweden

J.L.Feldman
Department of Physiology
Albert Einstein College of
Medicine of Yeshiva University
Bronx, N.Y., USA

B.Frankenhaeuser
Nobel Institute for Neuro-
physiology
Karolinska Institutet
Stockholm, Sweden

H.Gautier
Laboratoire de Physiologie
Faculté de Médecine Saint-Antoine
Paris, France

G.Gennser
Department of Obstetrics and
Gynaecology
Allmänna Sjukhuset
Malmö, Sweden

M.Głogowska
Laboratory of Neurophysiology
Polish Academy of Sciences
Medical Research Centre
Warszawa, Poland

L.Granholm
Clinics of Neurosurgery
Karolinska Sjukhuset
Stockholm, Sweden

R.Granit
Nobel Institute for Neuro-
physiology
Karolinska Institutet
Stockholm, Sweden

A.Grassino
Department of Physiology
McGill University
Montreal, Quebec, Canada

S.Grillner
Department of Physiology III
Karolinska Institutet
Stockholm, Sweden

F.S.Grodins
Biomedical Engineering
University of Southern
California
Los Angeles, Calif., USA

A.Guz
Department of Medicine
Charing Cross Hospital
Medical School
London, England

R.Harding
Nuffield Institute for Medical
Research
Oxford, England

M.K.S.Hathorn
London Hospital Medical
College
London, England

C.M.Hesser
Department of Environmental
Medicine
Karolinska Institutet
Stockholm, Sweden

A.Holmgren
Department of Clinical Physiology
Clinics of Thoracic Medicine and
Surgery
Karolinska Sjukhuset
Stockholm, Sweden

I.Homma
Department of Physiology
The Jikei University
Tokyo, Japan

T.Hukuhara
Department of Pharmacology
The Jikei University
Tokyo, Japan

P.Johnson
Nuffield Institute for Medical
Research
Oxford, England

M.Kalia
Department of Physiology and
Biophysics
Hahnemann Medical College &
Hospital of Philadelphia
Philadelphia, Pa., USA

F.F.Kao
Department of Physiology
State University of New York
Downstate Medical Center
Brooklyn, N.Y., USA

W.A.Karczewski
Laboratory of Neurophysiology
Polish Academy of Sciences
Medical Research Centre
Warszawa, Poland

P.Karlberg
Department of Pediatrics
Östra Sjukhuset
Göteborg, Sweden

M.Katz-Salamon
Nobel Institute for Neuro-
physiology
Karolinska Institutet
Stockholm, Sweden

G.W.King
Department of Physiology
Medical School
University of Minnesota
Minneapolis, Minnesota, USA

C.K.Knox
Department of Physiology
Medical School
University of Minnesota
Minneapolis, Minnesota, USA

H.P.Koepchen
Physiologisches Institut der
Freien Universität Berlin
Berlin,BRD

H.Lagercrantz
Department of Physiology
Karolinska Institutet
Stockholm, Sweden

S.Lahiri
Institute for Environmental
Medicine
University of Pennsylvania
Philadelphia, Pa., USA

D.Linnarsson
Department of Clinical
Physiology
Karolinska Sjukhuset
Stockholm, Sweden

J.Lipski
Department of Physiology
Medical Faculty
Warszawa, Poland

H.H.Loeschcke
Institut für Physiologie
Ruhr-Universität Bochum
Bochum-Querenburg, BRD

E.Lugaresi
Clinica delle Malattie Nervose
e Mentali della Università di
Bologna
Bologna, Italy

S.Majcherczyk
Department of Physiology
Institute of Physiological
Sciences
Medical Academy
Warszawa, Poland

I.Marttila-Löwgren
Nobel Institute for Neuro-
physiology
Karolinska Institutet
Stockholm, Sweden

E.G.Merrill
Department of Anatomy and
Embryology
University College London
London, England

J.Milic-Emili
Department of Physiology
McIntyre Medical Building
McGill University
Montreal, Quebec, Canada

F.Paleček
Department of Pathophysiology
Charles University
Faculty of Pediatrics
Prag, Czechoslovakia

P.L.Parmeggiani
Istituto di Fisiologia Umana
Università di Bologna
Bologna, Italy

B.Pernow
Department of Clinical Physiology
Karolinska Sjukhuset
Stockholm, Sweden

E.S.Petersen
University Laboratory of
Physiology
Oxford, England

H.F.R.Prechtl
Department of Developmental
Neurology
University Hospital
Groningen, Netherlands

M.J.Purves
Department of Physiology
School of Veterinary Science
University of Bristol
Bristol, England

J.E.Remmers
Department of Physiology
University of Texas Medical
Branch
Galveston, Texas, USA

D.W.Richter
Physiologisches Institut der
Universität
Heidelberg, BRD

H.Rigatto
Health Sciences Center
Winnipeg, Manitoba, Canada

G.Rooth
Laboratory of Neonatal Research
Clinics of Obstetrics and
Gynaecology
Akademiska Sjukhuset
Uppsala, Sweden

M.E.Schlaefke
Institut für Physiologie
Ruhr-Universität Bochum
Bochum-Querenburg, BRD

T.A.Sears
Sobell Department of Neuro-
physiology
The National Hospital
London, England

S.J.G.Semple
Department of Medicine
The Middlesex Hospital
Medical School
London, England

D.C.Shannon
Pediatric Intensive Care Unit
Massachusetts General Hospital
Boston, MA, USA

M.Stahlman
Department of Pediatrics
Neonatal Center
Vanderbilt University
Nashville, Tennessee, USA

U.Söderberg
Laboratory of Neurophysiology
Ulleråkers Sjukhus
Uppsala, Sweden

B.T.Thach
Department of Pediatrics
St.Louis Children's Hospital
St.Louis, Mo., USA

R.W.Torrance
St.John's College
Oxford, England

T.Trippenbach
Department of Physiology
McIntyre Medical Building
McGill University
Montreal, Quebec, Canada

J.Widdicombe
Department of Physiology
St.Georges Hospital Medical
School
London, England

P.Willshaw
Department of Physiology
University of Birmingham
Birmingham, England

J.Winberg
Department of Pediatrics
Karolinska Sjukhuset
Stockholm, Sweden

S.M.Yamashiro
Biomedical Engineering
University of Southern
California
Los Angeles, Calif., USA

R.Zetterström
Department of Pediatrics
S:t Görans Sjukhus
Stockholm, Sweden

Y.Zotterman
The Conference Secretariate
Wenner-Gren Center
Stockholm, Sweden

OPENING REMARKS

YNGVE ZOTTERMAN

Wenner-Gren Center, 113 46 Stockholm, Sweden

When can you say that respiratory physiology started? This morning Professor Kao told me that breathing and prenatal respiration was analysed in China by Hsi and Tai already 500 years B.C. Here in Europe it started, I think, with Michael Serveto who was burnt on stake by Calvin in Geneva in 1553. There is no doubt that Serveto discovered the circulation of the lungs and its purpose. I have read his original story in his book De Restitutio Christianismi, Vienne, 1553, in two of the four existing copies which I have hold in my hands. The first one was the copy kept in the Hofburg Library in Vienna; the other one in the Vatican Library. The first time I asked for it in the Vatican Library I got a reprinted version from Nürnberg from 1647. That copy may be still more rare than the four original copies at Vienna, Paris, Edinburgh and Rome.

When I started studying medicine the professors in the physiological disciplines anyhow used to start with a historical review when they started each series of lectures. They had plenty of time as it took the professor two years to cover all the sections of physiology in his lectures. I think it is a shame that medical history is so very neglected in the medical education nowadays.

But I have to stop my lamentation now as it is my pleasant duty to welcome you to Wenner-Gren Center and Curt von Euler´s symposium on Central Nervous Control Mechanisms in Regular, Periodic and Irregular Breathing (Physiological and clinical aspects in the adult and perinatal states).

When in 1918 I attended my first lecture in physiology Professor J.E. Johansson talked about the oxygen secretion defended by old Haldane of Oxford and Christian Bohr of Copenhagen and the new physical diffusion theory launched by Joseph Barcroft of Cambridge and August and Marie Krogh of Copenhagen. One morning

in the summer of 1920, when I was working in Adrian's room in Cambridge,
Joseph Barcroft came down and asked me to accompany him to a meeting of the
Physiological Society in London. He wanted me to help him to transport two
huge Douglas' bags filled with gas mixtures for his demonstration. When we
came out of King's Cross Station an old lady sitting in a corner of the street
asked Barcroft the way to Euston Station. Barcroft immediately handed over his
big Douglas bag to me and took the woman's very huge and heavy suitcase and
so all three of us rushed away to Euston Station which was rather out of our way.
Thus we arrived somewhat late to the meeting in London Medical School for
Women. I believe that we just missed the tea.

It was a most remarkable meeting as the meetings of the Physiological Society
often are. It was close after the first world war.   Joseph Barcroft and the
August and Marie Krogh presented the results of their recent experiments. Krogh
had just constructed his famous microtonometer with which he and Marie Krogh
had given the crucial proof that oxygen was taken up in the lungs entirely accordingly to physical laws, disapproving the old theory of oxygen secretion ardently
launched by Christian Bohr in Copenhagen and John Scott Haldane in Oxford. I
was impressed by the way in which the protagonists conducted the debate on such
a controversial subject in an atmosphere of mutual respect.

When I returned to Cambridge for the winter 1925-26 Barcroft had just started
his work on sheep foetuses and I was often up in his rooms where he made his
experiments together with Baron whom I later met in 1940 at Yale where he continued his research on prenatal physiology.

Another turning point in respiratory physiology was when Heymans in Ghent in
the 1930s discovered the carotid chemoceptors and their role in the control of
respiration. In 1935 simultaneously and quite independently of each other Pierre
Rijlandt in Brussels, Guilio Stella in Padova and I could present records of
impulses of chemoceptive fibres from the carotid body and show how they increased
in frequency, when the oxygen tension of the arterial blood was lowered. Actually
it became a turning point because hitherto many respiratory physiologists were
very much in doubt about Heymans' theory. When in 1935 at a meeting of our
Physiological Society in Stockholm I had presented my paper on the carotid
chemoceptor impulses Göran Liljestrand gave up and he and Ulf von Euler later
in 1939 joined me in my experiments. When in 1940 Yandel Henderson at Yale
had listened to my   gramophone records[x] he gave up too. Schmitt in Philadelphia,

---

x) One of these gramophone discs produced in 1939 was played to the
   audience.

however, did not give up his resistance until 1959 when he as chairman of a section of respiration at the Montreal International Congress of Physiology publically withdrew his opposition.

In one of his earlier papers in the 1890s my teacher Professor J.E. Johansson, who was a leading man in energy metabolism and the physiology of man in exercise, brought to discussion the regulation of the pulmonary ventilation in exercise particularly the question of what brings about the immediate increase of the ventilation when you start muscular work. He concluded that impulses must irradiate from the descending motor path ways stimulating the bulbar respiratory center. The question was later debated to great extent by Bainbridge in his monography Muscular Exercise in the 1930s. I wonder whether that hypothesis have been experimentally proven to be correct?

Another interesting story I remember from my young days was that in his doctorial thesis in 1917 Göran Liljestrand found that a naturally induced increase of ventilation — raised CO_2 pressure in the inspiratory air — was performed with a higher efficiency than when the same ventilation was induced voluntarily. This illustrated how well the respiratory mechanisms function.

I feel sure that to day and during the next two days you will give us further example of how beautifully all these mechanisms fit in with each other or the disharmony which will occur when they don't.

SESSION I

DRIVES FOR BREATHING

A. Chemical and Non-chemical Drives for Ventilation in the Adult Organism

WHAT DO WE BREATHE FOR?

M. J. PURVES

*Department of Physiology, School of Veterinary Sciences, Park Row,
Bristol BS1 5LS, U.K.*

The straightforward answer to this question, given in most textbooks, is that we breathe in order to supply oxygen in adequate amounts to metabolizing tissue, to assist in the elimination of CO_2 and in so doing, to regulate the pH of extracellular fluid to constancy. However, it is clear that through processes of evolution, respiration has acquired other functions. It forms an important part of a number of purely behavioural reactions such as anger, fright and sexual excitement. It is involved in communication, particularly in man, whether in talking, singing or the playing of musical instruments. Respiratory muscles are also involved in the maintenance of posture. Furthermore, it would seem that these differing respiratory functions operate through different neural pathways. (Mitchell & Berger, 1975). Behavioural or voluntary reactions involve pathways originating in the forebrain which descend to the spinal cord and which can be distinguished from the aggregations of neurones in the pons and medulla which represent the central organization of vagal and chemoreceptor reflexes concerned with the automatic component of respiratory control. It is probable that these pathways interact at a number of levels, including the spinal cord, so that activity in the final motor pathway involving phrenic and intercostal motor neurones, vagal efferent fibres to accessory respiratory muscles and bronchial smooth muscle will give rise to a series of patterned responses.

This ambiguity of the respiratory act is widely appreciated: but I believe equally widely ignored. Thus I have yet to see a model of respiratory control which includes the behavioural components of respiration in any but the most general terms. Alternatively, behavioural variations are deliberately suppressed so that for experimental purposes, 'pure' chemical or other reflex responses may be studied in isolation. Although this approach is, of course, perfectly justified, it has meant that our view of what we breathe for in our waking and sleeping hours, in infancy and in maturity, has become distinctly unbalanced. On a more practical plane it is probable that a whole variety of respiratory adaptations, many of which are to be discussed at this symposium, simply cannot be explained except in terms of interaction between the automatic and behavioural components of respiration.

The purpose of this introductory contribution, then, is an attempt to redress this balance. I consider two themes: respiratory aims and respiratory compromise.

Respiratory Aims

There would probably be little dissent from the view that the prime and
continuing function of respiration is to satisfy the metabolic demand. The
major constraint is this should be done as efficiently as possible, that is,
for any level of metabolism, the respiratory controller seeks the perfect or
ideal gas exchange in the lungs with the minimum expenditure of energy. It is
not difficult to determine theoretically what the ideal level of gas exchange
should be for any metabolic rate either in terms of the total volumes of O_2
taken up and CO_2 evolved or the exchange of these gases in blood. It is also
possible to draw up a comprehensive list of variables - respiratory, cardiovascular and in blood itself - which are concerned in pulmonary gas exchange
and to accord these variables levels of importance as has been done, for example,
by Hill, Power & Longo (1973). From this, it is evident that alveolar ventilation is only one of a number of variables which are concerned with optimum
gas exchange and that it is continuously having to adjust to small changes in
the other variables, notably the partial pressures of O_2 and CO_2 in mixed venous
blood and in pulmonary capillary blood flow. If this adjustment is imperfect,
the fact is signalled almost certainly in arterial blood; and ventilation is
then readjusted. Because this adjustment must be as economical as possible,
the respiratory controller must presumably take note of the arterial signal as
well as information about the current performance of the respiratory muscles
and it must then work out over the next two or three breaths, a new pattern of
respiration. That this pattern, in terms of respiratory frequency and tidal
volume, is economically determined has been amply documented, possibly most
neatly by Milic-Emili & Petit (1960) who showed that at four levels of metabolic
demand, the appropriate level of alveolar ventilation was achieved by a frequency of respiration which invariably coincided with that involving minimum
expenditure of energy. How this is achieved is imperfectly understood. It
clearly must involve information about current muscle performance from muscle
spindles and proprioceptors (Nathan & Sears, 1960), integration of this with a
CO_2 signal which is a function of metabolic demand (Bainton, Kirkwood & Sears,
1978), possibly at spinal level (Aminoff & Sears, 1971) while the resulting
activation of respiratory muscles is scanned by a process involving the fusimotor (γ -loop) system.

It is also unclear how the respiratory controller knows whether pulmonary
gas exchange is optimum or not and therefore whether its adjustments are appropriate. Originally, it was thought that imperfect gas exchange could be signalled simply by an alteration in the mean level of arterial blood gas tensions.
This could signal, for example, either that $\dot{V}_A$ and $\dot{Q}$ were mismatched or that
both were mismatched with the levels of $\dot{V}CO_2$ or $\dot{V}O_2$. More recently, attention
has focussed upon fluctuations of Po_2 (Purves, 1966d), pH (Band, Cameron & Semple,
1969) and PCO_2 (Carruthers, Ponte & Purves, 1978) in arterial blood which have
the same period as respiration. Since the amplitude of these fluctuations will
be a function of the mixed venous-to-alveolar gradients for O_2 and CO_2, of tidal
volume, FRC and other factors, such fluctuations could yield potentially important information about gas exchange. However, it has recently been shown by
direct measurement that, as predicted, the amplitude of these fluctuations
varies inversely with respiratory frequency and at normal frequencies in the cat
(ca 30 breaths per minute), the fluctuations are so attenuated as to be indistinguishable from noise (Carruthers, Ponte & Purves, 1978). This conclusion is
consistent with that arrived at following a study of the respiratory modulation
of carotid body chemoreceptor discharge at various respiratory frequencies
(Ponte & Purves, 1978). At normal respiratory frequencies in the cat, such modulation disappeared. In view of this evidence, it is difficult to see how
fluctuations of blood gas tensions could significantly contribute to respiratory

control at normal frequencies. However, as was originally pointed out by Priban & Fincham (1965), these fluctuations could be important in a negative sense, that is, if they are present, they indicate that gas exchange is less than perfect. The respiratory controller therefore always attempts to keep the amplitude of these fluctuations at a minimum.

An additional form of signal in arterial blood which may be of importance has recently been demonstrated by Carruthers, Ponte & Purves (1978). They have shown that $PaCO_2$, measured in the carotid artery of cats approximately 1.5-2.0 seconds away from the end of the pulmonary capillary, decays by up to 5 mmHg in approximately 10 seconds. The reason for this decay is unknown and is being studied intensively at present. It is further clear that the rate and size of this decay is affected by a number of factors notably, the degree of oxygenation of haemoglobin, the levels of mixed venous and alveolar CO_2 and the pulmonary transit time. Since the peripheral and central chemoreceptors are separated in time, they will thus sense a gradient rather than a mean level of $PaCO_2$ and since this gradient is a function of gas exchange, rather precise information is continuously available to the respiratory controller about disturbances to gas exchange and the accuracy of its adjustment to them. Of equal importance, in the present context, is the fact that if a negative (a-A) CO_2 gradient is developed and is maintained, gas exchange can be achieved with a lower level of alveolar ventilation than would otherwise be the case. This could be important at rest and even more so in exercise.

So far, I have considered respiration solely in its role of optimizing pulmonary gas exchange. However, it is probable that in every day life, it is always being frustrated because of the intervention of other factors which have an equal claim on the respiratory act. For example, if the subject changes his posture, a new combination of respiratory mechanical variables will have to be worked out and put into effect but the aim of the controller does not change. It aims for the appropriate level of alveolar ventilation with maximum economy only now, the level of respiratory work may be greater than before. This raises a question of great importance. If the claims of the automatic and behavioural components of respiration conflict, how does the respiratory controller respond? Does the final respiratory response simply reflect the sum of these claims; or is there evidence of genuine interaction? In other words, is the chemical control of respiration immutable or is there some degree of compromise?

Respiratory Compromise

This question has been answered fairly clearly by Phillipson et al (1978). They have shown that when such a conflict arises, in this case when a subject adjusts his expiratory flow rate in order to converse or to read aloud, the respiratory response to CO_2 is rather less than one third of that seen under control conditions. It appears that this reduction in respiratory sensitivity is not due to the thought processes associated with reading but with the act of phonation itself. How this is achieved is unknown but it is reasonable to suppose that activation of the forebrain structures associated with speech depresses the automatic respiratory pathways, possibly at spinal level. And although this might be classed as a voluntary act, it does not in fact involve a willed action; that is, a conscious effort to underbreathe or to suppress any sensation of dyspnoea. It is as automatic as the hyperpnoea which occurs with exertion.

A further example of interaction between the behavioural and automatic components of respiratory control is afforded by the adaptations which occur in sleep (Phillipson, 1978). In REM sleep, respiration is rapid and irregular;

sensitivity to CO_2 in reduced compared to that seen in slow wave sleep (SWS) or
when the subject is awake; the duration of apnoea elicited by the Hering Breuer
inflation reflex is reduced and the level of hypercapnia and hypoxia which cause
arousal is very considerably increased. By contrast, in SWS, breathing is slower
and more regular and in the absence of those non-specific factors which excite
respiration when the subject is awake, respiration appears to be wholly dependent
upon vagal and chemoreceptor input for if the subjects (dogs) have their vagi
cooled and are made alkalotic and hyperoxic, ventilation is markedly reduced or
abolished. These observations suggest that in REM and SWS, the behavioural and
automatic components dominate respectively while in REM sleep the automatic
component is suppressed in some way, possibly by a similar mechanism to that
seen during phonation.

These observations are of great interest by themselves but they have clear
relevance to the question of how breathing is regulated in the foetus and in the
newborn and the changes which occur at birth. Dawes et al (1972) showed that in
the mature sheep foetus, respiratory movements were made only when the e.e.g.
was desynchronized and of low voltage and in the presence of rapid eye movements.
This state has a number of features similar to that seen in REM sleep in the
adult. Thus, the respiratory movements are of relatively high frequency and
are irregular; their incidence is unaffected by changes in blood gas tensions
and pH and they occur whether the vagus is intact or not. This is consistent
with the observation made by Bystrzycka et al (1975) that although pulmonary
stretch receptors discharge tonically in the foetus (Ponte & Purves, 1974), electrical stimulation of the vagus or inflation of the foetal lungs affects neither
respiratory movements nor the discharge characteristics of medullary respiratory
neurones.

This pattern of respiratory activity alternates with periods of apnoea
associated with a synchronized, slow wave e.e.g. pattern. Not only is the foetus
apnoeic, but it is also atonic and neither respiratory nor more general movements
can be elicited by such stimuli as electrical stimulation of the sciatic nerve,
loud noise or bright light. The only consistent stimulus which is effective is
temporary occlusion of the umbilical cord. This is very remarkable because if
the SWS pattern seen in the foetus corresponds to that seen in the adult, then
as mentioned above, breathing movements should be present and almost entirely
regulated by vagal and chemoreceptor input. Since the foetus is apnoeic, we
must suppose that either these inputs are inhibited at receptor level or else
centrally. We do not have information adequate to distinguish between these
possibilities at present. Certainly, there is good evidence that the carotid
body chemoreceptors are inactive in the foetus (Biscoe, Purves & Sampson, 1969):
but the pulmonary stretch receptors are certainly active and there is reason to
believe that the central chemoreceptors are also active since, certainly during
REM sleep, respiratory activity is excited by CO_2 in the absence of a peripheral
chemoreflex. We may also suppose that the apnoea is not due to the suppression
of the automatic component by behavioural factors in view of the e.e.g. pattern.

The mechanism of apnoea during SWS in the foetus therefore remains a complete mystery. However, whatever mechanism is involved must clearly be reversed
at or very shortly after birth because now, in the vast majority of full-term
infants, breathing is continuous during REM sleep and SWS alike. There has not
yet been as systematic a study of respiratory adaptations in sleep in the newborn
as has been achieved in the adult, but again, it is reasonable to assume that in
SWS in the newborn, breathing is maintained mainly by vagal and chemoreceptor
input. Thus we know that the Hering Breuer inflation reflex is now active -
probably more so than at any other time in life - the carotid body chemoreceptors
are now active and, in approximately quantitative terms, the reflex respiratory

response to hypoxia and hypercapnia is similar to that seen in the adult, certainly in the lamb (Purves, 1966 a,b,c) and newborn infant (Brady & Ceruti, 1966).
This must mean that the automatic component of respiratory regulation is functioning and although, superficially, respiration appears to be steady or tolerably
so in the newborn, it is worth enquiring how efficient the automatic or metabolic
control is, as defined earlier in this paper.

Such evidence as there is suggests that in the foetus, the levels of
PaO_2 and $PaCO_2$ are adjusted through the aortic group of chemoreceptors which
initiate a series of cardiovascular responses which in effect direct a greater
or lesser proportion of blood flow through the ductus arteriosus and from the
aorta to the placenta. As far as can be judged, there is no respiratory contribution to this adjustment whatever. Furthermore, we may reasonably suppose that
in the foetus, the respiratory controller does not have to respond to non-specific stimuli, such as changes in environmental temperature, because such stimuli
are markedly attenuated. Quite suddenly, then, at birth the respiratory controller has to cope with an entirely new set of circumstances. Does it in some
fashion make the correct responses straight away or is there, as in other systems
e.g. the visual system, a period of learning? We do not know the answer to this
question yet: but there are clear indications that in the newborn, respiratory
control is somewhat precarious. Thus, apnoeic spells and periodic respiration
are not uncommon, especially in premature infants: there is evidence that respiratory sensitivity to CO_2 is increasing in the days or weeks before birth
(Rigatto, Brady & Verduzco, 1975) while respiration is rather easily depressed
by moderate hypoxia. Moreover, an increasing number of infants exhibiting
hypoventilation during sleep, specifically during SWS, are being reported in the
literature (Shannon et al, 1976). These infants undoubtedly represent the more
extreme examples of impaired sensitivity to CO_2 or delayed maturation. If so,
then it would be important to know the spectrum of CO_2 sensitivity displayed by
a large sample of normal, newborn infants. This is an important question to
answer because if CO_2 sensitivity is impaired to any degree in normal infants
then these infants will be most vulnerable to the effects of hypoventilation
during SWS when the normal waking stimuli are withdrawn. And in this context, it
may be significant that the incidence of sudden death during sleep in otherwise
normal infants increases markedly a week or so after birth when the proportion
of SWS to REM sleep suddenly and markedly increases.

What do we breathe for? I have suggested that we breathe in order to
satisfy a number of requirements, some metabolic, some behavioural and some postural. The relative importance of these requirements is constantly changing and
the evidence suggests that the respiratory controller recognises the priority
of the moment. In heavy exercise, the behavioural component is negligible: for
the clarinettist playing Mozart's quintet, metabolic control is relaxed. Possibly
the most interesting question to be answered is how the metabolic control of
respiration, suppressed in utero, is activated at birth and how soon and how
effectively the respiratory controller in the newborn learns the appropriate
adjustments. That it does in the majority of infants is fortunate since it
allows all of us to contribute to this symposium.

REFERENCES

M.J. Aminoff & T.A. Sears, Spinal integration of segmental, cortical and breathing inputs to thoracic respiratory motoneurones, J. Physiol. (Lond) 215,
   557-575 (1971).
C.R. Bainton, P.A. Kirkwood & T.A. Sears, On the transmission of the stimulating
   effects of carbon dioxide to the muscles of respiration, J. Physiol. (Lond)
   280, 249-272 (1978).
D.M. Band, I.R. Cameron & S.J.G. Semple, Oscillations in arterial pH with breathing in the cat, J. appl. Physiol. 26, 261-267 (1969).
T.J. Biscoe, M.J. Purves & S.R. Sampson, Types of nervous activity which may be
   recorded from the carotid sinus nerve in the sheep foetus, J. Physiol.
   (Lond) 202, 1-23 (1969).
J.P. Brady & E. Ceruti, Chemoreceptor reflexes in the newborn infant: Effects of
   varying degrees of hypoxia on the heart rate and ventilation in a warm
   environment, J. Physiol. (Lond) 184, 631-645 (1966).
E. Bystrzycka, B.S. Nail & M.J. Purves, Central and peripheral neural and respiratory activity in the mature sheep foetus and newborn lamb, Respir. Physiol.
   25, 199-215 (1975).
B. Carruthers, J. Ponte & M.J. Purves, Observations on the partial pressure of
   CO_2 in carotid arterial blood in cats (Communication to the Physiological
   Society, Cambridge, July 1978).
G.S. Dawes, H.E. Fox, B.M. LeDuc, G.C. Liggins & R.T. Richards, Respiratory movements and rapid eye movement sleep in the foetal lamb, J. Physiol. (Lond)
   220, 119-143 (1972).
E.P. Hill, G.G. Power & L.D. Longo, Mathematical stimulation of pulmonary O_2 and
   CO_2 exchange, Am. J. Physiol. 224, 904-917 (1973).
G. Milic-Emili & J.M. Petit, Mechanical efficiency of breathing, J. appl. Physiol.
   15, 359-362 (1960).
R.A. Mitchell & A.J. Berger, Neural regulation of respiration, Rev. Resp. Dis.
   111, 206-224 (1975).
P.W. Nathan & T.A. Sears, Effects of posterior root section on the activity of
   some muscles in man, J. Neurol. Neurosur. Psychiat. 23, 10-22 (1960).
E.A. Phillipson, Respiratory adaptations in sleep, Ann Rev. Physiol. 40, 133-156
   (1978).
E.A. Phillipson, P.A. McClean, C.E. Sullivan & N. Zamel, Interaction of metabolic
   and behavioural respiratory control during hypercapnia and speech, Am. Rev.
   resp. Dis. 117, 903-909 (1978).
J. Ponte & M.J. Purves, Types of afferent nervous activity which may be measured
   in the vagus nerve of the sheep foetus, J. Physiol. (Lond) 229, 51-76 (1974).
J. Ponte & M.J. Purves, Carbon dioxide and venous return and their interaction
   as stimuli to ventilation in the cat, J. Physiol. (Lond) 274, 455-476 (1978).
I.P. Priban & W.F. Fincham, Self adaptive control and the respiratory system,
   Nature, 208, 339-343 (1965).
M.J. Purves, Respiratory and circulatory effects of breathing 100% oxygen in the
   newborn lamb before and after denervation of the carotid chemoreceptors,
   J. Physiol. (Lond) 185, 42-59 (1966a).
M.J. Purves, The effects of hypoxia in the newborn lamb before and after denerv-
   ation of the carotid chemoreceptors, J. Physiol. (Lond) 185, 60-77 (1966b).
M.J. Purves, The respiratory response of the newborn lamb to inhaled CO_2 with
   and without accompanying hypoxia, J. Physiol. (Lond) 185, 78-94 (1966c).
M.J. Purves, Fluctuations of arterial oxygen tension which have the same period
   as respiration, Respir. Physiol. 1, 281-296 (1966d).
H. Rigatto, J.P. Brady & R. de la Torre Verduzco, Chemoreceptor reflexes in pre-
   term infants: the effect of gestational and postnatal age on the ventilatory response to inhaled CO_2 Pediatrics 55, 614-621 (1975).
D.C. Shannon, D.W. Marsland, J.B. Gould, B. Callahan, I.D. Todres & J. Dennis,
   Central hypoventilation during quiet sleep in two infants, Pediatrics, 57
   342-346 (1976).

FUNCTIONAL ASPECTS OF CENTRAL
CHEMOSENSITIVITY

H. H. LOESCHCKE

Institut für Physiologie, Ruhr-Universität Bochum, F.R.G.

The functional aspects of central chemosensitivity are twofold. There is the aspect of the function of the single element and the population of elements and there is also the aspect of the involvement of central chemosensitivity in the drive of respiration and in the control of acid-base homeostasis, i.e. the function in the context of the whole organism. In this paper it will be tried to contribute to both aspects. The last review on this field has been presented by Loeschcke and Schläfke, 1976 to the Krogh Centenary Symposium in Srinagar.

Contributions to the mechanism of chemosensory excitation

There seems to be agreement that central chemosensitivity reacts to the extracellular hydrogen ion concentration (Loeschcke et al., 1958, Mitchell et al., 1963, Pappenheimer et al., 1965, 1967). The fact that there is not much difference between the actions of a pH shift in a superfused buffer by a change of pCO_2 (respiratory acidosis) and a pH shift by fixed acid (metabolic acidosis) as long as the superfusion flow is rapid enough to replace diffusing CO_2 argues strongly against an important role of intracellular pH which should be much more influenced by the pCO_2 change. The old experiments would, however, not exclude a determining role of the H^+ gradient of the intracellular to the extracellular phase as has been discussed by Loeschcke and Katsaros, 1959. It remains, however, obscure how the hydrogen ion interacts with the cell with the consequence of variation of impulse generation. Recent experiments of Dev and Loeschcke, 1978 a, b, Schläfke and See, 1978 and of Fukuda and Loeschcke, 1978 may at least give a hint in which direction to look. They also give new information about the type of the cell structures involved in central chemosensitivity.

Dev and Loeschcke, 1978 a, b further elaborated on an observation of
Mitchell et al., 1963 that local application of <u>acetylcholine</u> to the at
that time discovered rostral field of chemosensitivity raised respiration
mainly increasing tidal volume. Dev and Loeschcke, 1978 a, b confirmed the
older experiments and demonstrated that acetylcholine acted preferentially
on two fields of the ventral medulla oblongata which corresponded reasonably
well with the fields where respiratory responses to H^+ are obtained. The
acetylcholine effect on respiration could be enhanced by locally applied
<u>physostigmine</u> and also physostigmine alone augmented resting ventilation.
<u>Atropine</u> locally applied diminished resting ventilation, abolished the
effect of local acetylcholine and also diminished the slope of the CO_2-
response curve (ventilation or tidal volume plotted against endtidal pCO_2).

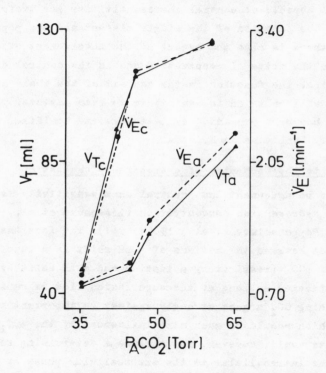

Fig. 1 Effect of atropine on the response of
the tidal volume (V_T) and the ventilation
($\dot{V}_E$) to increased endtidal P_{CO_2} ($P_{A CO_2}$).
V_{T_c} and $\dot{V}_{E_c}$ are the control values and V_{T_a}
and $\dot{V}_{E_a}$ are the values of V_T and $\dot{V}_E$
obtained after local application of
atropine ($10^{-2} g\ ml^{-1}$) to the chemosensory
areas of the medulla oblongata
(Experiment of N.B. Dev).

This in the end means that the atropine locally applied in fact interferes
with the respiratory chemosensitivity. Also <u>nicotine</u> on the same location
increases the respiratory drive. This effect could be counteracted by
intravenously given <u>hexamethonium</u>. These observations suggest that
cholinergic mechanisms with both muscarinic and nicotinic receptors are
involved in respiratory chemosensitivity as necessary links.

These observations were corroborated by Schläfke and See, 1978 who picked
up extracellular action potentials from the ventral surface layer of the
medulla oblongata in anaesthetized cats. Such neurons which increased their
impulse frequency if acid buffers were applied to the surface of if CO_2 was
inhaled also reacted with increased impulse frequency if acetylcholine was
applied to the surface. There were also neurons which did not react to acid
but still responded to acetylcholine. These neurons, however, responded to
drugs acting on arterial pressure. They seem not to have to do anything
with the respiratory system.

Fukuda et al., 1978 cut thin slices from the ventral surface of the
medulla oblongata of cats and rats and mounted them in a perfusion chamber.
Neurons which discharged spontaneously and which increased their discharge
when the perfusion fluid was made more acid were observed in this surviving
in vitro preparation. These same cells also reacted to acetylcholine added
to the perfusion fluid with increased discharge in a time course which was
similar to that of the reaction to acidity. Atropine though increasing the
discharge prevented the action of acetylcholine on the discharge and so did
hexamethonium. Physostigmin enhanced it. Atropine also made the cell
insensitive to hydrogen ion. Furthermore mecamylamine, an acetylcholine
antagonist, completely stopped the discharge making the cell insensitive
to H^+ and to acetylcholine. These experiments more directly show the effect
of cholinergic and anticholinergic drugs on hydrogen ion sensitive cells.
The effect of hydrogen ion on the cellular discharge seems to depend on a
cholinergic mechanism. There are several possibilities, how this may be the
case. It is for example known that the activity of acetylcholinesterase
depends on pH and therefore H^+ may modulate the destruction of acetylcholine.
It is also possible that H^+ acts on the release of acetylcholine. Finally
H^+ could interfere with the action of acetylcholine as a transmitter.

Other experiments of Fukuda and Loeschcke, 1977 also allowed further
conclusions about the kind of neurons implied in the action of hydrogen ion.

If the magnesium concentration in the perfusion fluid was increased and the calcium concentration decreased the reaction to H^+ was lost and finally the discharge of the cells was depressed by increased H^+. It was assumed that increase of magnesium and decrease of calcium concentrations would interfere with synaptic transmission. If this is so it should be concluded that the hydrogen ion effect is bound to synaptic transmission. This now suggests that central chemosensitivity resides in a process of synaptic transmission and therefore should depend on some synaptic input. I shall leave this question to Dr. Schläfke for further discussion. It should be mentioned, however, that in Dr. Fukudas slices the neural input at least should be strongly diminished because the tracts are cut. A 'spontaneous' origin of impulses which also may be influenced by cholinergic drugs therefore cannot be excluded. On the other hand impulses may originate on the cut surfaces and impinge on the hydrogen ion sensitive cells, their transmission being modified by the hydrogen ion concentration.

Hydrogen ion sensitive cells in the experiments of Fukuda and Loeschcke, 1977 were not restricted to the chemosensitive areas on the ventral side of the medulla. Such cells also were observed in dorsal slices. Their density, however, was much higher in the ventral site. Speckmann et al., 1970 described cells in the spinal cord which were excited by increased H^+ calling them E-neurons and other cells which were inhibited by increased H^+ which were called I-neurons. The same two types were found in Fukudas ventral and dorsal slices the difference being in the relative density of E and I neurons which on the ventral side was so much in favour of the E-neuron. The specificity for respiratory reactions therefore may not be a specificity of a certain cell type which does not occur elsewhere but a specificity of projection inasmuch as only the cells of the E type in the chemosensitive regions may be connected to the respiratory neural pathway and the influence of H^+ on the other cells cannot be observed by recording respiration.

Recent data on the environmental conditions of central chemosensitive structures

Objections have been raised against the concept of central chemosensitivity responding to interstitial pH. In the experiment of Lambertsen et al., 1965 the time course of pH in CSF samples was compared with the time course of ventilation if CO_2 was inhaled. Ventilation was faster. Of course in a transient state pH in a CSF sample is not representing pH in the inter-

stitial fluid and this objection therefore was not very serious. Still it
remained desirable to show the time relation between the interstitial pH
and the ventilation. This was tried recently by Cragg et al., 1977 using a
pH-microelectrode inserted into the ventral surface of the medulla oblongata.
There was an approximate agreement of the time courses of pH measured with
this method and the tidal flow in respiratory acidosis. The authors, however,
did not succeed to obtain a change of ventilation if they superfused the
medullary surface with buffers of varying pH. This is probably nothing more
than an indication that the experiment is difficult. There are also a number
of pitfalls of the technique of pH measurement. Microelectrodes of course
are extremely sensitive to disturbances because of their high resistance.
They also probably measure DC potentials between electrode and reference.
Some of these may be caused by injury. Furthermore it must be assumed that
the electrodes interfere with local circulation and therefore exert themselves some influence on local pH. This may be additionally dangerous
because the tissue moves with pulse and respiration.

   Ahmad et al., 1976, Ahmad et al., 1978 in their experiments used a
different technique of pH measurement which also may have its shortcomings
which, however, avoids the sources of error mentioned. They used a surface
electrode with the reference electrode very closely attached. The flat H^+
sensitive membrane was rectricted to the part which touched the surface.
To insure constant minimal pressure to the surface the electrode was
balanced in such a way that it could move with the medullary movements.
This type of electrode gave stable readings. Its application for measurement the interstitial brain pH is based on the electron-microscopic
observation of Dermietzel, 1976 that the intercellular spaces of the
medulla open to the surface as has also been verified by the demonstration
that an indicator like horse raddish peroxidase easily enters the medulla
from the subarachnoid space. The pH changes measured in this way occurred
in a time course well correlated to the time course of ventilation. There
was a very small delay of ventilation in the order of magnitude of a few
seconds which also was reproducible. This could for example well be
demonstrated by plotting tidal volume against local pH while changing
arterial pCO_2 in an approximately rectangular way by having the cat inhale
a gas mixture of decreasing CO_2 concentration. In the resulting loop the
upstroke and the downstroke after the end of CO_2-inhalation indicated an
excellent correlation and a minimal delay only. The delay if the same
experiment was performed on the hemisphere was much more pronounced. This

experiment to us seems now to establish the excellent time correlation of
local interstitial pH and ventilation changes. The experiments of Ahmad et
al., 1976, 1978 also gave new information on the time courses of the ex-
changes of CO_2, bicarbonate and chloride ions and on the buffering properties of the cells in the CNS. The chloride concentration was measured with
a silver-silver chloride electrode. In respiratory acidosis the bicarbonate
increase was close to one to one with the chloride decrease in extracellular
fluid.

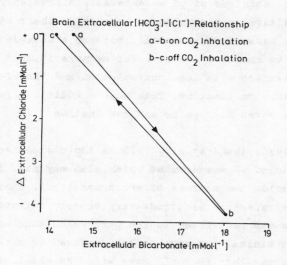

Fig. 2   Comparison of the increase of the
bicarbonate concentration with the
decrease of the chloride concentration
on the cortical surface in the steady
state before and during respiratory
acidosis. The ratio $-\Delta Cl^-/\Delta HCO_3^-$ is
approximately 1. This means that there
is a one to one exchange of these anions
similar to the Hamburger shift in blood.
(Experiment of H.R. Ahmad)

These investigations led to a new concept regarding the exchange processes of bicarbonate and chloride ions between blood plasma and interstitial fluid of the brain and between the cells of the CSN (glia) and
interstitial fluid. In respiratory acidosis the latter exchange is the
leading process in such a way that CO_2 from blood enters the interstitial
fluid and the brain cells without restriction, that it reacts with the

intracellular buffers forming HCO_3^- which in turn is exchanged against extracellular chloride ion much in analogy to the Hamburger shift in blood. This concept is based on the observation of opposite shifts of bicarbonate and chloride concentration in the interstitial fluid of the brain and on the observation that the increase of interstitial bicarbonate concentration in respiratory acidosis exceeds the increase in blood plasma and that it occurs also if blood bicarbonate is prevented from increasing by acid injection as has been shown by Pannier et al., 1971. If, however, a metabolic alkalosis is produced by i.v. injection of bicarbonate an exchange of bicarbonate against chloride takes place at the border between blood and interstitial fluid again an analogue of the Hamburger shift. If pCO_2 is maintained constant in this experiment by manipulation of the ventilation there is no reason for an exchange between cells and interstitial fluid and the complete change of bicarbonate and chloride concentrations in the interstitial fluid must be accounted for by this type of exchange. The concept described offers a new way of understanding the changes of CSF bicarbonate in respiratory and non-respiratory acidosis as described by Pappenheimer et al., 1965, 1967 and Pappenheimers assumption of an active transport process seems not to be necessary.

Some exchange of chloride against bicarbonate has also been reported under different conditions by Nattie and Romer, 1978. The exchange in these experiments was not one to one and the authors assumed that the difference was due to unmeasured anions. Nevertheless the exchange was interpreted as an exchange with brain cells analogous to the Hamburger shift and in so far in agreement with the conclusion of Ahmad et al., 1976, 1978.

The role of central chemosensitivity in respiratory control (reinvestigated)

Cooling of the intermediate area stops breathing when the peripheral chemosensitivity is eliminated. This is the case regardless whether or not CO_2 is inhaled (Schläfke and Loeschcke, 1967). This was interpreted as meaning that the impulse traffic of the central chemosensitivity was blocked and since ventilation failed completely it was assumed that this impulse traffic is the only chemosensitive one except peripheral chemosensitivity. Cherniack et al., 1977 meanwhile demonstrated that cooling can be counteracted by an increased stimulus of inhaled CO_2. Since the thermode was not applied to the rostral or caudal chemosensitive areas this observation has probably not to do with an interaction of temperature with the chemosensitive mechanism but

may be an indication that cooling is not so much acting on fiber tracts
than on synaptic transmission. The cooling experiment was repeated by
Loeschcke et al., 1978 under different conditions. It seemed necessary to
exclude the possibility that after blockade of the major source of chemosensory impulses minor contributions from other sources might not any more
be effective if a minimum threshold input would be necessary. This time,
while the intermediate areas on both sides were cooled after cutting the
sinus and the aortic nerves the central ends of the sinus nerves were
stimulated and some respiration was thus maintained. It turned out that
also in this experiment inhalation of CO_2 remained completely <u>ineffective</u>.
This again and with more clarity shows that no other chemosensitivity to
inhaled CO_2 is left.

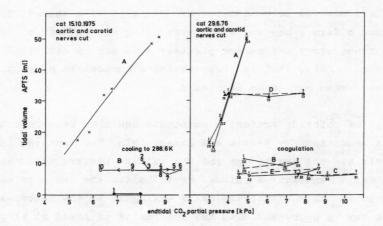

Fig. 3 Response of tidal volume to increased endtidal
P_{CO_2} in the steady state before and after
elimination of central chemosensitivity by
cooling (left) or by coagulating (right) the
intermediate area. A control, B, C, D and E
several runs while cooling or after coagulation
under maintenance of respiration by stimulation
of the central ends of the cut sinus nerves
either with a continuous sequence of impulses
(B, C, E) or with trains of impulses (D) imposing
the respiratory frequency. Only in the latter case
it was possible to produce tidal volumes above
control. The serial number and in the right diagram
also the respiratory frequencies are written to the
points. The aortic nerves are cut. In no case any response
to elevated CO_2 was observed after elimination of the
intermediate area.

A comparison between the central and the peripheral chemosensitivities to CO_2 (H^+) in the steady state

Middendorf and Loeschcke, 1976 published a mathematical model of the respiratory control system. This model takes into account peripheral and central chemosensitivity and the brain circulation and it also introduces delays between lung and peripheral and lung and central chemosensitivity. It allows to investigate the influences of alteration of the gas composition in the inhaled air and also the influence of changes of the buffer base in blood. The effects of respiratory and of non-respiratory acidosis-alkalosis can be simulated. This model was applied by Middendorf and Loeschcke, 19 for a comparison of central and of peripheral chemosensitivity to CO_2 (H^+) in the steady state. Several experiments of the literature could be used which showed that the pH changes in the CSF after i.v. injection of acid or base in the steady state were minimal. There was only one ratio between central to peripheral chemosensitivities which was compatible with this result. The sensitivity to H^+ of the central chemosensors turned out to be 25 times the sensitivity of the peripheral chemosensors to H^+. This result is restricted to the steady state and to a situation when pO_2 is normal that is high enough not to act appreciably on peripheral chemosensitivity. It does not describe the responses of the two chemosensitivities in transient states. As a matter of fact in a transient state the contribution of the pCO_2 (H^+) sensitivity of the peripheral chemosensor must be expected to be much higher than in the steady state.

Ahmad, H.R., Berndt, J. and Loeschcke, H.H.: Bicarbonate exchange between
    blood, brain extracellular fluid and brain cells at maintained pCO_2.
    Pages 19-27 in Acid-Base Homeostasis of the Brain Extracellular Fluid
    and the Respiratory Control System. Ed. Loeschcke, H.H., Thieme Verlag,
    Stuttgart (1976)

Ahmad, H.R., Loeschcke, H.H. and Woidtke, H.H.: Three compartments model
    for the bicarbonate exchange of the brain extracellular fluid with
    blood and cells. Pages 195-209 in Regulation of Respiration during
    Sleep and Anaesthesia. Ed. Fitzgerald R.S., Lahiri, S. and Gautier, H.
    Plenum Press, New York (1978)

Cherniack, N.S., von Euler, C., Homma, I. and Kao, F.F.: Effects of graded
    changes in central chemoreceptor input by local temperature changes on
    the ventral surface of medulla. Pages 397-402 in Regulation of Respira-
    tion during Sleep and Anaesthesia. Ed. Fitzgerald, R.S., Lahiri, S. and
    Gautier, H. Plenum Press, New York (1978)

Cragg, P., Patterson, L. and Purves, H.J.: The pH of brain extracellular
    fluid in the cat. J. Physiol. 272, 137-166 (1977)

Dermietzel, R.: Central chemosensitivity, morphological studies. Pages
    52-65 in Acid-Base Homeostasis of the Brain Extracellular Fluid and the
    Respiratory Control System. Ed. Loeschcke, H.H., Georg Thieme Publishers,
    Stuttgart (1976)

Dev. N.B.: Wirkung neurotroper Substanzen auf die an der Regulation von
    Atmung und Vasomotorik beteiligten Gebiete der ventralen Oberfläche der
    Medulla oblongata der Katze. Dissertation Abt. Biol. Ruhr-Universität
    Bochum (1977)

Dev, N.B. and Loeschcke, H.H.: Topography of the respiratory and circulatory
    responses to acetylcholine and nicotine on the ventral surface of the
    medulla oblongata. Pflüg. Arch. (subm.)

Dev, N.B. and Loeschcke, H.H.: Cholinergic mechanism implied in the respira-
    tory chemosensitivity of the medulla oblongata in the cat. Pflüg. Arch.

    (subm.)

Fukuda, Y. and Loeschcke, H.H.: Effect of H^+ on spontaneous neuronal
    activity in the surface layer of the rat medulla oblongata in vitro.
    Pflüg. Arch. 371, 125-134 (1977)

Fukuda, Y. and Loeschcke, H.H.: Cholinergic mechanism involved in the neuronal excitation by H^+ in the respiratory chemosensitive structures of the ventral medulla oblongata of rats in vitro. Pflüg. Arch.(subm.)

Lambertsen, C.I., Gelfand, R. and Kemp, R.A.: Dynamic response characteristics of several CO_2-reaction components of the respiratory control system. In Cerebrospinal Fluid and the Regulation of Ventilation. Ed. McC. Brooks, C., Kao, F.F. and Lloyd, B.B. Pages 211-240, Blackwell Sci. Publ. Oxford (1965)

Loeschcke, H.H., Koepchen, H.P. and Gertz, K.H.: Über den Einfluß von Wasserstoffionenkonzentration und CO_2-Druck im Liquor cerebrospinalis auf die Atmung. Pflüg. Arch. 266, 569-585 (1958)

Loeschcke, H.H. and Katsaros, B.: Die Wirkung von in den Liquor cerebrospinalis eingebrachten Ammoniumchlorid auf Atmung und Vasomotorik. Pflüg. Arch. 270, 147-160 (1959)

Loeschcke, H.H. and Schläfke, M.E.: Central chemosensitivity. Pages 282-298 in: Morphology and Mechanisms of Chemoreceptors. Ed. by Paintal, A.S., Vallabhdhai Patel Chest Institute, University of Delhi (1976)

Loeschcke, H.H., Schläfke, M.E., See, W.R. and Herker-See, A.: Does CO_2 act on the respiratory centers? Pflüg. Arch. (subm.)

Middendorf, T. and Loeschcke, H.H.: Mathematische Simulation des Respirationssystems. J. Math. Biol. 3, 149-177 (1976)

Middendorf, T. and Loeschcke, H.H.: Cooperation of the peripheral and central chemosensitive mechanisms in the control of the extracellular pH in brain in non-respiratory acidosis. Pflüg. Arch. 375, 257-260 (1978)

Mitchell, R.A., Loeschcke, H.H., Massion, W. and Severinghaus, J.W.: Respiratory response mediated through superficial chemosensitive areas on the medulla. J. Appl. Physiol. 18, 523-533 (1963)

Nattie, E.E. and Romer, C.: The role of chloride and other anions in cerebrospinal fluid bicarbonate regulation. Pages 211-218 in: Regulation of Respiration during Sleep and Anaesthesia. Ed. Fitzgerald, R.S., Lahiri, S. and Gautier, H. Plenum Press, New York (1978)

Pannier, J.L., Weyne, J. and Leusen, I.: The CSF/blood potential and the regulation of the bicarbonate concentration of CSF during acidosis in the cat. Life Sciences 10, 287-300 (1971)

Pappenheimer, J.R.: The ionic composition of cerebral extracellular fluid and its relation to control of breathing. Harvey Lectures 61, 71-94 (1967)

Pappenheimer, J.R., Fencl, V., Heisey, S.R. and Held, D.: Role of cerebral fluids in control of respiration as studies in unanaesthetized goats. Am. J. Physiol. 207, 436-450 (1965)

Schläfke, M.E. and Loeschcke, H.H.: Lokalisation eines an der Regulation von Atmung und Kreislauf beteiligten Gebietes an der ventralen Oberfläche der Medulla oblongata durch Kälteblocke. Pflüg. Arch. 297, 201-220 (1967)

Schläfke, M.E. and See, W.R.: Ventral surface stimulus response in relation to ventilatory and cardiovascular effects.Pages 97-104 in Central Interaction between Respiratory and Cardiovascular Control Systems. Eds. Koepchen, H.P., Hilton, S.M. Trzebski, A., Springer Verlag, Berlin, Heidelberg, New York (1974)

Speckmann, E.J., Caspers, H. and Sokolov, W.: Aktivitätsänderungen spinaler Neurone während und nach einer Asphyxie. Pflüg. Arch. 319, 122-138 (1970)

DISCUSSION

Loeschcke was asked whether the results suggesting the involvement of synaptic transmission in central chemoceptive control of respiration and circulation had given rise to any change in his concepts concerning the basis for the central chemosensitivity. Loeschcke replied that he used to prefer to talk about 'chemosensory structures' rather than 'chemoreceptors'.

In this connection attention was drawn to the fact that sensory receptors form a very heterogeneous group with respect to morphology and receptor mechanisms. Several of the well studied sensory receptors include synaptic transmission between receptor cell and the primary afferent endings and, in the cases where efferent, centrifugal, control is present this is mediated by synaptic mechanisms.

ORIGIN AND AFFERENT MODIFICATION OF RESPIRATORY DRIVE FROM VENTRAL MEDULLARY AREAS

M. E. SCHLAEFKE, W. R. SEE and J. F. KILLE

Institute für Physiologie, Ruhr-Universität, 4630 Bochum, F.R.G.

Berndt et al. (1) suggested that the central H^+ion sensitivity of ventilation should be located at about 250 to 300 μm below the ventral medullary surface. Schwanghardt et al. (2), who used novocain to abolish the drive from chemosensitive areas on the ventral medullary surface, assumed that a block of the most superficial 50 μm of tissue is sufficient for an elimination of rhythmic respiratory center output under the condition of cut peripheral chemoreceptors. The observations coincide with former experiments in which the central chemosensitive drive could be eliminated by bilateral cold block or by bilateral superficial coagulation of an area described by Schlaefke and Loeschcke (3), the area S or intermediate area (4, 5, 6). In more recent approaches central chemosensitivity was studied by extracellular action potential recording and histological techniques, as well as by neurophysiological methods in vitro (7, 8, 9, 10, 11, 12). In the following a recently developed hypothesis and some new data will be discussed, based on formerly obtained results (13). Four groups of experiments mainly will be taken into consideration: 1. Elimination of central chemosensitive drive and the role of peripheral chemoreceptors. 2. Elimination of central chemosensitivity and muscular exercise as respiratory stimulus. 3. 'Chemosensitive' neurones and stimulation of peripheral chemoreceptors. 3. 'Chemosensitive' neurones and stimulation of afferents from the muscles.

Survey of methods

1. Cats were anaesthetized with ketamine hydrochloride and chloralose urethane (acute experiments) or with sodium pentobarbital (for surgery in chronic experiments). In anaesthetized or awake cats ventilation was measured by the excursions of a spirometer, which was connected to a linear displacement transducer, endtidal PCO_2 was analyzed by infrared absorption. In acute experiments arterial pressure was measured through a femoral catheter leading to a strain gauge. Arterial blood samples were withdrawn from the femoral artery (acute and chronic experiments), pH, PCO_2, and PO_2 were analyzed by a blood microsystem with electrodes (Astrup). The ventilatory response to hypoxia and hypercapnia was observed; for this the cats inhaled gas mixtures containing varying concentrations of O_2, N_2 and CO_2. After control measurements the area S was bilaterally coagulated. The measurements were repeated in acute experiments 20 minutes after the coagulation, and in the chronic studies once a day up to 12 days after the

25

coagulation.

2. In anaesthetized cats the area S was bilaterally cold blocked (8 - 10°C; after peripheral chemoreceptors had been cut. Both caudal ends of the cut ventral roots of L7 were stimulated electrically which elicited movements of both hind limbs. The respiratory effect was observed before and during cold block of both areas S (14).

3. In anaesthetized and spontaneously breathing cats floating glass micro-electrodes, filled with procion yellow and connected to the preamplifier by a 50 μm thick silver wire, were used to measure action potentials extra-cellularly from neurones 0 - 1800 μm below the surface of the area S. The ventral medullary surface was continuously superfused with artificial cere-brospinal fluid of pH 7.4, 7.6 or 7.0 (5). The surface pH was indicated by a floating H^+ion sensitive glass electrode placed on the area M (rostral area, 15). The ipsilateral sinus nerve was stimulated electrically with a bipolar steel electrode. In other experiments the oxygen concentration was lowered or 0.2 ml NaCN (0.1 %) was injected intravenously. In some experiments i.v. injections of 3 ml $NaHCO_3$ (1M) or inhalation of CO_2 were used to change the medullary pH.

4. In anaesthetized and artificially ventilated cats, paralyzed with gala-mintriethiodid, the efferent discharge of the cut phrenic nerve was recor-ded. Analogous to 3. the neuronal response to changes of the H^+ion concen-tration was tested. The rostral end of a femoral or tibial nerve was sti-mulated electrically for 30 seconds. The action potentials per second of single medullary neurones were counted by a computer over 60 seconds of steady state when pH or pCO_2, or PO_2 were varied, and before and during the electrical stimulation of the peripheral nerves or the injection of NaCN. Interspike-interval histograms either free running or stimulus-triggered were determined by a computer. The electrode position was histo-logically verified by fluorescence of procion yellow (iontophoresis with 600 nA, 10 min) or the tip of the electrode trace was localized after silver impregnation (16) of the 40 μm thick freeze sectioned slices.

Survey of results

1. After elimination of the superficial structure of the area S the venti-latory response to CO_2 was reduced or abolished in anaesthetized as well as in awake cats. This was correlated with the complete loss of marginal nerve cells (17) and with degenerations within the ventral pole of the nucleus paragigantocellularis (NPG) (18). Under hyperoxic conditions venti-lation was about 17 % of the control. Cutting of the peripheral chemore-ceptors was followed by a complete loss of respiratory drive. In the cats with intact peripheral chemoreceptors the arterial blood indicated a res-piratory acidosis of 7.09 (control pH 7.30) and a PCO_2 of 8.17 kPa (control 4.28 kPa) in the average of 6 cats. In addition in the awake cats after chronic central chemodenervation periodic breathing was observed as well as irregular increases of the ventilatory volume, the latter evidently pro-voked by nonchemical stimuli causing an arousal reaction as well. A reduc-tion of the arterial PO_2 e.g. to 15 kPa and below stimulated respiration, however the ventilatory response to hypoxia remained less than 50 % of the control (13).

2. In cats with cut peripheral chemoreceptors, bilateral cold block of the area S causes apnea (4, 19). Bilateral electrical stimulation of the ventral roots of L7 produces an increase of ventilation. Combined with cold block of the areas S no effective drive could be observed. This means

that apnea occurs in spite of the continuation or the onset of the stimulation (14). The movements of the hind limbs are not affected by the cold
block.

3. Neuronal discharge recorded extracellularly from the superficial layer
of the area S reveals a significant dependence of the impulse discharge
in specific neurones upon the pH of the artificial cerebrospinal fluid
superfused on the ventral medullary surface. Such variations of the surface pH are accompanied by ventilatory reactions as formerly described (1).
The neurones can be clearly discriminated from other, non chemosensitive
neurones, e.g. from neurones involved in the regulation of arterial pressure (20). 'Chemosensitive' as well as neurones involved in the regulation
of arterial pressure were located within the NPG (see fig. 3 below, compare 21).

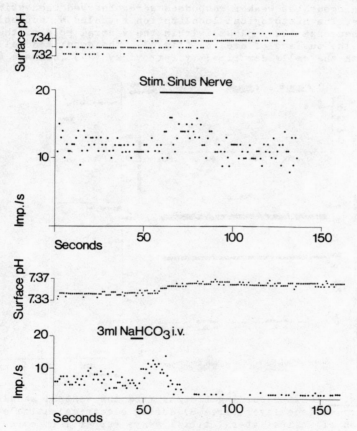

Fig. 1 Single unit response from 450 μm below area S
to i.v. injection of 1M NaHCO₃ (lower part) and to
stimulation of an ipsilateral sinus nerve 1ms, 40 Hz,
1 V (upper part). Top traces: surface pH measured
2 mm rostral of the recording site. Bottom traces:
unit discharge [Imp/s].

Within the superficial structure of the area S and partly within the NPG
we now found neurones which drastically increased their impulse frequency
when NaCN was injected i.v. or when the O_2 partial pressure was lowered,
or when the sinus nerve was stimulated electrically (22). The discharge
frequency of some of these neurones can also be modulated by pH changes
on the surface or in the blood (fig. 1). The cell type responding to sinus
nerve stimulation could not yet be clearly identified.

4. After identification of 'chemosensitive' neurones within the superficial
layer of the area S by their response to pH changes it could be shown that
afferent stimulation of the tibial nerve affected the tonic discharge frequency of the same neurones. The latency between the stimulus onset at the
tibial nerve and the response of a chemosensitive medullary neurone was 22
msec, that between the increase or decrease of neuronal discharge and the
corresponding increase or decrease of phrenic nerve activity another 22 msec
(fig. 2). Analogous but weaker responses were observed when stimulating the
femoral nerve. The histological localization revealed a 'subnucleus' of
small-sized neurones (22 - 31 µm) within the ventral pole of the NPG (200 -
450 µm below the surface of area S) (fig. 3). The described cells are not
identical with the cells described by Petrovicky (17) (compare 6).

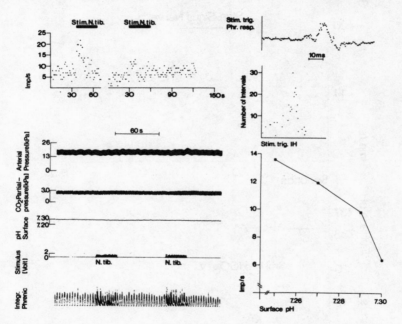

Fig. 2 Unit recording (Imp/s) from the ventral medullary surface layer (area S) during electrical stimulation of an ipsilateral tibial nerve (upper left corner).
Stimulus triggered intervall histograms (IH) of unit
(lower) and phrenic (upper) activity (upper right corner); note the different latencies (unit 22 ms; phrenic
44 ms). pH-response curve of unit (lower right corner)
to changes of CSF pH on the ventral surface . Original
recording of P art, endexp. PCO_2, surface pH, electrical
stimulus of tibial nerve, and integrated phrenic activity (from top to bottom, lower left corner). Artificially ventilated cat.

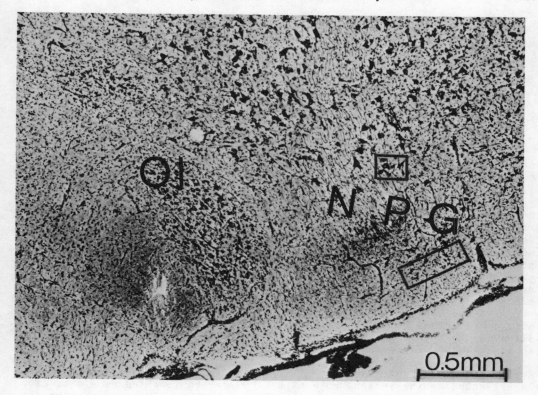

Figure 3 Transverse freeze section of the medulla
oblongata 5.95 mm caudal of the foramen coecum. Eager
stain. Rectangle: small cell type (see text). Square:
medium sized cell type (see text). OI: Oliva inferior;
NPG: Nucleus paragigantocellularis.

DISCUSSION

Central chemosensitivity and its modification by peripheral chemoreceptors

The block or coagulation of a circumscribed structure on the ventral medullary surface, which is not the site of a respiratory center, eliminates
the central chemosensitive drive of respiration. The result is an insensitivity to CO_2, periodic or irregular breathing and a severe respiratory
acidosis due to hypoventilation. The peripheral chemoreceptors deliver
sufficient drive to guarantee rhythmic respiratory center output, however,
the respiratory response to hypoxia is diminished by about 50 % (13). This
observation raised the question whether or not peripheral chemoreceptor
input would reach the respiratory center deprived of an input from central
chemosensitivity, or whether or not in addition the structure of the areas
S would receive information from peripheral chemoreceptors directly. See
and Schlaefke (22) suggest the possibility of a confluence of both, central
chemosensitive impulses and impulses induced or modified by peripheral
chemoreceptor activation within the structure of the area S. This assumption of a 'sideway' of peripheral chemoreceptors is supported by recent

results of Kille and Schlaefke (23) who described, besides the known pathway to the region of the nucleus tractus solitarii, degenerated fibers
within the NPG after intracranial section of the glossopharyngeal nerve
(23 days survival time). These new and not yet accomplished studies stand
in contrast to the view we have today from the findings of Biscoe and
Sampson (24), Lipski et al. (25) and Cottle (26). Their data give no evidence for peripheral chemoreceptor projections in nuclei of the ventral
reticular formation. More data are necessary to clarify the functional
role of the NPG in the regulation of ventilation.

Central chemosensitivity and its modification by muscular exercise

Spode and Schlaefke (14) found that an increase of respiratory drive induced by muscular exercise does occur only as long as the incoming impulses
from the muscles meet sufficient respiratory activity, which, when peripheral chemoreceptors are cut, is guaranteed by the central chemosensitive
mechanism (27). The idea of H^+ion dependent tonic drive arising within
the ventral part of the NPG being influenced by afferents from the muscles,
could give one reason why the cold block of the areas S does not allow
any respiratory drive during muscular exercise. Furthermore the same
possible characteristics of H^+ion responsive neurones should be taken into
consideration when discussing the problem of how the enormous ventilatory
drive during muscular exercise may arise. From the results of our experiments in cats we conclude that under resting conditions and in hyperoxia
87 % of the ventilatory drive can be attributed to the central chemosensitive mechanism. Under the condition of muscular exercise this type of
drive may be increased which would be reflected in an increase of the
tonic activity of chemosensitive neurones.

Applying the model of Fukuda et al. (12) the ventral medullary surface
layer including the ventral pole of the NPG may be regarded as a site of
synaptic transmission including signals from peripheral chemoreceptors
as well as from afferents from the working muscles to neurones leading to
the respiratory centers. Since the synapses are of cholinergic nature the
role of the actual H^+ concentration would consist in an influence on the
transmitter release and the cholinesterase activity, as well as on the Ca^{++}
concentration (12)For such a functional concept of central chemosensitivity
the structure of the described location may provide favourizing conditions.
The ultrastructure presents multisynaptic contacts and a 'glia spongiosa'
containing multiple capillaries with adjacent nerve cells.

There are objections against a general H^+ion sensitivity of the NPG.
Schlaefke and See (22) found neurones, also belonging to the NPG lying
in close vicinity to H^+ion responding neurones, which do not react when
the surface pH is changed but which increase their tonic discharge when
an antihypertensive drug (imidazoline derivative) is applied on the surface. The elevation of activity is followed by a decrease of splanchnic
nerve activity with a latency of 20 msec and a fall of arterial pressure
later on. We were able to discriminate both types of neurones, both being
of cholinergic nature, but the tonic discharge of only one type was modulated by H^+ions. The latter was traced to a group of small cells in a short
distance from the surface, the former to a medium-sized type deeper below
the surface (600 - 1200 µm) (fig. 3, square). In connection with the data
of Berndt et al. (1) the location of H^+ion modulated units within 200 -
450 µm below the surface corresponds with the theoretically determined
site of H^+ion sensitivity.

We cannot tell at the moment whether the synaptic model covers the secret of central chemosensitivity completely or whether specialized neurones may contribute to the H^+ion-sensitive mechanism also; for example a specialization could exist in neurones of the NPG sending dendrites to the chemosensitive areas M and L. By such a neuronal arrangement we could explain the ventilatory responses to local pH changes as well as the effect of cold block or coagulation (5, 6). The findings of Schwanghardt et al. (2) would rather be in favour of the second model. A combination of both models may be conceivable.

CONCLUSIONS

The findings that peripheral chemoreceptor activation, as well as stimulation of afferents from the muscles, are used by neurones underneath the area S for a modification of their tonic discharge which is dependent upon pH, coincide with the former results obtained by bilateral cold block or coagulation of the area S during peripheral chemoreceptor activation and during exercise. We may conclude that the central chemosensitive mechanism is modified by peripheral chemoreceptors and by muscular exercise. According to Fukuda et al. (12) the central chemosensitive mechanism may be a characteristic of cholinergic synapses formed by different afferents. Here now, we may add, within the NPG underneath of the area S respiratory afferents may converge, including those from the chemosensitive areas on the medullary surface, and may be constituting tonic afferent respiratory drive. How much acetylcholine is allowed to act on the synapses in order to form the tonic drive would be a matter of the acute H^+ion concentration. Thus the ventral medullary surface may serve as a site of origin and modification of respiratory drive.

SUMMARY

Bilateral cold block or coagulation of the area S (intermediate area) on the ventral medullary surface, which eliminates the central CO_2 drive of respiration, leads to a diminished ventilatory response to hypoxia, and abolishes the respiratory drive induced by muscular exercise, the latter in absence of peripheral chemoreceptors. Extracellular recordings of tonically discharging neurones within the superficial layer of the area S revealed a dependence of the impulse frequency upon the surface pH. The tonic discharge of some of these neurones was modified by sinus nerve stimulation, systemic hypoxia or i.v. injection of NaCN. A small cell type within the ventral pole of the nucleus paragigantocellularis (220 - 450 μm below the surface of the area S) showed a strong dependence of discharge frequency on the surface pH, and in addition, was influenced by stimulation of the tibial or femoral nerve. It is concluded that the area S acts as a site of confluence of chemosensitive signals from the medullary surface and afferents from different sources, forming cholinergic synapses.

REFERENCES

(1) J. Berndt, W. Berger, K. Berger, and M. Schmidt; Untersuchungen zum
     zentralen chemosensiblen Mechanismus der Atmung. II. Die
     Steuerung der Atmung durch das extracelluläre pH im Gewebe der
     Medulla oblongata. Pflüg. Arch. 332, 146-170 (1972).

(2) F. Schwanghardt, R. Schröter, D. Klüssendorf, and H.P. Koepchen
     (1974), The influence of novocaine block of superficial brain
     stem structures on respiratory and reticular neurones. In:
     Central Rhythmic and Regulation. W. Umbach and H.P. Koepchen
     (Eds.). Stuttgart: Hippokrates (pp. 10-210).

(3) M.E. Schlaefke and H.H. Loeschcke; Lokalisation eines an der Regula-
     tion von Atmung und Kreislauf beteiligten Gebietes an der ven-
     tralen Oberfläche der Medulla oblongata. Pflüg. Arch. 297,
     201-220 (1967).

(4) M.E. Schlaefke, W.R. See, W.H. Massion, and H.H. Loeschcke, Die Rolle
     spezifischer und unspezifischer Afferenzen für den Antrieb der
     Atmung, untersucht durch Reizung und Blockade von Afferenzen an
     der decerebrierten Katzen. Pflüg. Arch. 312, 189-205 (1969).

(5) M.E. Schlaefke, W.R. See, and H.H. Loeschcke, Ventilatory response
     to alterations of H^+ion concentration in small areas of the
     ventral medullary surface. Resp. Physiol. 10, 198-212 (1970).

(6) M.E. Schlaefke, J.F. Kille, and H.H. Loeschcke, Elimination of cen-
     tral chemosensitivity by coagulation of a bilateral area on the
     ventral medullary surface. Studies in awake cats. Pflüg. Arch.
     (in press).

(7) M. Pokorski, M.E. Schlaefke, and W.R. See, Neurophysiological studies
     on the central chemosensitive mechanism (rostral area). Pflüg.
     Arch. Suppl. 335: R 33 (1975).

(8) R.K. Prill, M. Pokorski, W.R. See, and M.E. Schlaefke, Neurophysiolo-
     gical studies on the central chemosensitive mechanism (caudal
     area). Pflüg. Arch. Suppl. 255: R 33 (1975).

(9) M.E. Schlaefke, M. Pokorski, W.R. See, R.K. Prill, and H.H. Loeschcke,
     Chemosensitive neurones on the ventral medullary surface. Bull.
     Physio-pathol. resp. 11, 277-284 (1975).

(10) Y. Fukuda, and Y. Honda, pH sensitivity of cells located at the ventro-
     lateral surface of the rat medulla oblongata in vitro. Pflüg.
     Arch. 364, 243-247 (1976).

(11) Y. Fukuda, and H.H. Loeschcke, Effect of H^+ on spontaneous neuronal
     activity in the surface layer of the rat medulla oblongata in
     vitro. Pflüg. Arch. 371, 125-134 (1977).

(12) Y. Fukuda, Y. Honda, M.E. Schlaefke, and H.H. Loeschcke, Effect of
     H^+ on the membrane potential of silent cells in the ventral and
     dorsal surface layers of the rat medulla in vitro. Pflüg. Arch.
     376, 229-235 (1978).

(13) M.E. Schlaefke (1976), Central chemosensitivity: Neurophysiology and
     contribution to regulation. In: Acid Base Homeostasis of the
     Brain Extracellular Fluid and the Respiratory Control System.
     H.H. Loeschcke (Ed.). Thieme, Ed. Publ. (pp. 66-69).

(14) R. Spode, and M.E. Schlaefke, Influence of muscular exercise on res-
     piration after central and peripheral chemodenervation. Pflüg.
     Arch. 359, R 49 (1975).

(15) R.A. Mitchell, H.H. Loeschcke, W.H. Massion, and J.W. Severinghaus,
     Respiratory responses mediated through superficial chemosensitive
     areas on the medulla. J. appl. Physiol. 18, 523-533 (1963).

(16) R.P. Eager, Selective staining of degenerating axons in the central
     nervous system by a simplified silver method: spinal cord pro-
     jections to external cuneate and inferior olivary nuclei in the
     cat. Brain Res. 22, 137-141 (1970).

(17) R. Petrovický, Über die Glia marginalis und oberflächliche Nerven-
     zellen im Hirnstamm der Katze. Z. Anat. Entw. 127, 221-231
     (1968).

(18) E. Taber, The cytoarchitecture of the brain stem of the cat I. Brain
     stem nuclei of cat. J. Comp. Neurol. 116, 27-70 (1970).

(19) W.R. See, Die Rolle chemischer und nichtchemischer Afferenzen des
     Nervus vagus als Atmungsantriebe. Diplomarbeit Abt. Biologie,
     Ruhr-Universität (1973).

(20) M.E. Schlaefke, and W.R. See, Ventral surface stimulus response in
     relation to ventilatory and cardiovascular effects. In: Central
     Interaction between Respiratory and Cardiovascular Control
     Systems. Symp. Berlin (in press).

(21) R.E. Dermietzel, A. Leibstein, I. Willenberg, W.R. See, and M. E.
     Schlaefke, In vivo labelling of neurones in the chemosensitive
     fields of the ventral surface of the medulla oblongata with
     horseraddish peroxidase. Proc. Int. Un. Physiol. Sci. XIII,
     521 (1977).

(22) W.R. See, and M.E. Schlaefke, The influence of sinusnerve stimulation
     on neuronal activity of ventral medullary neurones. Neurosci.
     Letters, Suppl. 1, S 19 (1978).

(23) J.F. Kille, and M.E. Schlaefke, Histological studies on the medullary
     chemosensitive areas after chronic denervation of a carotid body.
     Neurosc. Letters, Suppl. 1, S 16 (1978).

(24) T.J. Biscoe, and S.R. Sampson, Responses of cells in the brain stem
     of the cat to stimulation of the sinus, glossopharyngeal aortic
     and superior laryngeal nerves. J. Physiol. 209, 359-373 (1970).

(25) J. Lipski, R.M. McAllen, and K.M. Spyer: The sinus nerve and baro-
     receptor input to the medulla oblongata of the cat. J. Physiol.,
     251, 61-78 (1975).

(26) M.K. Cottle, Degeneration studies of primary afferents of IXth and
          Xth cranial nerves in the cat. J. comp. Neurol. 122, 329-345
          (1964).

(27) M.E. Schlaefke, 'Specific' and 'non-specific' stimuli in the drive of
          respiration. Acta Neurobiol. Exp. 33, 149-154 (1973).

DISCUSSION

Commenting on the conclusion by Schlaefke that carotid sinus nerve
(CSN) afferents projects onto the nucleus paragigantocellularis
Lipski pointed out that 1) CSN is only a small branch of the glossopharyngeal nerve, 2) the responses might well be polysynaptic, 3)
according to earlier results (Lipski et al., J.Physiol. 251, 61, 1975)
the CSN afferents terminate exclusively in nucleus tractus solitarius.
In this connection Euler called attention to their findings (Cherniack
et al., p35, this volume) that the afferent inputs from CSN afferents
and from other glossopharyngeal afferents are treated quite differently by the central reflex mechanisms and that the reflex effects
mediated by the CSN afferents are not influenced by moderate focal
cooling of the 'intermediate' areas.

Schlaefke was asked whether she had evidence that the neurons which
were said to "belong to the cardiovascular system" do have a direct
action on this system or whether they merely exhibit a discharge
pattern in parallel with changes in cardiovascular or sympathetic
activities. Schlaefke stated that activation of these neurons in the
nucleus paragigantocellularis was followed by an inhibition of
splanchnic and cervical sympathetic efferent activity, a fall in
arterial blood pressure, and a decrease in the plasma - renin activity. She also referred to the recent work of Amendt et al. (Pflügers
Arch. 375, 289, 1978) showing projections of cells of the nucleus
paragigantocellularis onto the intermediolateral neuron pools of
thoracic spinal segments.

INTERACTIONS BETWEEN A CENTRAL CHEMOCEPTIVE SYSTEM AND OTHER VENTILATORY DRIVES

N. S. CHERNIACK, C. VON EULER, I. HOMMA and F. F. KAO

Nobel Institute for Neurophysiology, Karolinska Institutet, Stockholm, Sweden

During the last few decades a considerable amount of evidence has accumulated in favour of the concept that the central chemoceptive drive for ventilation does not arise from brainstem respiratory neurons but from specific intracranial chemoreceptive structures (Refs 1,2)

Mitchell and Herbert (3) for instance, in their intracellular studies of medullary respiratory neurons, showed that an increase in PCO_2 caused only hyperpolarization indicating a reduced excitability of these neurons. It was further shown that iontophoretically applied hydrogen ions extracellularly in the vicinity of the investigated neurons failed to produce any signs of excitation of these neurons. However, recent work suggests that the stimulating effect of (CO_2, H^+) on ventilation is not due solely to excitatory effects but also to inhibitory processes. Thus, it has been shown that the central effects of an increase in PCO_2 on ventilation is due both to an excitatory effect on the rate of rise of the central inspiratory activity, CIA, and to an inhibitory effect causing a more or less 'matching' increase in the thresholds of the inspiratory 'off-switch' mechanisms (Ref. 4). This might provoke the question whether the inhibitory action on the 'off-switch' mechanism could possibly be the result of a direct hyperpolarizing action of (CO_2, H^+) on neurons involved in these mechanisms in contrast to the excitatory effect on the generation of CIA which apparently emanates from the intracranial chemoceptive structures.

Largely through the extensive work of the Bochum school there has been much progress in defining the localization of the intracranial chemoreceptors to circumscribed areas on the ventral surface of medulla and determining the adequate stimuli for these receptors (see *e.g.* Loeschcke in this volume). Relatively little is known, however, about the characteristics and location of the neural structures subserving the interactions between the afferent inputs from the intracranial chemoceptive structures, on the one hand, and from the peripheral chemoreceptors and other reflex and central sources on the other.

In a recent paper (Ref. 5) we have attempted to elucidate the problems mentioned above *i.e.* 1) whether the central effects on ventilation of changes in PCO_2 are all due to the afferent input from specific cen-

tral chemoceptive structures, or whether there are any significant
effects on respiratory regulation exerted directly on neurons involved
in any of the sub-mechanisms of the respiratory pattern generator and
2) concerning the features of the interactions between the central
chemoreceptor input and some other ventilatory drive inputs. To this
end we have tried to modulate, in a direct way, the input from the
intracranial (CO_2, H^+)-receptors.

Results of the Bochum group suggest that the afferent input from the
intracranial chemoceptive structures to the respiratory pattern generator might be influenced directly at the 'intermediate' or 'S' area
(here denoted $I_{(S)}$ area) *e.g.* by means of cooling these areas.

The method of focal cooling of certain neural structures has proved
a very useful analytical tool in the neurophysiology of the central
nervous system to induce a rapid and fully reversible block of synaptic transmission within a narrow region in the brain. At a tissue
temperature of about 20° C all synaptic transmission is selectively
blocked; much lower temperatures are required to block impulse conduction in nerve fibres. An advantageous feature of this method is
the high spatial selectivity of the focal temperature effects which
depends on the steep temperature gradients in brain tissue around a
'cryogenic' probe inserted in subcortical structures or beneath a
thermode applied on the brain surface. The gradient has been found to
be in the order of 5 to 10° C per mm (see *e.g.* Refs. 6,7).

Employing this method we have been able to produce rapid and graded
modulations of the input from the intracranial chemosensitive structures and to study the effects of such procedures on the timing and
amplitude parameters of the breathing pattern and its neural correlates at various levels of PCO_2 and PO_2 with and without functional
chemostatic feedback. For the detailed account of methods and results
we refer to the original paper (Ref. 5). In the present communication
we will only make brief mention of some of the main results and
discuss some of their implications.

We have confirmed the general finding of the Bochum school that strong
bilateral cooling of the $I_{(S)}$ areas can cause apnoea. In our experiments, however, apnoea occurred even at a surface temperature of these
areas of about 20° C in normoxic and normocapnic conditions. We
further found that the temperature effect on respiration was graded:
In the range between 26° to 43° C the relationships between surface
temperature and the effects on the respiratory parameters were almost
linear, though different at different PCO_2 levels, with enhancements
of $\dot{V}$, V_T, and Phr_T by focal warming and depressions by cooling to a
temperature below 37° C (see Fig. 1A).

Moderate focal cooling or heating (28° to 43° C) of the $I_{(S)}$ areas
caused an almost parallel shift of the whole CO_2-response (V_T, Phr_T)
curves to the right with little or no change in slope (see Fig. 1B).
Also the 'apnoea point', (the PCO_2 threshold for manifest respiratory
activity) was shifted. Accordingly it was found that these temperature
effects could be compensated by corresponding changes in PCO_2. The
effects of moderate focal cooling of the $I_{(S)}$ areas to various temperature resembled in detail the effects of hypocapnia and the effects
of warming mimicked precisely the effects of increased PCO_2. Thus,
the proportional relationships between the effects on the time course
of the inspiratory trajectory and on the inspiratory 'off-switch'

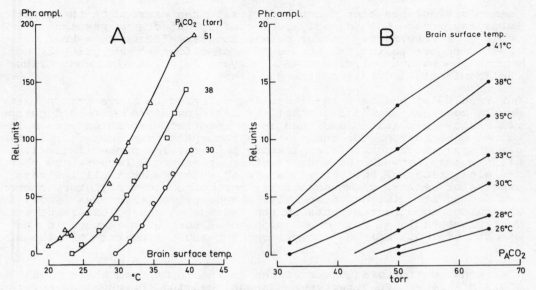

Fig. 1. Effects on tidal phrenic amplitude (*i.e.*
peak amplitude of the moving average of efferent
phrenic activity) of focal I$_{(S)}$ area temperatures
at different P$_A$CO$_2$ levels (A) and of P$_A$CO$_2$ at
different I$_{(S)}$ area temperatures (B).

mechanisms were the same in response to focal cooling at constant
PCO$_2$ as in response to alterations of PCO$_2$ (cf. Ref. 4). The Hering-
Breuer volume - time relationships were not affected by cooling the
I$_{(S)}$ areas nor by changing PCO$_2$. Moderate cooling of the I$_{(S)}$ areas
caused only minor effects on systemic blood pressure. It should be
emphasized that the results of focal cooling of I$_{(S)}$ areas are quite
different from those reported for whole body hypothermia and also
from those obtained in response to local temperature changes of the
'thermosensitive' structures deep in the bulbar brainstem.

Several lines of evidence have permitted us to conclude that the
effects of moderate focal cooling (above 28° C) are mediated by
structures located very superficially at the I$_{(S)}$ areas. With stronger
cooling, however, also other structures, probably located somewhat
deeper beneath the surface, are affected and cause some additional
type of effects which can *not* be mimicked neither by local application of procaine (which only penetrates to a depth of less than 100
µm) nor by lowering of PCO$_2$; nor could they be fully compensated by
hypercapnia. The occurrence of complex effects, probably of multiple
origin, in response to cooling to temperatures below 28° C is an indication of the danger of relying on results only from severe cooling
and the importance of employing moderate temperature changes when
trying to evaluate the specific effects of changes in the input from
the central chemoceptive structures. It should be recalled that the
structures in close approximation to and partly overlapping with the
'chemoceptive' areas are structures which appear to be quite hetero-
genous in function (see *e.g.* Ref. 8, and the presence of noradrenergic
and 5-HT neurons, Ref. 9) and of subst. P cells (T.Hökfelt, personal

communication) has been described. Influences exerted on these structures may induce both direct and secondary effects on respiration. A
variety of respiratory and/or cardiovascular effects have been obtained in response to topical application of different synaptically active
substances such as glycine, GABA, strychnine, clonidine and various
cholinomimetic and anticholinergic drugs.

Our results of moderate focal cooling referred to above were obtained
during constant artificial ventilation (in paralysed cats and peripheral chemo-denervation) and thus in an open loop situation with maintained constancy of the chemical environment of the deeper brainstem
structures which control respiratory pattern. The close similarity in
all respects between the effects of moderate focal temperature changes
and alterations of PCO_2 provides strong evidence that all the main
aspects of central chemosensitivity for metabolic ventilatory control
are due to stimulation of specific chemoceptive structures (Refs. 1,
2) and not to direct effects on the neurons of the bulbar respiratory
control mechanisms. This conclusion holds both with respect to the
effects of (CO_2, H^+) on 'off-switch' thresholds and rate of rise of
CIA.

The technique for graded variations in the input from the central
(CO_2, H^+)-receptive structures without changing the chemical environment of the respiratory neurons proved a valuable tool in the analysis
of the interactions between the central chemo-drive and the drives
from the peripheral chemoreceptors and other non-chemical sources.
Both 'multiplicative' and 'additive' types of interaction were encountered. Possibly these two types could appear in various combinations.
Examples of the multiplicative or 'gain-changing' type of interaction
are provided by the reflex increase in inspiratory activity which can
be provoked by the lung deflation reflex (Ref. 10) or by stimulation
of pharyngeal afferents. These reflexes showed a marked CO_2-dependence
with little response effect at, or close to, the CO_2-threshold for
manifest breathing ('apnoea point') but with progressively stronger
reflex effects at increasing levels of PCO_2. The CO_2-effect on these
reflexes was closely mimicked by focal cooling of the $I_{(S)}$ areas.
This is shown in Fig. 2A which further illustrates that at a given
PCO_2 focal cooling causes a decrease, or even a nullification of the
responsiveness to the stimulus merely by shifting the CO_2-response
curve to the right. This means that a depression or extinction of
such reflexes in response to focal cooling can *not* be taken as evidence that the superficial structures of these areas are involved in
the pathways of these reflexes but should be regarded merely as consequences both of the effect of the focal cooling on the CO_2-response
and of the 'multiplicative' character of the interaction between these
reflexes and the central chemoceptive afferents.

In contrast hypoxia or electrical stimulation of the carotid sinus
nerve (CSN) showed little or no CO_2-dependence (see Fig. 2B). These
reflexes caused almost the same absolute increase of V_T or Phr_T at
all PCO_2 levels and at all focal temperatures of the $I_{(S)}$ areas. This
suggests an additive or 'threshold- and recruitment-changing' type of
interaction between the afferent inputs from the central and the peripheral chemoreceptors. With this type of interaction the reflex responses cause a shift also of the 'apnoea point' to lower PCO_2 values.
Thus these reflexes caused not only a shift upwards of the CO_2-response
curves to higher response values for a given CO_2-value. They also
caused an extension of the curves to the left into a range of PCO_2

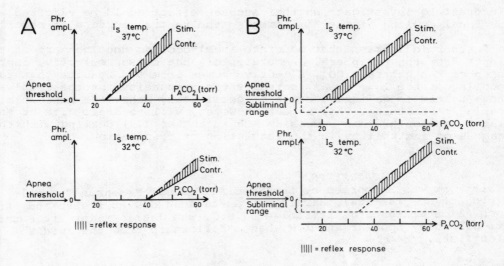

Fig. 2. To show two main types of interaction between reflex and central chemo-drive. A: 'additive' or 'threshold- and recruitment-changing' interaction at two different $I_{(S)}$ area temperatures. B: 'multiplicative' or 'gain-changing' interaction at two different $I_{(S)}$ area temperatures.

values which, in the 'unstimulated' condition, was below the 'apnoea point'. This implies that the central (CO_2, H^+)-sensors have an operational range far below the CO_2-threshold for *manifest* respiratory output activity. Below the 'apnoea point' there seems to be a considerable range in which sub-threshold processes and interactions can occur (cf. Eldridge & Gill-Kumar in this volume), and where summation of subliminal excitatory inputs from the central and peripheral chemoreceptors and from other additively-acting reflex sources can lead to that the threshold gets exceeded and breathing resumed. Exercise (cf. Kao in this volume), the ventilatory stimulus from the hypothalamic thermoregulatory mechanisms (Ref. 11), and probably also some components of the complex 'wakefulness' drive may serve as further examples of respiratory stimuli of mainly additive character. By employing the method of graded focal cooling of the $I_{(S)}$ areas we could show that the structures responsible for the integration between the peripheral chemoreceptors and the central chemoreceptors were *not* located superficially at this area. Only further research can determine whether some other additively-acting respiratory stimuli of reflex or central origin might be affected by moderate cooling of those superficial structures of the $I_{(S)}$ areas which transmit the input from the central chemoceptive structures.

Majcherczyk and Willshaw (12) have studied another type of interaction between central and peripheral chemoreceptors. They have shown that a decrease of PCO_2 by hyperventilation can induce an increased centrifugal activity in the carotid sinus nerve combined with corresponding diminution of the afferent chemoreceptive input from the carotid body. As mentioned earlier (Ref. 5) it would be of great interest to investigate whether such an effect could be elicited also by focal cooling of the $I_{(S)}$ area on the ventral surface of medulla.

A further indication that moderate focal cooling does not affect the input from the peripheral chemoreceptors but causes selective depression of the central (CO_2, H^+)-drive comes from our results that focal cooling of the $I_{(S)}$ areas increases the preponsity for the respiratory system to go into a state of oscillatory behaviour and exhibit periodic breathing. This aspect, however, will be dealt with at the later session of this symposium (Cherniack *et al.*) dealing with the causes of instability in the regulation of respiration.

ACKNOWLEDGEMENTS

This work was supported by the Swedish Medical Research Council (project no. 14X-544), Harald och Greta Jeansons Stiftelse and Knut och Alice Wallenbergs Stiftelse. N.S.C. was Josiah Macey Jr. Foundation Faculty Scholar and I.H. had a fellowship from the Swedish Institute.

REFERENCES

(1) C.v.Euler & U.Söderberg, Medullary chemosensitive receptors, *J.Physiol*. 118, 545 (1952).

(2) A.Åström, On the action of combined carbon dioxide excess and oxygen deficiency in the regulation of breathing, *Acta physiol.scand*. 27, Suppl. 98 (1952).

(3) R. Mitchell & D.A.Herbert, The effect of carbon dioxide on the membrane potential of medullary respiratory neurons, *Brain Res*. 75, 345 (1974).

(4) C.v.Euler & T.Trippenbach, Excitability changes of the inspiratory 'off-switch' mechanism tested by electrical stimulation in nucleus parabrachialis in the cat, *Acta physiol.scand*. 97, 175 (1976).

(5) N.S.Cherniack, C.v.Euler, I.Homma & F.F.Kao, Graded changes in central chemoceptor input by local temperature changes on the ventral surface of medulla, *J.Physiol*. 287, 191 (1979).

(6) H.H.Jasper, D.G.Shacter & J.Montplaisir, The effect of local cooling upon spontaneous and evoked electrical activity of cerebral cortex, *Canad.J.Physiol.Pharmacol*. 48, 640 (1970).

(7) M.Bénita & H.Condé, Effects of local cooling upon conduction and synaptic transmission, *Brain Res*. 36, 133 (1972).

(8) W.Feldberg & P.G.Guertzenstein, Vasodepressor effects obtained by drugs acting on the ventral surface of the brain stem, *J.Physiol*. 258, 337 (1976).

(9) A.Dahlström & K.Fuxe, Evidence for the existence of monoamine-containing neurons in the central nervous system. I. Demonstration of monoamines in the cell bodies of brain stem

neurons, *Acta physiol.scand.* 62, Suppl. 232 (1964).

(10) C. von Euler, M.Glogowska & I.Homma, Inspiratory-facilitatory
     reflexes provoked by inflations and deflations in cats.
     Proc. IUPS XIII, 792 (1977).

(11) W.R.See, Über den Beitrag des Hypothalamus zur Atmung nach Aus-
     schaltung der chemischen Atemantriebe. Thesis, Bochum,
     123 pp (1976).

(12) S.Majcherczyk & P.Willshaw, The influence of hyperventilation on
     efferent control of peripheral chemoreceptors, *Brain Res.*
     124, 561 (1977).

DISCUSSION

Referring to the fact that important blood vessels perfusing the core
of medulla penetrate from the ventral surface areas questions were
raised whether the effects of cooling, application of drugs and
coagulation to the regions of the ventral surface of medulla might
not be referred to alterations in the circulation of deep bulbar
structures rather than to direct effects on superficial chemoceptive
structures.

Euler replied that with respect to the effects of moderate focal
cooling there were several lines of evidence of which a detailed
account was given in the full paper by Cherniack et al. (J.Physiol.
287, 191, 1979) showing that the reported effects of moderate cooling are mediated by superficial structures and cannot be explained
on the basis of spread of temperature changes from the surface to
neural mechanisms located in the depth of medulla, neither by con-
vection by the circulating blood nor by conduction through the
tissues.

ROLE OF MEASURABLE CHEMICAL STIMULI IN CHRONIC VENTILATORY ADAPTATIONS

J. A. DEMPSEY

*Pulmonary Physiology Laboratory, Department of Preventive Medicine,
University of Wisconsin, Madison, Wisconsin 53706, U.S.A.*

ABSTRACT

We evaluated the role of arterial PO_2 and pH and CSF pH as mediators of ventilatory
acclimatization to and deacclimatization from chronic hypoxia and hypocapnia in
awake humans and animals. The data were consistent in showing that these variables
changed as <u>functions</u> of the time-dependent ventilatory change in both normoxic and
hypoxic states, during increasing or decreasing ventilation and regardless of
whether the chemical stimuli were increasing, decreasing or remaining unchanged.
Further, the relative insensitivity of CSF pH as a chronic ventilatory stimulus was
demonstrated in patients with COPD by comparing it's effects with those of a "non-
chemical" hormonal stimulus. Simple algebraic summation of measurable chemical
stimuli in the plasma and CSF does not account for chronic ventilatory adaptation.
The potential role of $[H^+]$ in other cerebral fluids and of other "non-chemical"
stimuli in the CNS were discussed.

In assessing factors contributing to a given level of ventilation in any condition,
a first order of consideration is given to the so-called "chemical" stimuli--tradi-
tionally defined as pH and PO_2 acting at peripheral and/or central chemosensitive
reflex receptors. While many other factors may influence breathing in various
physiologic states, these "chemical" drives are conventionally assigned crucial
roles in normal air-breathing eupnea and are believed to explain all of the adaptive changes in ventilation which occur during acclimatization to various chronic
states such as hypoxia or acid-base derangements. The data we have obtained during
ventilatory acclimatization to several different states question this role of
"chemical" stimuli. Further, we believe these data question the more basic concept
and practice of assigning changing contributions of chemoreceptors to total ventilatory drive, based on observed or implied changes in plasma PO_2 and pH or brain pH.

Role of "Measurable" Chemical Stimuli in Plasma and CSF

During sojourn at high altitudes, humans show a time-dependent hyperventilation
over the initial 10-14 days. In Table 1 are the accompanying levels of measurable
chemical stimuli in arterial blood and lumbar or cisternal CSF at selected time
points of acclimatization (1-4). The following points are made against a role for
chemical stimuli.

TABLE 1 Measurable "Chemical" Stimuli during Acclimatization to Chronic Hypoxia in Awake Humans and Ponies

	A. Humans (at 4300 m) 1 Hr to 2 Wks	Δ	B. Humans (at 3100 m) 1 Hr to 8 Hrs to 3 Wks	Δ	C. Humans (at 3200 m) Control vs. NaHCO₃**	Δ	D. Ponies (at 4300 m) 1 Hr to 1-2 Days to 5-10 Days	Δ
$PaCO_2$ (mmHg)	36 to 24	↓	39 to 36 ↓ to 32	↓	33 vs. 33	↔	36 to 28 ↓ to 33	↑
pH ⎰ −art.	7.42 to 7.45	↑	7.39 to 7.42 ↑ to 7.42	↔	7.44 vs. 7.49	↑	7.47 to 7.45 ↔ to 7.44	↔
pH ⎱ −CSF*	7.34 to 7.38	↑	7.32 to 7.34 ↑ to 7.34	↔	7.34 vs. 7.34	↔	7.35 to 7.39 ↑ to 7.35	↓
PaO_2 (mmHg)	40 to 48	↑	50 to 52 to 60	↑	55 vs. 55	↔	41 to 44 ↑ to 45	

*−Lumbar CSF in humans and cisternal CSF in ponies.

**−Two groups of 5 subjects each were studied before and throughout 5 days' sojourn at 3200 m: a "control" group ($[HCO_3^-]$ = 22.2 mEq/ℓ plasma and 23.2 CSF at 5 days) and a group with continuous NaHCO₃ ingestion ($[HCO_3^-]$ = 25.6 plasma and 23.0 CSF at 5 days).

−Arrows (under Δ) indicate those differences between means which were significantly different (P < .05) or indicate no significant change or difference (↔) (P > .05). Note, that in each example shown here (and in Table 2) the direction of change in $PaCO_2$ (and in V_A/VCO_2) is not positively correlated with concomitant changes in plasma pH, CSF pH or PaO_2.

1. In humans, as ventilation increases between 1 hr and 2 wks hypoxia
    (see A), arterial and CSF pH and arterial PO_2 all increase. Simi-
    larly, as hyperventilation increases from 1 to 8 hrs to 3 wks of
    moderate hypoxia (see B), CSF and arterial alkalinity either in-
    crease (1-8 hrs) or remain constant. These examples simply show
    no positive correlation of $\dot{V}_A/\dot{V}CO_2$ to changes in "chemical stimuli"
    and suggest, instead, that the levels of chemical stimuli at both
    peripheral and central chemoreceptors are resultant from the ven-
    tilatory changes.

2. Example C shows that experimental manipulation of plasma $[HCO_3^-]$
    and $[H^+]$ and therefore the gradient between CSF and plasma $[HCO_3^-]$
    (via $NaHCO_3$ ingestion) also had no significant effect on human
    ventilatory acclimatization over 5 days at 3200 m.

3. In example D, advantage is taken of the pony's characteristic (also
    shown by some other non-human species) of showing increasing hyper-
    ventilation during the first 3-4 days in hypoxia followed by a
    gradual decrease in ventilation and relative CO_2 retention over the
    subsequent few days in hypoxia. Note that--as in humans--the in-
    crease in ventilation over the first 2 days of sojourn is accom-
    panied by increased plasma and CSF alkalinity and PaO_2; and that
    as $\dot{V}_A$ falls and $PaCO_2$ rises with further time in hypoxia, a sig-
    nificant acid shift occurs in cisternal CSF. Measurable chemical
    stimuli clearly <u>follow</u> an increasing <u>or</u> decreasing ventilation in
    chronic hypoxia.

Another hallmark of ventilatory acclimatization to chronic hypoxia occurs when normoxia is suddenly restored. Hyperventilation continues at only a slightly reduced
level below that in chronic hypoxia and this hyperventilation gradually diminishes
with further time in normoxia. An examination of measurable chemical stimulus
levels during these periods of normoxic "deacclimatization" from chronic hypoxia
also shows that they follow rather than lead the ventilatory changes (Table 2)
(5,6).

1. Examples A and B compare control sea-level with one hour return to
    normoxia following acclimatization to hypoxia. Note that the sus-
    tained hyperventilation following acclimatization is accompanied
    by a CSF pH which is either the same (human lumbar CSF) or signif-
    icantly alkaline (pony cisternal CSF) to that obtained under con-
    trol normoxia at sea-level prior to sojourn.

2. As normoxic conditions are maintained for many hours, V_A gradually
    falls toward normal sea-level control levels and $PaCO_2$ rises (see
    C); but pH in both arterial blood and CSF become increasingly acid.
    Hence, neither the continued hyperventilation following acclimati-
    zation nor its gradual dissipation with time are compatible with
    measurable chemical stimuli.

3. An analogous situation to "deacclimatization" is seen following
    prolonged voluntary hyperventilation and hypocapnia (see D) where
    spontaneous hyperventilation persists for many hours and this level
    of spontaneous hyperventilation is greater if the preceding period
    of voluntary hyperventilation was carried out in hypoxia. As shown
    by the comparisons in Table 2-D, this extra effect of the accom-
    panying hypoxia on the subsequent spontaneous hyperventilation in
    normoxia was contrary to that expected from the accompanying
    measurable chemical stimuli in CSF and arterial blood.

TABLE 2 Measurable "Chemical" Stimuli in Normoxia following Acclimatization to Chronic Hypoxia and/or Hypocapnia (Note: All values are in normoxia [PaO_2 > 90 mmHg])

	A. Human Prior to vs. 1 Hr (Following 3 days' sojourn to 4300 m)				B. Pony Prior to vs. 1 Hr (Following 3 days' sojourn to 4300 m)				C. Human 1 Hr vs. 12 Hrs (Following 3 days' sojourn to 4300 m)				D. Human At 1 Hr of spontaneous breathing in normoxia (Following 26 Hrs of voluntary hyperventilation* in) Normoxia vs. Hypoxia			
				Δ				Δ				Δ				Δ
$PaCO_2$ (mmHg)	40	vs.	32	↓	39	vs.	28	↓	32	vs.	36	↑	36	vs.	33	↓
pH { -art.	7.44	vs.	7.44	↑	7.43	vs.	7.41	↓	7.44	vs.	7.41	↓	7.45	vs.	7.48	↑
-CSF	7.32	vs.	7.32	↔	7.33	vs.	7.35	↑	7.32	vs.	7.29	↓	7.32	vs.	7.36	↑
PaO_2 (mmHg)	95	vs.	98	↔	88	vs.	98	↑	98	vs.	99	↔	94	vs.	98	↑

*-The same group of 7 subjects were studied for 26 hours of voluntary hyperventilation in normoxia (PaO_2 ~ 95, $PaCO_2$ 31 mmHg) and in hypoxia (PaO_2 55, $PaCO_2$ 31 mmHg). The mean values shown here were obtained during spontaneous ventilation in normoxia, 60 minutes following each of these conditions of voluntary hyperventilation.

-Arrows (under Δ) indicate those differences between means which were significantly different (P < .05).

We think these data demonstrate that measurable chemical stimuli in arterial blood
and in bulk CSF are not mediators of ventilatory acclimatization to nor deacclimatization from chronic hypoxia. To the contrary, changes in [H⁺] in plasma and especially CSF appear as a <u>function</u> of ventilatory change. It appears, then, as if
the normally potent, high gain feedback of alveolar ventilation to changes in brain
ECF [H⁺] seen under normal conditions with ventricular-cisternal perfusion is no
longer operative during both acclimatization to and deacclimatization from chronic
hypoxia and/or hypocapnia.

The question remains--are we really seeing a relative depression in sensitivity of
central chemoreception overridden by other as yet undefinable regulators <u>or</u> are the
usual chemical stimuli still essential mediators of the ventilatory changes but we
have failed to detect their appropriate changes in the true environment of the
chemoreceptors. We present two further considerations which bear on this question.

<u>Relative Insensitivity to [H⁺]</u>

The data in Fig. 1 examine this question by demonstrating the following points in
patients with COPD and chronic CO_2 retention (7). Chronic hypoventilation persists

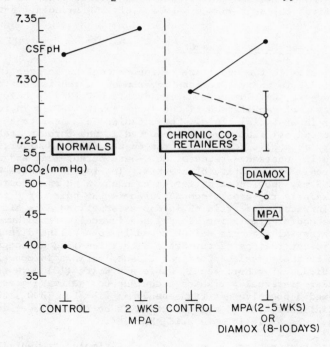

Fig. 1.

Chronic ventilatory response: 1) in 6 normals to oral medroxyprogesterone acetate
(MPA) (60 mg, day); and 2) in 9 patients with COPD and chronic CO_2 retention to MPA
and to DIAMOX. In addition to the changes shown in CSF pH, arterial pH fell significantly with DIAMOX (7.40 to 7.34) and rose with MPA (to 7.42). Arterial PO_2 remained in the 50-60 mmHg range. A sustained ventilatory response occurred in all 9
patients receiving MPA (-5 to -12 mmHg $\Delta PaCO_2$) and in 4 of the same patients receiving DIAMOX. The range of the CSF pH response to DIAMOX is indicated.

in the presence of an acid CSF $[H^+]$. Further, if a carbonic anhydrase inhibitor is given over an 8-10 day period which restores plasma $[HCO_3^-]$ (-5 to 10 mEq/ℓ) back to normal levels and reduces plasma and CSF pH, ventilation either remains unaffected (in 4 of the 9 patients) or shows a moderate increase. Why do these patients fail to respond or to respond adequately to these self-imposed or experimentally imposed forms of acidosis in plasma and CSF? Conventionally, the documented mechanical load on the pulmonary system would be implicated as the primary cause. However, it does not appear that these patients are incapable of responding to a chronic ventilatory stimulus, as shown by their correction of CO_2 retention upon administration of a synthetic progestin (medroxyprogesterone acetate or MPA). Note further that MPA produces only a moderate chronic ventilatory stimulus as shown in normal subjects (-5 mmHg PaCO$_2$) and that the sustained ventilatory response to MPA in normals or patients occurs and is sustained despite an accompanying alkalosis in CSF (and plasma).

Undoubtedly the ventilatory control system in these patient models is a highly complex one involving as yet undiscovered interactions among mechanical, neural and chemical stimuli acting at numerous levels of integration. Yet these patients do present another example, consistent with that previously shown in normals in chronic hypoxia, of a "responsive" control system which either fails or at least is "relatively insensitive" to the feedback between $[H^+]$ and alveolar ventilation.

Role of $[H^+]$ at Other Sites in the CNS

Chemosensitive cells in the medullary region respond to changes in the pH of interstitial fluid (ISF) in their immediate environment which is some distance below the medullary surface (9,10). Hence, the measurable CSF $[H^+]$ is only meaningful as a potential effector of ventilation if the large cavity CSF is in ionic equilibrium with the deeper interstitial fluid. These fluids do appear to be in equilibrium based on transependymal flux studies conducted in the chronic steady-states of normoxia or primary metabolic acid-base derangements (11). However, this equilibrium is not achieved in nonsteady-states of acid-base derangement and may not be present even in the chronic steady-state of hypoxia. Two recent studies whow that other areas of the CNS may show quite different changes in pH in chronic hypoxia than the progressive alkalosis repeatedly demonstrated in the bulk CSF. Pelligrino, et al. (12) measured intracellular brain pH in N_2O anesthetized dogs after 1 and 5 hours of hypoxic hypocapnia, simulating blood gases in acclimatizad humans at 4300 m (Fig. 2). As arterial and bulk CSF pH moved in an alkaline direction, intracellular pH in four different regions of the brain either remained unchanged or fell slightly below normoxic control levels. Cortical tissue lactic acid coneentrations increased by about two-thirds. Further, Fencl, Gable and Wolfe (13) have recently applied their ventricular-cisternal perfusion technique to the awake goat after 5 days at 4300 m and showed a positive net transependymal flux for $[HCO_3^-]$ to such an extent that interstitial fluid $[HCO_3^-]$ was estimated to be 25-30% lower in ISF than CSF and thus ISF pH was substantially more acid than CSF.

Thus, these data suggest that a potential $[H^+]$ stimulus to ventilation is available during hypoxia. Most convincing here is the finding of acidity in the brain ISF, which, while not an exact quantitative representation of the $[HCO_3^-]$, PCO$_2$ and thus $[H^+]$ affecting the chemosensitive cells (10), certainly reflects a more realistic stimulus level than that measurable in bulk CSF. Brain intracellular pH also undergoes appropriate changes to qualify as a potential chemoreceptor stimulus in hypoxic hypocapnia, but we are not at all sure that changes in pH$_i$--in addition to Δ ISF pH or by itself--affects the output of medullary chemosensitive cells. We know of no systematic investigations which have definitively ruled out this potential mediator role for changes in brain intracellular pH.

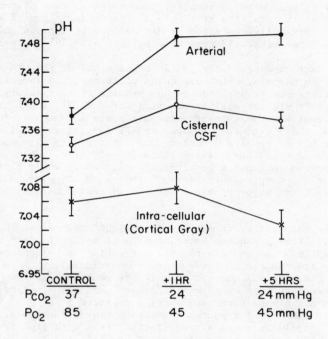

Fig. 2.

Effects of short-term hypoxic hypocapnia on arterial CSF and brain intracellular pH (pH_i) in anesthetized dogs. Each data point for brain pH_i represents the mean of 3 methods of measurement (DMO, CO_2 and CPK equilibrium techniques) and includes a correction for measured brain extracellular fluid space. The constancy of slightly acidic changes in pH_i shown here for cortical gray matter was also observed in 2 other brain regions--paraventricular white matter and the floor of the 4th ventricle.

SUMMARY

The role of chemical stimuli and of cerebral fluid [H+] in the control of breathing in general and specifically in the mediation of ventilatory acclimatization remains unresolved, although some progress has been made. First, it seems clear on the basis of evidence such as that presented in Tables 1 and 2 that measurable chemical stimuli in the arterial blood and bulk CSF simply do not explain and in fact are incompatible with observed ventilatory changes in a variety of conditions. This conclusion was consistently upheld across a variety of species, in both normoxic and hypoxic states, during increasing or decreasing ventilation and regardless of whether chemical stimuli were increasing, decreasing or remaining unchanged. We propose, then, that the practice of simple algebraic summation of measurable chemical stimuli, as originally conceived by Mitchell, Severinghaus and colleagues to account for many forms of ventilatory adaptation (14,15,16) is no longer acceptable.

The evidence to date showing pH changes in other areas of the CNS and most notably in the brain ISF in hypoxia, which are quite different than those in bulk CSF, presents an exciting new perspective on the problem of ventilatory acclimatization. For sure, these data caution against assuming CSF-ISF [H+] equilibrium only on the basis of an apparent steady-state of acid-base status. Whether, in turn, we can also presume that these estimated changes in ISF pH are truly reflective of changes in chemoreceptor ECF pH remains untested (10). These data also show that ventilation is up at a time when interstitial fluid [H+] is acid. Hence, it is enticing to immediately presume a cause:effect relationship which would place [H+] back into its seemingly logical compensatory feedback role with alveolar ventilation. However, we think at least three major problems must be addressed before this conclusion is tenable.

First, and at the very least, it must be established that a reasonable correlation does exist between time-dependent ventilatory acclimatization and deacclimatization vs. changes in ISF pH. An analogy to this suggestion is evident in the series of negative correlations (based on time-course measurements) which were necessary to adequately test the original concept of bulk CSF pH and plasma PO_2 and pH as mediators of acclimatization (see examples in Tables 1 and 2). In fact, these previously obtained data point to many occasions where a positive Δ ISF pH:Δ $\dot{V}_A$ may be in doubt. For example, it would not be expected that brain tissue lactic acid production (12) and thus ISF [H+] would increase as ventilation rises with time from acute to chronic hypoxia. Nor would an alkalotic shift in ISF be predicted in such non-human species, as pony and goat, as ventilation falls back and $PaCO_2$ rises toward normal beyond the first few days of continued hypoxia. But this skepticism is only theoretical and it does require thorough testing.

Secondly, it is important to question the meaning--in functional terms--of any measured change in brain ISF pH. Can one readily apply the (very substantial) gain of $\dot{V}_A$ vs. ISF pH as established by ventricular-cisternal perfusion techniques in normal animals at sea-level to metabolically induced changes in ISF pH in the chronically hypoxic animal? We think not, because the methods of inducing changes in cerebral pH are markedly different; and because the actual output or gain of either the peripheral or central chemoreceptors may be markedly affected by changes in the activity of or stimulus to either one. For example, Majcherczyk, et al. (17) have demonstrated marked changes in the anesthetized cat's carotid sinus nerve efferent and afferent activities in response to acutely induced changes in medullary ECF pH. Further, the examples in awake humans and animals shown in Tables 1 and 2 and Fig. 1 indicate, with as yet only very indirect data, that the relative contributions of the "central" [H+] stimulus to total ventilatory drive may be depressed or "overridden" in conditions such as chronic hypoxia or long-standing respiratory acid-base derangements.

A third factor to consider in assessing the relative contributions of measured changes in potential chemical stimuli to total ventilatory drive is some recent work demonstrating important physiologic influences on ventilatory control which are independent of [H$^+$]. Carotid and aortic body denervation has been shown to eliminate much of the time-dependent ventilatory response to chronic hypoxia in awake animals (18). CNS lesioning in cats revealed significant influences from supra-pontine regions on ventilatory responses to acute and chronic hypoxia (19). Pharmacologic blockade of tryptophan hydroxylation has shown that serotonin depletion removes a moderately strong inhibitory influence on air-breathing eupnea in awake rats (20)--an influence which may have significance if it is also triggered by the time-dependent physiologic depletion of brain monoamines in hypoxia (21).

In short, we have proposed that a new model for the mediation of ventilatory adaptation is required. If such a scheme incorporates straightforward interplay between central and peripheral chemoreception, this simplicity would be refreshingly welcome in an otherwise highly complex control system. On the other hand, it also seems clear that an inadequate data base exists currently to propose such a model and that the recent discovery of "nonchemical" effectors of ventilatory drive in the CNS caution against traditional simplicity.

ACKNOWLEDGMENTS

The collaboration of many colleagues was essential to the original results reported here including Drs. H. Forster, G. Bisgard, J. Orr, D. Pelligrino, T. Musch, J. Skatrud, and L. Chosy. I also thank Ms. Barbara Dahlen and Ms. Naomi Wells for the manuscript preparation. This work was supported by NIH (Grant No. HL-15469 and RCDA No. HL-00149), the U.S. Army MRDC and the University of Wisconsin Graduate School.

REFERENCES

(1) J. A. Dempsey, H. V. Forster, and G. A. doPico, Ventilatory acclimatization to moderate hypoxemia in man: The role of spinal fluid [H$^+$], J. Clin. Invest. 53, 1091 (1974).

(2) J. A. Dempsey, H. V. Forster, L. W. Chosy, P. G. Hanson, and W. G. Reddan, Regulation of CSF [HCO$_3^-$] during long-term hypoxic hypocapnia in man, J. Appl. Physiol.: Respir. Environ. Exercise Physiol. 44, 175 (1978).

(3) H. V. Forster, J. A. Dempsey, and L. W. Chosy, Incomplete compensation of CSF [H$^+$] in man during acclimatization to high altitude (4300 m), J. Appl. Physiol. 38, 1067 (1975).

(4) J. A. Orr, G. E. Bisgard, H. V. Forster, D. D. Buss, J. A. Dempsey, and J. A. Will, Cerebrospinal fluid alkalosis during high-altitude sojourn in unanesthetized ponies, Respir. Physiol. 25, 23 (1975).

(5) H. V. Forster, G. E. Bisgard, J. A. Dempsey, and J. A. Orr, Role of intracranial [H$^+$] receptor in physiologic regulation of ventilation in ponies, Chest 73(Suppl), 253 (1978).

(6) J. A. Dempsey, H. V. Forster, N. Gledhill, and G. A. doPico, Effects of moderate hypoxemia and hypocapnia on CSF [H$^+$] and ventilation in man, J. Appl. Physiol. 38(4), 665 (1975).

(7) J. B. Skatrud, J. A. Dempsey, P. Bhansali, and C. G. Irvin, Chronic ventilatory response to medroxyprogesterone acetate (MPA) in COPD, Fed. Proc. 37, 714 (1978) (Abstract).

(8) J. B. Skatrud, J. A. Dempsey, and D. G. Kaiser, Ventilatory response to medroxyprogesterone acetate in normal subjects: Time course and mechanism, J. Appl. Physiol. 44(6), 939 (1978).

 (9) J. R. Pappenheimer, V. Fencl, S. R. Heisey, and R. D. Held, Role of cerebral
      fluids in control of respiration as studied in unanesthetized goats, Am.
      J. Physiol. 208, 436 (1965).

(10) P. Cragg, L. Patterson, and M. J. Purves, the pH of brain extracellular fluid
      in the cat, J. Physiol. (London) 272, 137 (1977).

(11) V. Fencl, T. Miller, and J. R. Pappenheimer, Studies on the respiratory re-
      sponse to disturbances of acid-base balance, with deductions concerning
      ionic composition of cerebral interstitial fluid, Am. J. Physiol. 210, 459
      (1966).

(12) D. A. Pelligrino, T. I. Musch, J. A. Dempsey, and F. J. Nagle, Brain pH$_i$:
      Interregional differences, comparison of methods, and effects of hypoxic
      hypocapnia, Fed. Proc. 37(3), 532 (1978) (Abstract).

(13) V. Fencl, R. Gable, and D. Wolfe, Cerebral fluids in goats at high altitude,
      Fed. Proc. (Abstract) (in press, 1979).

(14) Mitchell, R. A. (1966) Advances in Respiratory Physiology, Williams and
      Wilkins, Baltimore.

(15) J. W. Severinghaus, R. A. Mitchell, B. W. Richardson, and M. M. Singer,
      Respiratory control at high altitude suggesting active transport regulation
      of CSF pH, J. Appl. Physiol. 18, 1155 (1963).

(16) R. D. Crawford, and J. W. Severinghaus, CSF pH and ventilatory acclimatization
      to altitude, J. Appl. Physiol. 45, 275 (1978).

(17) S. Majcherczyk, A. Trzebski, and P. Szvkzyk, The effect of changes of pH of
      CSF on the ventral surface of the medulla oblongata on the efferent dis-
      charge in carotid sinus and aortic nerves in the rat, Acta Med. Pol. 15,
      11 (1974).

(18) H. V. Forster, G. E. Bisgard, B. Rasmussen, J. A. Orr, D. D. Buss, and M.
      Manohar, Ventilatory control in peripheral chemoreceptor denervated ponies
      during chronic hypoxemia, J. Appl. Physiol. 41, 878 (1976).

(19) S. M. Tenney, and L. C. Ou, Hypoxic ventilatory response of cats at high alti-
      tude: An interpretation of 'blunting', Respir. Physiol. 30, 185 (1977).

(20) D. R. McCrimmon, E. B. Olson, Jr., and J. A. Dempsey, The role of serotonin
      in the control of ventilation in awake rats, Fed. Proc. 37(3), 904 (1978)
      (Abstract).

(21) J. N. Davis, Adaptation of brain monoamine synthesis to hypoxia in the rat,
      J. Appl. Physiol. 39, 215 (1975).

DISCUSSION

In the discussion of Dempsey's paper Loeschcke and Cunningham commented that the strategy of investigations in this field would have
to be to try to study one mechanism at a time in isolation, and then
to try to find out how the different parts are interacting with each
other under various conditions.

Cunningham further commented that in the interactions between the
different components and submechanisms of the controller also the
mechanisms of re-setting may be of great importance in changing sensitivity and thresholds under various conditions.

INTEGRATIVE ASPECTS OF HYPOTHALAMIC INFLUENCES ON RESPIRATORY BRAIN STEM MECHANISMS DURING WAKEFULNESS AND SLEEP

P. L. PARMEGGIANI

Istituto di Fisiologia umana, Università di Bologna,
Piazza di Porta San Donato 2, 40127 Bologna, Italy

ABSTRACT

In recent years the study of the somatic and vegetative phenomenology of sleep has revealed that homeostatic regulation is a discontinuous process being periodically replaced by a poikilostatic mode of operation. The contrasting sets of sleep events appear to be basically the result of a reversible release of brain stem mechanisms from hypothalamic regulatory influences. This temporary suspension of hypothalamic homeostatic activity occurring during desynchronized sleep implies that the instability of effector functions is the more marked the less they are endowed with autoregulation and/or controlled by reflex mechanisms. The latter are variably modified, during desynchronized sleep, as a consequence of the suspension of hypothalamic homeostatic regulation. The functional dichotomy of sleep may be utilized for experiments appraising the respective roles of reflex and central mechanisms in respiratory regulation.

The concept of physiological homeostasis (Cannon 1929) has underlain the development of operational models in many fields of Physiology, including respiratory functions. This conceptual trend was recently supported by the mathematical tools of control theory and particularly by the results of the analysis of feedback mechanisms (cf. Grodins 1963). So, the properties of open and closed loop operations of control mechanisms have become increasingly clear and the corresponding mathematical models more suitable for the description of physiological regulations. It does not appear necessary to stress the notion that the actuation of physiological homeostasis is strictly dependent on the action of feedback mechanisms.

In recent years the study of the somatic and vegetative phenomenology of sleep has revealed that homeostatic regulation is a discontinuous process being periodically replaced by a poikilostatic mode of operation during desynchronized sleep (REM sleep). In other words, according to the principles of the control theory, this phase of sleep is characterized by a functional change that consists in the prevalence of open loop vs. closed loop operations. This appears to depend on a reversible release, during desynchronized sleep, of brain stem control mechanisms from hypothalamic homeostatic influences, which are active during wakefulness and synchronized sleep (Parmeggiani 1968). This functional condition implies that the instability of effector functions is the more marked the less they are endowed with autoregulation and/or controlled by reflex mechanisms. The latter too, however, are variably modified, during desynchronized sleep, as a consequence of the suspension of hypothalamic homeostatic regulation.

Summing up, as far as vegetative and postural adjustements are concerned, closed loop operations represent the rule during wakefulness and synchronized sleep, whereas open loop operations are specific of desynchronized sleep. In contrast, "voluntary" (cortically driven) activity may not respect the principle of closed loop and may occur, during wakefulness, according to the open loop mode. It is clear nevertheless, that any open loop operation during wakefulness implies changes in variables that must be successively compensated by closed loop operations.

Concerning respiration, current concepts indicate the existence of two control mechanisms, one voluntary (or behavioural) and the other automatic (or metabolic), arising in the cortex and the brain stem, respectively (Mitchell and Berger 1975). This distinction has important functional implications that will be examined in the next paragraphs concerning the regulation of respiration during wakefulness (a), synchronized sleep (b), and desynchronized sleep (c).

(a) Wakefulness. Respiratory regulation during wakefulness is characterized by the interaction of voluntary and automatic mechanisms. This complex function, including open loop and closed loop operations, underlies the adaptability of breathing patterns to the needs of both behavioural expression and metabolic homeostasis.

Voluntary (more precisely cortical) influences appear to exert excitatory effects on brain stem respiratory structures, as shown both in man (Fink 1961, Mitchell and Berger 1975) and in the dog (Phillipson 1977, Phillipson et al. 1976b). Probably, the only observation of facilitatory effects depends on the experimental conditions. Other conditions may lead to the detection of inhibitory effects as well.

As the voluntary control of breathing operates also according to the open loop mode, the importance is clear of the closed loop operation of the automatic control mechanism for resetting drifts of respiratory variables within the normal range. The interaction between voluntary and automatic control mechanisms of breathing is assumed to occur primarily at brain stem and spinal levels (Mitchell and Berger 1975). However, the elaboration of complex behavioural patterns involving both somatic and vegetative effectors implies the integration of respiratory activity also at higher levels. In this respect, the functional relationships between driving cortical structures and homeostatic hypothalamic mechanisms appear to be necessary. This view is supported by experimental results showing that hypothalamic thermoceptive structures influence both gamma motor activity and EEG patterns (von Euler and Söderberg 1957). Moreover, there is evidence of a powerful hypothalamic control of vegetative mechanisms (Hess 1938, 1947). On this basis and on the ground of experimental

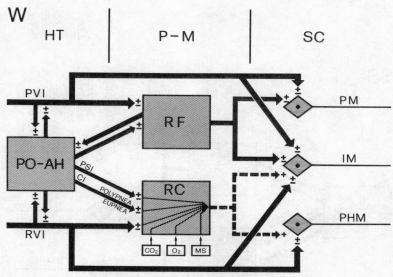

VOLUNTARY (OPEN LOOP) and AUTOMATIC (CLOSED LOOP)

Fig. 1. Voluntary and automatic control mechanisms of respira-
         tion during wakefulness (W).

In this and Figs. 2 and 3: a) Plus and minus signs indicate excitatory and inhibitory net influences, respectively, regardless of the specific synaptic organization; b) Abbreviations: CI, chronotropic influences; CO_2, capnoceptive inputs; HT, hypothalamus; IM, intercostal motoneurons; MS, mechanoceptive inputs; O_2, oxyceptive inputs; P-M, pons and medulla; PHM, phrenic motoneurons; PM, postural motoneurons; PO-AH, preoptic region and anterior hypothalamus; PSI, phase switching influences; PVI, postural voluntary influences; RC, respiratory centres; RF, reticular formation; RVI, respiratory voluntary influences; SC, spinal cord. The simplified scheme shows functional relationships among voluntary and automatic control mechanisms of both respiration and posture underlying the phenomenology of wakefulness.

results presented in the next paragraphs the hypothalamus is viewed as a substantial part of the automatic control mechanism of breathing in normal conditions (Fig. 1).

(b) <u>Synchronized sleep</u>. The transition from wakefulness to synchronized sleep consists in the progressive inactivation of the voluntary control mechanism and the release of the automatic control mechanism. This transition during stages 1 and 2 of synchronized sleep is
characterized by breathing instability (Duron 1972, Gillam 1972,
Reite et al. 1975, Snyder et al. 1964, Specht and Fruhmann 1972,
Webb 1974) and the appearance of respiratory and circulatory periodic
phenomena (Bülow 1963, Duron 1972, Lugaresi et al. 1972). Such
events appear to be the necessary result of the resetting of feedback
mechanisms (set point, gain , threshold) controlling effector activities according to the functional state of late synchronized sleep
(stages 3 and 4).

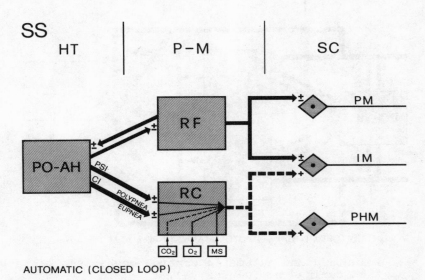

Fig. 2. Automatic control mechanism of respiration during syn-
        chronized sleep (SS).

The simplified scheme shows functional relationships between
automatic control mechanisms of respiration and posture and
hypothalamic structures. Note the slight depression of capnoceptive respiratory responses.

Regular breathing sets in with stages 3 and 4 of synchronized sleep.
At this point, breathing is driven by the automatic control mechanism. Ventilation decreases in both man (Birchfield et al. 1959,
Bülow 1963, Bülow and Ingvar 1961) and animals (Orem et al. 1977b,
Phillipson et al. 1976b) according to the metabolic rate. A concomitant increase in $PACO_2$ in man (Bülow 1963, Bülow and Ingvar 1971)
and animals (Phillipson et al. 1976b, Wurtz and O'Flaherty 1967)
and in $PaCO_2$ in man (Birchfield et al. 1958 and 1959) and cats
(Guazzi and Freis 1969) associated with a decrease in PAO_2 and PaO_2
in man (Robin et al. 1958) and cats (Guazzi and Freis 1969) was observed. Total airway resistance is decreased (Robin et al. 1958)
being the upper airway beancy normal (Orem et al. 1977a). These

changes in respiratory variables are in good agreement with a state
of rest at minimum energy expenditure such as synchronized sleep.
Although the operation of the automatic control mechanism appears
to be tuned to a lower activity level, it maintains all compensatory physiological responses. In fact, respiratory chemosensitivity
to CO_2 is only moderately reduced (Bellville et al. 1959, Birchfield
et al. 1959, Bülow 1963, Reed and Kellog 1958, Robin et al. 1958),
whereas the hypoxic response is unaffected in man (Reed and Kellog
1960) as well as in the dog (Phillipson et al. 1978). Moreover,
pulmonary inflation and deflation reflexes are active during synchronized sleep in both infants (Finer et al. 1976) and animals
(Farber and Marlow 1976, Phillipson et al. 1976b). The responses
to a mechanical respiratory load (airway occlusion, inspiration
from a rigid container) are also practically identical to those
observed during wakefulness (Phillipson et al. 1976a), therefore
showing that proprioceptive reflexes of intercostal muscles (cf.
Pengelly et al. 1974) are normal during synchronized sleep.

The preservation of homeostatic activity during synchronized sleep
regards not only the automatic control mechanism of breathing but
also other basic functions as circulation (Baust and Bohnert 1969,
Coccagna et al. 1971, Guazzi and Zanchetti 1965, Mancia et al. 1971,
Snyder et al. 1964) and thermoregulation (Heller and Glotzbach 1977,
Glotzbach and Heller 1976, Parmeggiani et al. 1971, 1973, 1976,
1977, Parmeggiani and Rabini 1967, Parmeggiani and Sabattini 1972)
in man and animals.

Experimental evidence in unrestrained cats shows that during synchronized sleep hypothalamic structures exert a negative and a positive chronotropic influence on brain stem respiratory mechanisms
in eupnea and polypnea, respectively (Parmeggiani 1978, Parmeggiani
and Sabattini 1972). Other results in cats point to the existence
of such hypothalamic influences under different experimental conditions. Either an increase or a decrease in respiratory frequency
was elicited by selective electrical stimulation of hypothalamic
structures (Hess 1938, 1947, Hess and Müller 1946). Lesions in the
lateral and anterior hypothalamus produced decrease and increase in
respiratory rate, respectively (Redgate and Gellhorn 1958). Polypnea
was induced by precollicular decerebration (Fink et al. 1962) and
hypocapnic polypnea abolished by intercollicular decerebration
(Cohen 1964). A recent study in the cat has evidentiated the respiratory driving power of anterior hypothalamic structures after
abolition of peripheral and central chemoceptive inputs (See 1976a
and b). In such a condition, anterior hypothalamic electrical or
thermal stimulation reactivates and maintains rhythmical respiratory activity. However, the ensuing respiratory acidosis indicates
that hypothalamically driven respiration is insufficient to preser-
ve the metabolic homeostasis. In conclusion, it is justified to
include hypothalamic structures in the automatic control mechanism
of respiration in order to explain not only full homeostatic regulation but also complete integration of all input variables influencing respiration in normal conditions (Fig. 2).

(c) Desynchronized sleep. The phenomenology of desynchronized sleep
points to a profound alteration in the activity of the automatic
control mechanism of respiration. In fact, the respiratory rhythm
in man and animals is very irregular (Aserinsky 1965, Aserinsky and

Kleitman 1953, Duron 1972, Phillipson 1978, Snyder et al. 1964),
the average frequency being increased or decreased with respect to
the rate attained during synchronized sleep in eupnea or polypnea,
respectively (Parmeggiani 1978, Parmeggiani and Sabattini 1972).
The respiratory activity of intercostal muscles is diminished in
cats and lambs (Duron 1969, Henderson-Smart and Read 1978, Islas-
Marroquin 1966, Parmeggiani and Sabattini 1972) and infants
(Tusiewicz et al. 1977). However, ventilation increases in man
(Bolton and Herman 1974, Bülow 1963, Fagenholz et al. 1976, Finer
et al. 1976, Hathorn 1974, Purcell 1976) and dogs (Phillipson et

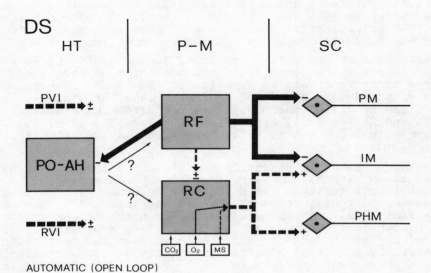

AUTOMATIC (OPEN LOOP)

Fig.3.   Automatic control mechanism of respiration during de-
         synchronized sleep (DS).

The simplified scheme shows inhibitory influences on postural
and intercostal motoneurons and on hypothalamic homeostatic
mechanisms arising in brain stem structures effecting desynchronized sleep phenomenology. Note the strong depression of
capnoceptive and of some mechanoceptive respiratory responses.

al. 1977) mostly in temporal relation to myoclonic twitches
(Orem et al. 1977b, Wurtz and O'Flaherty 1967). During desynchronized sleep, alveolar ventilation may be variable too as
shown by either a decrease (Bülow 1963, Phillipson et al. 1976b,
Wurtz and O'Flaherty 1967) or no change (Fagenholz et al. 1976,
Guazzi and Freis 1969, Remmers et al. 1976) in $PACO_2$. It is important to stress that such disturbances are of central origin as
they persist after vagotomy (Dawes et al. 1972, Phillipson et al.
1976b, Remmers et al. 1976), section of the spinal cord at T_{1-2}
(Puizillout et al. 1974, Thach et al. 1977), afferent denervation
of mid-thoracic chest wall (Phillipson 1977), denervation of carotid and aortic chemo- and baroreceptors (Guazzi and Freis 1969),

hypercapnia (Phillipson et al. 1977) and hypoxia (Phillipson et al. 1978). Upper airway resistance increases (Orem et al. 1977a) and

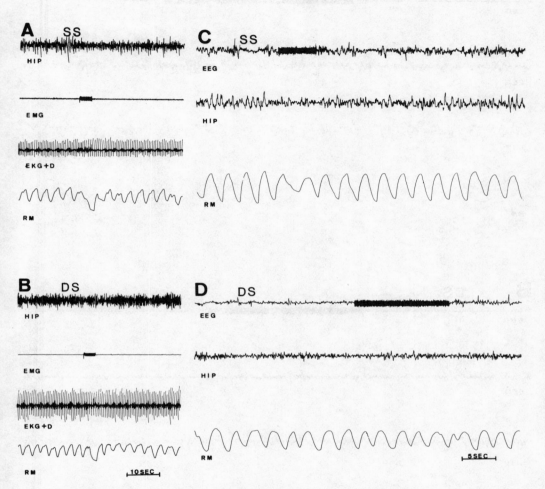

Fig. 4.   Respiratory effects of vagal electrical stimulation in the unrestrained cat.

During synchronized sleep, pulmonary inflation (A) and deflation (C) -like responses are elicited by stimulation of the central and of the left vagus nerve (A: 30/sec, 4 V, 0.5 msec; C: 100/sec, 3 V, 0.5 msec). During desynchronized sleep, the same stimulation is less effective (B) or fails to evoke the response (D). Abbreviations of this and Figs. 5 and 6: D, diaphragmatic electrogram; DS, desynchronized sleep; EEG, electroencephalogram; EKG, electrocardiogram; EMG, neck muscle electrogram; HIP, hippocampogram; RM, respiratory movements; SS, synchronized sleep.

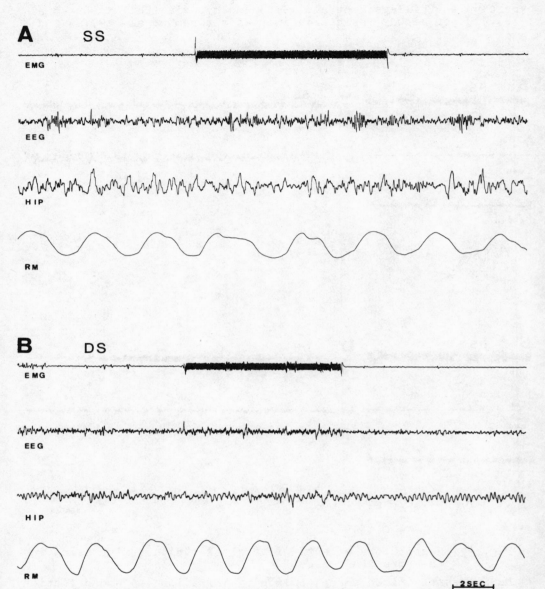

Fig. 5. Respiratory effects of hypothalamic electrical stimulation in the unrestrained cat.

Stimulation of the preoptic region (80/sec, 2.8 V, 5 msec)
elicits phase switching and a negative chronotropic effect
during synchronized sleep (A) and is ineffective during desynchronized sleep (B).

respiratory load compensation is irregular and weak in infants (Frantz et al. 1976, Knill et al. 1976, Purcell 1976) and lambs (Henderson-Smart and Read 1978) during desynchronized sleep. The alteration of the automatic control mechanism of respiration is shown also by other phenomena. In dogs and infants, respira-

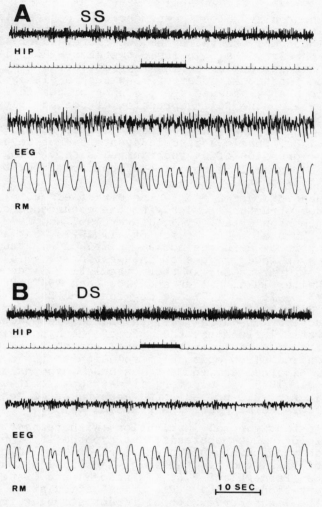

Fig. 6. Respiratory effects of hypothalamic electrical stimulation in the unrestrained cat.

Stimulation of the preoptic region (60/sec, 2.5 V, 2 msec) elicits a positive chronotropic effect during synchronized sleep (A) and is ineffective during desynchronized sleep (B).

tory responses to hypercapnia are depressed (Bryan et al. 1976, Phillipson et al. 1977),while those to hypoxia are unchanged (Bolton and Herman 1974, Fagenholz et al. 1976, Phillippson et al. 1978). Pulmonary deflation and inflation reflexes persist in the opossum, although they are more variable than during synchronized sleep (Farber and Marlow 1976). In contrast, the inflation reflex is practically abolished during desynchronized sleep in dogs (Phillipson et al. 1976b) and infants (Finer et al. 1976).

In general, desynchronized sleep phenomenology is classified under the criteria of tonic (e.g. postural atonia, neocortical desynchronization, hippocampal theta rhythm, thermoregulatory inactivation, etc.) and phasic (REMs, myoclonic twitches, PGO spikes, irregularities of cardiac and breathing rhythms, etc.) development. However, from the functional point of view such a distinction should not be too sharp, because the presence of phasic events may not be associated with the full depression of the activity underlying tonic events. Rather, phasic events build up on the background of tonic activity, which presumably is necessary for their free occurrence. So, phasic and tonic events cannot be considered as a dichotomic expression of desynchronized sleep, being the former only the paroxysmal climax of the open loop mode of operation typical of this phase of sleep.

The described phenomena are not only the direct effect of the activity of brain stem structures underlying the occurrence of desynchronized sleep (Hobson et al. 1974, Jouvet 1967 and 1972, McCarley and Hobson 1975, Moruzzi 1972, Netick et al. 1977), but also the result of the suppression in the normal animal of hypothalamic regulatory influences on lower levels of integration (Fig. 3). This is particularly evident as far as thermoregulation is concerned (Glotzbach and Heller 1976, Heller and Glotzbach 1977, Parmeggiani et al. 1971, 1973, 1976 and 1977, Parmeggiani and Rabini 1967, Parmeggiani and Sabattini 1972). Although it may be surmised that hypothalamic inactivation during desynchronized sleep depends on ascending brain stem influences, the role of the hypothalamus is not simply passive. In fact, in the normal animal the occurrence of the desynchronized sleep episode in relation to the conditions of internal and external environments is under hypothalamic control (Parmeggiani et al. 1975). Moreover, it was shown that a change in hypothalamic unit activity precedes the appearance of desynchronized sleep phenomenology (Parmeggiani and Franzini 1973).

Owing to its important general implications with respect to the concept of physiological homeostasis, the hypothesis of brain stem release during desynchronized sleep was further studied by means of experiments of vagal and hypothalamic electrical stimulation in unrestrained cats (Parmeggiani P.L., Calasso M. and Cianci T., Unpublished observations, 1978). Electrical stimulation of the central end of the vagus nerve with different stimulus frequencies and intensities (cf. Wyss 1943) elicits responses similar to those of pulmonary inflation or deflation during synchronized sleep (Figs. 4A and 4C). In contrast, during desynchronized sleep the same stimulation is less effective (Fig. 4B) or fails to evoke the response (Fig. 4D). Taking into account the different experimental conditions, these results are practically in agreement with those of previously quoted authors. Most interesting is, however, the fact that the electrical stimulation of the anterior hypothalamus, eliciting phase switching (Fig. 5A) or chronotropic effects (Figs. 5A and 6A) during synchronized sleep, is ineffective during desynchronized sleep (Figs. 5B and 6B). Such unresponsiveness of anterior hypothalamic structures during desynchronized sleep was also shown by means of thermal stimuli (Glotzbach and Heller 1976, Parmeggiani et al. 1973, 1976 and 1977).

On this basis, it may be surmised that the changes in chemoceptive and mechanoceptive respiratory reflexes during desynchronized sleep are different depending on the degree of their normal subordination to higher levels of integration. It is particularly interesting that during desynchronized sleep oxyceptive inputs maintain their influence with regard not only to breathing, but also to circulation, being baroceptive reflexes strongly depressed (Guazzi et al. 1968, Guazzi and Zanchetti 1965).

It is tempting to conclude that the functional condition of desynchronized sleep reveals phylogenetically determined levels of autonomy as a result of a temporary regression from the normal degree of diencephalization. This view partially disagrees with that considering the respiratory phenomenology of desynchronized sleep as depending on the activation of the voluntary control mechanism (Phillipson 1977 and 1978). Such activation is surely actual but is not necessary for the genesis of desynchronized sleep phenomenology (Jouvet 1965, Morrison and Pompeiano 1966). Emphasis is principally laid here on the changes occurring in the automatic control mechanism after inactivation of hypothalamic homeostatic functions. The prevalence of open loop operations in such a functional condition appears to underlie the instability of breathing patterns during desynchronized sleep.

REFERENCES

Aserinsky, E., Periodic respiratory pattern occurring in conjunction with eye movements during sleep, Science 150, 763 (1965).

Aserinsky, E. and Kleitman, N., Regularly occurring periods of eye motility and concomitant phenomena, during sleep, Science 118, 273 (1953).

Baust, W. and Bonhert, B., The regulation of heart rate during sleep, Exp. Brain Res. 7, 169 (1969).

Bellville, J. W., Howland, W. S., Seed, J. C. and Houde, R. W., The effect of sleep on the respiratory response to carbon dioxide, Anesthesiology 20, 628 (1959).

Birchfield, R. I., Sieker, H. O. and Heyman, A., Alterations in blood gases during natural sleep and narcolepsy, Neurology 8, 107 (1958).

Birchfield, R. I., Sieker, H. O. and Heyman, A., Alterations in respiratory function during natural sleep, J. Lab. clin. Med. 54, 216 (1959).

Bolton, D. P. G. and Herman, S., Ventilation and sleep state in the newborn, J. Physiol. (London) 240, 67 (1974).

Bryan, H. M., Hagan, R., Gulston, G. and Bryan A. C., CO_2 response and sleep state in infants, <u>Clin. Res.</u> 24, A689 (1976).

Bülow, K., Respiration and wakefulness in man, <u>Acta physiol. scand.</u> 59, suppl. 209 (1963).

Bülow, K. and Ingvar, D. H., Respiration and state of wakefulness in normals, studied by spirography, capnography and EEG, <u>Acta physiol. scand.</u> 51, 230 (1961).

Cannon, W. B., Organization for physiological homeostasis, <u>Physiol. Rev.</u> 9, 399 (1929).

Coccagna, G., Mantovani, M., Brignani, F., Manzini, A. and Lugaresi, E., Arterial pressure changes during spontaneous sleep in man, <u>Electroenceph. clin. Neurophysiol.</u> 31, 277 (1971).

Cohen, M. I., Respiratory periodicity in the paralyzed, vagotomized cat: hypocapnic polypnea, <u>Am. J. Physiol.</u> 206, 845 (1964).

Dawes, G. S., Fox, H. E., Leduc, B. M., Liggins, G. C. and Richards, R. T., Respiratory movements and rapid eye movement sleep in the foetal lamb, <u>J. Physiol. (London)</u> 220, 119 (1972).

Duron, B., Activité électrique spontanée des muscles intercostaux et de diaphragme chez l'animal chronique, <u>J. Physiol. (Paris)</u> 61, suppl. 2, 282 (1969).

Duron, B. La fonction respiratoire pendant le sommeil physiologique, <u>Bull. Physio-pathol. Resp.</u> 8, 1031 (1972).

Euler, C. von and Söderberg, U., The influence of hypothalamic thermoceptive structures on the electroencephalogram and gamma motor activity, <u>Electroenceph. clin. Neurophysiol.</u> 9, 391 (1957).

Fagenholz, S. A., O'Connell, K. and Shannon, D. C., Chemoreceptor function and sleep state in apnea, <u>Pediatrics</u>, 58, 31 (1976).

Farber, J. P. and Marlow, T. A., Pulmonary reflexes and breathing pattern during sleep in the opossum, <u>Respir. Physiol.</u> 27, 73 (1976).

Finer, N. N., Abroms, I. F. and Taeusch, H. W. Jr., Ventilation and sleep state in new born infants. <u>J. Pediatr.</u> 89, 100 (1976).

Fink, B. R., Influence of cerebral activity in wakefulness on regulation of breathing, <u>J. appl. Physiol.</u> 16, 15 (1961).

Fink, B. R., Katz, R., Reinhold, H. and Schoolman, A., Suprapontine mechanisms in regulation of respiration, <u>Am. J. Physiol.</u> 202, 217 (1962).

Frantz, I. D., Adler, S. M., Abroms, I. F. and Thach, B. T., Respiratory response to airway occlusion in infants: sleep state and maturation, <u>J. appl. Physiol.</u> 41, 634 (1976).

Gillam, P. M. S., Patterns of respiration in human beings at rest and during sleep, <u>Bull. Physio-pathol. Resp.</u> 8, 1059 (1972).

Glotzbach, S. F. and Heller, H. C., Central nervous regulation of body temperature during sleep, <u>Science</u> 194, 537 (1976)

Grodins, F. S. (1963) Control Theory and Biological Systems, Columbia University Press, New York.

Guazzi, M., Baccelli, G. and Zanchetti, A. Reflex chemoceptive regulation of arterial pressure during natural sleep in the cat, Am. J. Physiol. 214, 969 (1968).

Guazzi, M. and Freis, E. D., Sinoaortic reflexes and arterial pH, PO_2 and PCO_2 in wakefulness and sleep, Am. J. Physiol. 217, 1623 (1969).

Guazzi, M. and Zanchetti, A., Blood pressure and heart rate during natural sleep of the cat and their regulation by carotid sinus and aortic reflexes, Arch. ital. Biol. 103, 789 (1965).

Hathorn, M. K. S., The rate and depth of breathing in new-born infants in different sleep states, J. Physiol. (London) 243, 101 (1974).

Heller, H. C. and Glotzbach, S. F., Thermoregulation during sleep and hibernation, in Environmental Physiology II, D. Robertshaw (Ed.), International Review of Physiology, University Park Press, Baltimore 15, 206 (1977).

Henderson-Smart, D. J. and Read, D. J. C., Depression of intercostal and abdominal muscle activity and vulnerability to asphyxia during active sleep in the newborn, in Sleep Apnea Syndromes. C. Guilleminault and W. C. Dement (Eds.). Kroc Foundation Series, A. R. Liss, New York 11, 93 (1978).

Hess. W. R. (1938) Beiträge zur Physiologie des Hirnstammes. II Teil. Das Zwischenhirn und die Regulation von Kreislauf und Atmung, Thieme, Leipzig.

Hess, W. R., Vegetative Funktionen und Zwischenhirn, Helv. physiol. pharmacol. Acta, 5, suppl. IV (1947).

Hess, W. R. and Müller, H. R., Einflüsse des Mittel- und Zwischenhirns auf die Atmung, Helv. physiol. pharmacol. Acta 4, 347 (1946).

Hobson, J. A., McCarley, R. W., Pivik, R. T. and Freedman, R., Selective firing by cat pontine brain stem neurons during desynchronized sleep, J. Neurophysiol. 37, 497 (1974).

Islas-Marroquin, J., L'activité des muscles respiratoires pendant les différentes phases du sommeil physiologique chez le chat, Arch. Sci. physiol. 20, 219 (1966).

Jouvet, M., Paradoxical sleep: a study of its nature and mechanisms, Progr. Brain Res. 18, 20 (1965).

Jouvet, M., Neurophysiology of the states of sleep, Physiol. Rev. 47, 117 (1967).

Jouvet, M., The role of monoamines and acetylcholine containing neurons in the regulation of the sleep-waking cycle, Ergebn. Physiol. 64, 166 (1972).

Knill, R., Andrews, W., Bryan, A. C. and Bryan, M. H., Respiratory load compensation in infants, J. appl. Physiol. 40, 357 (1976).

Lugaresi, E., Coccagna, G., Mantovani, M. and Lebrun, R., Some

periodic phenomena arising during drowsiness and sleep in man,
Electroenceph. clin. Neurophysiol. 32, 701 (1972).

Mancia, G., Baccelli, G., Adams, D. B. and Zanchetti, A., Vasomotor regulation during sleep in the cat, Am. J. Physiol. 220,
1086 (1971).

McCarley, R. W. and Hobson, J. A., Discharge patterns of cat pontine
brain stem neurons during desynchronized sleep, J. Neurophysiol.
38, 751 (1975).

Mitchell, R. A. and Berger, A. J., Neural regulation of respiration,
Am. Rev. respir. Dis. 111, 206 (1975).

Morrison, A. R. and Pompeiano, O., Vestibular influences during sleep.
II. Effects of vestibular lesions on the pyramidal discharge
during desynchronized sleep, Arch. ital. Biol. 104, 214 (1966).

Moruzzi, G., The sleep-waking cycle, Ergebn. Physiol. 64, 1 (1972).

Netick, A., Orem, J. and Dement, W., Neural activity specific to rem
sleep and its relationship to breathing, Brain Res. 120, 197
(1977).

Orem, J., Netick, A. and Dement, W. C., Increased upper airway
resistance to breathing during sleep in the cat, Electroenceph.
clin. Neurophysiol. 43, 14 (1977a).

Orem, J., Netick, A. and Dement, W. C., Breathing during sleep and
wakefulness in the cat., Respir. Physiol. 30, 265 (1977b).

Parmeggiani, P. L., Telencephalo-diencephalic aspects of sleep
mechanisms, Brain Res. 7, 350 (1968).

Parmeggiani, P. L., Regulation of the activity of respiratory muscles
during sleep, in The Regulation of Respiration during Sleep and
Anesthesia, R. S. Fitzgerald, H. Gautier and S. Lahiri (Eds.),
Advances in Experimental Medicine and Biology, Plenum Press, New
York 99, 47 (1978).

Parmeggiani, P. L., Agnati, L. F., Zamboni, G. and Cianci, T.,
Hypothalamic temperature during the sleep cycle at different
ambient temperatures, Electroenceph. clin. Neurophysiol. 38, 589
(1975).

Parmeggiani, P. L. and Franzini, C., On the functional significance
of subcortical single unit activity during sleep, Electroenceph.
clin. Neurophysiol. 34, 495 (1973).

Parmeggiani, P. L., Franzini, C. and Lenzi, P., Respiratory frequency as a function of preoptic temperature during sleep, Brain Res.
111, 253 (1976).

Parmeggiani, P. L., Franzini, C., Lenzi, P. and Cianci, T., Inguinal
subcutaneous temperature changes in cats sleeping at different
environmental temperatures, Brain Res. 33, 397 (1971).

Parmeggiani, P. L., Franzini, C., Lenzi, P. and Zamboni, G.,
Threshold of respiratory responses to preoptic heating during
sleep in freely moving cats, Brain Res. 52, 189 (1973).

Parmeggiani, P. L. and Rabini, C., Shivering and panting during
sleep, Brain Res. 6, 789 (1967).

Parmeggiani, P. L. and Sabattini, L., Electromyographic aspects of postural respiratory and thermoregulatory mechanisms in sleeping cats, Electroenceph. clin. Neurophysiol. 33, 1 (1972).

Parmeggiani, P. L., Zamboni, G., Cianci, T. and Calasso, M., Absence of thermoregulatory vasomotor responses during fast wave sleep in cats, Electroenceph. clin. Neurophysiol. 42, 372 (1977).

Pengelly, L. D., Rebuck, A. S. and Campbell, E. J. M. (1974) Loaded Breathing, Longman, Don Mills, Ont.

Phillipson, E. A., Regulation of breathing during sleep, Am. Rev. respir. Dis. 115 (suppl.), 217 (1977).

Phillipson, E. A., Respiratory adaptations in sleep, Ann. Rev. Physiol. 40, 133 (1978).

Phillipson, E. A., Kozar, L. F. and Murphy, E., Respiratory load compensation in awake and sleeping dogs, J. appl. Physiol. 40, 895 (1976a).

Phillipson, E. A., Kozar, L. F., Rebuck, A. S. and Murphy, E., Ventilatory and waking responses to CO_2 in sleeping dogs, Am. Rev. respir. Dis. 115, 251 (1977).

Phillipson, E. A., Murphy, E. and Kozar, L. F., Regulation of respiration in sleeping dogs, J. appl. Physiol. 40, 688 (1976b).

Phillipson, E. A., Sullivan, C. E., Read, D. J. C., Murphy, E. and Kozar, L. F., Ventilatory and waking responses to hypoxia in sleeping dogs, J. appl. Physiol. 44, 512 (1978).

Puizillout, J. J., Ternaux, J. P., Foutz, A. S. and Fernandez, G., Les stades de sommeil chez la préparation encéphale isolé. 1. Déclenchement des pointes ponto-géniculo-occipitales et du sommeil phasique à ondes lentes. Rôle des noyaux du raphé, Electroenceph. clin. Neurophysiol. 37, 561 (1974).

Purcell, M., Response in the newborn to raised upper airway resistance, Arch. Dis. Child. 51, 602 (1976).

Redgate, E. S. and Gellhorn, E., Respiratory activity and the hypothalamus, Am. J. Physiol. 193, 189 (1968).

Reed, D. J. and Kellogg, R. H., Changes in respiratory response to CO_2 during natural sleep at sea level and at altitude, J. appl. Physiol. 13, 325 (1958).

Reed, D. J. and Kellogg, R. H., Effect of sleep on hypoxic stimulation of breathing at sea level and altitude, J. appl. Physiol. 15, 1130 (1960).

Reite, M., Jackson, D., Cahoon, R. L. and Weil, J. V., Sleep physiology at high altitude, Electroenceph. clin. Neurophysiol. 38, 463 (1975).

Remmers, J. E., Bartlett, D. Jr. and Putnam, M. D., Changes in the respiratory cycle associated with sleep, Respir. Physiol. 28, 227 (1976).

Robin, E. D., Whaley, R. D., Crump, G. H. and Travis, D. M.,

Alveolar gas tension, pulmonary ventilation and blood pH during physiologic sleep in normal subjects, J. clin. Invest. 37, 981 (1958).

See, W. R. (1976a) Ueber den Beitrag des Hypothalamus zur Atmung nach Ausschaltung der chemischen Atemantriebe, Ph. D. Thesis, University of Bochum.

See, W. R., Respiratory drive in hyperthermia, interaction with central chemosensitivity, in Acid Base Homeostasis of the Brain Extracellular Fluid and the Respiratory Control System, H. H. Loeschke (Ed.), Thieme, Stuttgart, 122 (1976b).

Snyder, F., Hobson, J. A., Morrison, D. F. and Goldfrank, F., Changes in respiration, heart rate, and systolic blood pressure in human sleep, J. appl. Physiol. 19, 417 (1964).

Specht, H. and Fruhmann, G., Incidence of periodic breathing in 2000 subjects without pulmonary or neurological disease. Bull. Physio-pathol. Respir. 8, 1075 (1972).

Thach, B. T., Abroms, I. F., Frantz, I. D., Sotrel, A., Bruce, E. N. and Goldman, M. D., REM sleep breathing pattern without intercostal muscle influence, Fed. Proc. 36, 445 (1977).

Tusiewicz,K., Moldofsky, H., Bryan, A. C. and Bryan, M. H., Mechanics of the rib cage and diaphragm during sleep, J. appl. Physiol. 43, 600 (1977).

Webb, P., Periodic breathing during sleep, J. appl. Physiol. 37, 899 (1974).

Wurtz, R. H. and O'Flaherty, J. J., Physiological correlates of steady potential shifts during sleep and wakefulness. 1. Sensitivity of the steady potential to alterations in carbon dioxide, Electroenceph. clin. Neurophysiol. 22, 30 (1967).

Wyss, O. A. M., L'interprétation du pneumogramme concernant les modifications du type respiratoire, Helv. physiol. pharmacol. Acta 1, 301 (1943).

DISCUSSION

Euler remarked that it would be of great interest to learn whether the operation of other homeostasis mechanisms such as the water- and electrolyte regulation is similarly readjusted to low regulatory efficiency. Also in the wake state homeostatic controllers can temporary be given lower regulatory efficiency. This seems to be the case, for instance, under conditions which cause rivalry to occur between different homeostatic mechanisms utilizing common effector mechanisms. Under such conditions priority is shifted presumably by adjustments of the set-points so that the regulatory function of the controller which at the occasion is of lesser vital importance is sacrified to some degree (see e.g. Euler, Pharmacol.Rev. 13, 361, 1961). This may certainly be purposeful for the whole organism. In the case

of REM sleep we have to admit that we do not understand the purpose
of this depression of the regulatory efficiency of some homeostatic
mechanisms in REM sleep. It would certainly be of great interest to
learn about the functional significance of this phenomenon and about
the neural mechanisms involved in changing the mode of operation of
the controllers.

The presence of ventilatory responses to hypoxia in REM sleep shows
that at least one important closed loop regulation is operating also
in this state.

It was argued that a maintained responsiveness to hypoxia together
with a decreased responsiveness to changes in PCO_2 in REM sleep should
lead to periodic breathing unless at the same time the overall 'gain'
of the oxystatic function is somewhat decreased by the peripheral
suppression of the non-diaphragmatic respiratory muscles and the
varying non-metabolic contributions to the drive of the diaphragm.

In his reply Parmeggiani emphasized that although some reflexes such
as the hypoxic reflex effects on blood pressure and respiration and
some autoregulatory functions are operating also in REM sleep it
seems presently justified to regard this state on the whole as a
'poikilostatic' condition. He further drew attention to the fact that,
as an emergency reaction, both hypoxia and hypercapnia will cause
arousal which, in turn, leads to resumption of the 'homeostatic' condition.

Remmers drew attention to the concept that in the REM sleep state
central motor control lung mechanisms are quite active although
blocked at the spinal levels. He raised the issue that if central
irradiation of the motor control activities onto respiration occurs
this might be contributing to the changes in respiration, in this
sleep state, in particular to the occurrence of the tachypneic ir-
regularitors. Parmeggiani replied that he expected that this could
be the case, and emphasized that there are indications showing that
the activities of the motor systems are characterized by a dominance
of open loop operation.

FACTS AND HYPOTHESIS CONCERNING
CORTICAL MODULATION OF MEDULLARY
REFLEX MECHANISMS

A. GUZ, P. MITCHELL-HEGGS, K. MURPHY and R. ROSSER

Departments of Medicine and Psychiatry,
Charing Cross Hospital Medical School, London W.6, U.K.

INTRODUCTION

The 'facts' in this paper arise from a preliminary study undertaken to examine the effects of diazepam in the breathlessness of the 'pink-puffer' syndrome. These patients with chronic obstructive airway disease keep a normal or slightly low P_aCO_2, and they are near normoxaemic. Their principal symptom is severe dyspnoea. The rationale for studying the effect of benzodiazepines was that they are said to depress ventilation and we thought that this might reduce breathlessness possibly at the expense of some rise in P_aCO_2. The 'facts' also stem from another study using diazepam in normal controls.

METHODS AND RESULTS

Four desperately breathless patients with severe airway obstruction were first studied; the P_aO_2 was always greater than 60 mmHg and the P_aCO_2 less than 45 mmHg. Diazepam (25 mg/day) was given in a single blind cross-over study in hospital; breathlessness at rest and with minimal exertion was relieved within 5 days. On placebo, breathlessness returned in 3 of the 4 subjects within 5 days. During the study, spirometry, arterial blood gases, CO_2 sensitivity (measured by a rebreathing method keeping PO_2 constant about 90 mmHg), the peak CO_2 tolerated during rebreathing and the serum diazepam and desmethyldiazepam levels were measured.

Spirometric readings and arterial gases at rest were <u>not</u> affected by diazepam. The patients were not made hypercapnoeic. The ventilatory sensitivity to CO_2 fell, and the peak CO_2 tolerated rose with diazepam; on placebo the values returned to control levels. These changes were reflected in the serum diazepam and desmethyldiazepam levels. Sedation with diazepam was minimal and lasted for only 48 hours after the drug was first given.

None of these patients had a chronic anxiety state; 3 out of the 4 were depressed by the incapacity resulting from their breathlessness.

These effects of diazepam on the ventilatory sensitivity to CO_2 and on the peak CO_2 tolerated during rebreathing have been seen in 3 normal subjects studied in an exactly similar way to that used for the patients. In spite of the depression of sensitivity the pattern of ventilation and the end-tidal CO_2 at rest did not change.

Diazepam can therefore reduce the ventilatory sensitivity to CO_2 in normal subjects and in patients with the 'pink-puffer' syndrome without affecting the 'set-point' for arterial PCO_2.

It should be noted that we did not study the effect of diazepam on the ventilatory sensitivity to exercise. We are currently trying to measure these responses.

HYPOTHESIS

Benzodiazepines bind specifically to receptors in the brain; this binding is uneven with much the greatest binding present in the frontal and occipital cortex. Binding in the pons and medulla is least, whereas in the hippocampus moderate binding is found (Squires and Braestrup, 1977). The action on the cortex is that of an inhibition which appears to be GABAmimetic.

Influences from the cerebral cortex can profoundly inhibit the behavioural functions of the respiratory act and also the metabolic functions (Plum, 1970). Patients with bilateral cerebral infarction have an increased responsiveness to ventilatory stimulation with CO_2 (Heyman, Birchfield and Sieker, 1958; Brown and Plum, 1961; Plum, 1970).

A cerebral respiratory-activating system is also clearly present and this is damped by natural sleep (Birchfield, Sieker and Heyman, 1958). We would like to propose that the GABAmimetic actions of diazepam result in an altered balance of the inhibiting and activating descending influences towards inhibition with resulting reduction in <u>gain</u> of the ventilatory response to CO_2 mediated at medullary level.

This type of mechanism has been previously analysed for the reflex vagal bradycardia elicited by electrical stimulation of the carotid sinus nerve; the response was inhibited by diazepam in dosages of 0.175 - 2.8 mg/kg (Hockman and Livingston, 1970). The inhibitory effect of the drug was not observed in the animal decerebrated either at midcollicular level or in such a way as to leave the diencephalon intact. These results suggested that the drug induced inhibition may arise at forebrain level.

REFERENCES

H. W. Brown and F. Plum, The neurological basis of Cheyne-Strokes respiration, Am. J. Med. 30, 849 (1961).

R. I. Birchfield, H. O. Sieker, and A. Heyman, Alteration in blood gases during natural sleep and narcolepsy, Neurology, Minneap. 8, 107 (1958).

A. Heyman, R. I. Birchfield and H. O. Sieker, Effects of bilateral cerebral infarction on respiratory center sensitivity, Neurology, Minneap. 8, 694 (1950).

C. H. Hockman and K. E. Livingston, Inhibition of reflex vagal bradycardia by diazepam, Neuropharmacology, 10, 307 (1971).

B. R. Kaada, Cingulate, posterior orbital, anterior insular and temporal pole
    cortex, Handbook of Physiology (Am. Phys. Soc.) Section 1, 2, 1345 (1960).

F. Plum, Neurological integration of behavioural and metabolic control of
    breathing, Breathing: Hering-Breuer Centenary Symposium (Ciba Fdn. Symp)
    159 (1970).

R. F. Squires and C. Braestrup, Benzodiazepine receptors in rat brain, Nature
    266, 732 (1977).

DISCUSSION

It was suggested that the main results might be explained on the
basis of two mechanisms: Firstly, an input from those parts of the
brain where the emotional colouring of perceptions and sensations
take place might provide some contribution to the drive for ventilation in a slope-or-gain-changing manner altering the PCO_2 - $\dot{V}$ relationship. Secondly, diazepam might act to depress and remove some of
the emotional and distressing overtones of perception, although it
has been found to have relatively little effect on the simplest
psychophysical relationships between stimulus intensity and magnitude
estimation for several sensory functions.

Semple commented on the problem why the level of PCO_2 was not found
to change despite the decrease of the slope of the CO_2 - $\dot{V}$ relationship. He referred to the work by Dejours et al. (J.appl.Physiol. 20,
890, 1965) showing that available methods do hardly make it possible
to pick up changes in PCO_2 around resting levels of ventilation when
the CO_2-response curve changes. He further expressed the opinion that
too much attention has been attached to reports on an absence of
changes in PCO_2 concomitant with changes in the slope of CO_2 - $\dot{V}$
curve.

Cunningham remarked that this investigation as well as many other
recent papers in the literature (e.g. Asmussen, Acta physiol.scand.
99, 85, 1977) indicate the importance to define the level of wakefulness and alertness of the individuals when trying to make inter-
or intraindividual comparisons of the so-called CO_2-'sensitivity'.

Cunningham commented on the degree of long term constancy of human
resting alveolar PCO_2 throughout adult life. He said that this constancy may be temporary disturbed in a variety of conditions such as
pregnancy, metabolic acidosis, and at altitude but after the disturbances have passed alveolar PCO_2 comes back to its old value.

Bryan and several other participants emphasized, however, that in a
short term perspective, PCO_2 may exhibit great fluctuations, especially in REM-sleep, and during wake conditions at relative rest when
there may be some rivalry for priority between the metabolic regulation of ventilation on the one hand and various behavioural demands
or demands from other homeostasis mechanisms on the ventilatory
system on the other.

INTERACTION BETWEEN NEUROGENIC
EXERCISE DRIVE AND CHEMICAL DRIVE

F. F. KAO, S. S. MEI and M. KALIA

Departments of Physiology, Downstate Medical Center,
State University of New York, Brooklyn, New York, and
Hahnemann Medical College and Hospital, Philadelphia, Pa., U.S.A.

Long before the end of the nineteenth century, physiologists had evidence that ventilation can respond to a number of stimuli, yet it was not until 1945, that Gray
definitely described the pluralistic concept of the regulation of ventilation
(Gray,1950). It will perhaps never be known whether the pluralism of the development of the socio-philosophical concepts in the beginning of the twentieth century
is related to the discovery of scientific theories, however, it can be stated with
some certainty that Gray's multiple factor theory has strongly influenced the field
of research in the regulation of respiration for the past three decades.

Since respiration responds to a number of stimuli, such as chemical drive, afferents
from the chest wall and the vagi, influences from supramedullary structures and
exercise drive, a great deal of experimental work has been done in recent years
concerning the mode and mechanism of action of each of these stimuli which affect
ventilation. Physiologists working on chemical drive alone, i.e., Po_2 and Pco_2-pH
complex, have been impressed by their complexity and importance of these inputs and
hence have euphemized this area of investigation as chemical control of ventilation.

It is interesting to point out that with all the effort made by so many investigators for so many years, the sites of action for the chemical drive had not been
worked out. Moreover, the pathways involved in transmitting these stimuli from
the receptor sites to the central control mechanisms in the brain are vague. Without
the definitive anatomical identification of the pathways and the nature of the
receptor involved,it is not possible to fully understand the mechanisms responsible
for the interaction between two or more stimuli that are involved in a physiological
response!

It has been known to neurophysiologists since the time of Sherrington that the
phenomena of summation, facilitation, and occlusion must occur at each level of
the central interaction of various stimuli. It would be natural to assume that
such a system must exist in the central respiratory controller and make possible
a variety of responses when varying inputs are received from different regions.Kao
and Mei have recently referred to this phenomenon in ventilatory control as multiple interaction (Kao & Mei, 1978).

The problem becomes even more intriguing when the interaction between exercise drive
and chemical drive are considered simultaneously, because at the present time, a
difference of opinion still exists regarding the nature of the exercise drive. Not
knowing the nature of this stimulus, how can a physiologist study the interaction

(summation or multiplicative interaction) of exercise drive with chemical drive?

It is, therefore, necessary to approach the study of the interaction of exercise drive with chemical drive systematically in three steps: 1. The existence of the exercise stimulus must be demonstrated. Do we need a separate stimulus for exercise hyperpnea? Can any one or would a combination of the presently known chemical stimuli be sufficient to account for exercise hyperpnea? 2. If there is an exercise stimulus(i) responsible for the ventilatory increase in muscular activity, then, what is the exact nature of this stimulus? Where does it originate? How does it operate? And how does it influence the central regulatory mechanisms, so that that stimulus specifically is finally integrated into the neuronal circuitry for the augmentation of ventilation? 3. How does this exercise drive interact with chemical drive? And where are the sites of interaction?

EVIDENCE IN REGARD TO THE EXISTENCE OF THE NEUROGENIC EXERCISE STIMULUS

Venous Chemoreceptor

It had been a priori logic in the past to postulate that since many kinds of chemicals are known to be produced during muscular activity, any one or a combination of these chemical products can be candidate for the stimulus of exercise hyperpnea (cf Geppert & Zuntz, 1888). For example, CO_2 production in the muscles during exercise is increased and CO_2 does stimulate ventilation, therefore, it has been proposed that the venous Pco_2 produced during exercise should stimulate ventilation. Several types of experiments had been performed in the past to demonstrate the effect of an increase in venous CO_2 on ventilation. These have included the perfusion of CO_2-rich blood without exercise and the identification of CO_2 receptors in the venous circulation which might alter ventilation (Cropp & Comroe, 1961; Wasserman et al, 1975; Gonzalez et al, 1977; Ponte & Purves, 1978). This work seems to have produced some new information regarding the perfusion blood flowrate relationship to ventilation (Ponte & Purves, 1978), however, it has never been shown that the effect of perfused CO_2 on ventilation could account for the exercise hyperpnea. The increase in ventilation during CO_2 perfusion is the result of an elevation of arterial Pco_2 and its stimulation of chemoreceptor on the arterial side. It is well known that during moderate exercise, arterial Pco_2 does not change. As far as gas exchange functions are concerned, it seems obvious that the primary duty of the respiratory system is directed toward the arterialization of the blood. It is, therefore, illogical to expect some venous receptors to be involved in regulating the arterial gas composition! There is no evidence to support the existence of venous chemoreceptors involved in the regulation of arterial blood gas compositions. Thus, although the venous CO_2 does rise during muscular exercise, it does not play a 'stimulating' role in the regulation of ventilation during muscular exercise.

Arterial Chemoreceptor

The next question to be raised is: are there any chemical constituents in the arterial blood produced during exercise which could cause exercise hyperpnea? Perfusion of arterialized exercising blood to a resting animal caused no change in ventilation (Kao, 1956). This experiment also ruled out the possibility of the existence of the mysterious respiration X (Haggard & Henderson, 1920). This finding further verified the inadequacy of Heymans' experiment in which the frequency of the twitching of the larynx (used as an index of ventilatory response) of an isolated dog's head was increased when it received exercising arterialized blood from a donor dog (Heymans et al, 1947). Our experiments in perfusing arterialized exercising blood to a second animal were limited to an exercise of moderate intensity as judged by the degree of oxygen consumption increment. In severe exercise where arterial acidemia exists, a perfusion of such blood would increase ventilation via its hydrogen ion effect (Grodins, 1950).

Artificial CO_2-Rich Blood Perfusion, and Perfusion of Venous Exercising Blood

Recently, there has been a revived interest in perfusion experiments in which the CO_2-rich venous blood was artificially introduced into an animal with the intent of, in some way, mimicking the venous blood from an animal under conditions of muscular activity (Yamamoto & Edwards, 1960; Wasserman et al, 1975; Ponte & Purves, 1978). It must be noted, however, that there is no evidence whatsoever to indicate that artificially introduced venous blood, in any way, simulates the venous blood of exercise. Thus, the basic surmise of the validity of the experiments mimicking exercise is open to question.

Furthermore, it has been shown that perfusion of venous exercising blood into a second animal, using cross-circulation techniques, produced only a curvilinear relationship of $\dot{V}$-$\dot{V}co_2$ (Kao, 1963; Kao et al, 1964). In a single intact animal induced to exercise and in exercising man, within a metabolic change of no more than 10 times of its resting values, $\dot{V}$-$\dot{V}co_2$ relationship is always rectilinear (Asmussen & Nielsen, 1957; Kao et al, 1964). This curvilinear relationship of $\dot{V}$-$\dot{V}co_2$ is an important finding and indicates that the arterial blood CO_2 increment is not sufficient to account for the total increment of exercise hyperpnea. Furthermore, this curvilinear relationship was what observed in the humoral dog which received exercising blood and which had its neural signals of exercise totally removed or inactivated. Here we touch a point of another philosophical question in physiological research. In the cross-circulation experiments (Kao, 1963), eventhough we were able to separate the humoral and the neural components, can we say that the ventilatory responses in the two animals individually must be equally summated in the single intact animal?

Oscillation Hypothesis

The oscillation hypothesis of Yamamoto and Edwards (1960) regarding exercise hyperpnea was indeed an intriguing idea, and it stimulated a considerable amount of research work in the field. It was proposed that the steady state Pco_2 was not as effective as the oscillating Pco_2 which supposed to occur during muscular activity, and that this oscillation could be responsible for the increase in ventilation during exercise. Experimental observations to support this hypothesis were difficult to make, and those investigators, who succeeded in designing certain experimental procedures in oscillating the arterial Pco_2, were unable to find a difference in ventilatory response (Cunningham et al, 1965; Perkins et al, 1966).

The Neurogenic Exercise Drive

The concept of the neurogenic exercise stimulus is neither new nor a recent one. Definite ideas regarding this were formulated and published in literature as early as 90 years ago by Geppert and Zuntz (1888). Because of the inherent difficulty involved in identifying an exercise stimulating factor to ventilation in the absence of exercise during an experimental situation, evidence was not available until appropriate experimental techniques were developed (Comroe & Schmidt, 1943; Comroe, 1944). According to Cunningham, the most convincing evidence supporting the existence of the neurogenic exercise stimulus was obtained from the cross-circulation experiments (Cunningham, 1974). Denervation experiments, ischemia experiments, passive exercise experiments, and venous blood perfusion experiments, all have certain drawbacks with regard to obtaining valid physiological data, therefore, they do not help in making definitive interpretation about exercise hyperpnea (Kao,1963). Yet, in spite of these obvious uncertainties we still see the resurgence of the relatively useless experiments appearing in the literature from time to time.

The existence of the neurogenic stimulus was originally a mere hypothesis, subsequently has been supported by experimental results, and we have been able to demonstrate that the neurogenic exercise stimulus is the one which is responsible for the ventilatory change during moderate exercise (Kao, 1963). From the triad arrangement of cross-circulation experiments which we performed some years ago, it was clearly demonstrated that as long as the head of an animal was maintained in an isocapnic state, the neurogenic exercise stimulus could account for the total exercise hyperpnea (Kao, 1963, Kao et al, 1963).

If a neurogenic exercise drive does, indeed, exist, then, theoretically and logically, stimulation of muscle nerve should effect a state of hyperpnea. In recent years, using electrophysiological techniques (Eccles & Lundberg, 1959; Douglas & Ritchie, 1962), it has been possible to demonstrate the existence of this phenomenon in experimental animal and to identify the nature of the neurogenic exercise stimulus (Kao, 1963; Kalia, 1973; Kao et al, 1978).

THE NATURE OF THE NEUROGENIC EXERCISE DRIVE

Experiments performed in the past decades have produced a vast amount of data to support the neurogenic exercise drive which is responsible for the exercise hyperpnea. A logical question now arises - What is the nature of this neurogenic drive?

Skeletal muscle is rich in sensory nerve endings (Granit, 1955). Exhaustive work has been done on the muscle spindle and its afferent and efferent innervation. It seems, at the first glance, that the muscle spindle must be the most likely candidate for the neurogenic stimulus in exercise hyperpnea. However, the work of Hodgson and Matthews (1968), using vibration as a specific stimulus for muscle spindles has shown that the muscle spindles do not play any role in increasing of ventilation. This, therefore, excludes the possibility of these receptors being involved in exercise hyperpnea. It has been shown by Bessou et al (1959) that electrical stimulation of group I and group II fibers of muscle nerve increased ventilation. In muscle nerve, there are large numbers of unmyelinated fibers (Ranson & Davenport, 1931; Rexed & Therman, 1948), yet, there are surprisingly few reports available regarding the electrophysiological activity and the function of these fibers. The only published report available so far is a brief communication by Iggo (1961), who has reported activity in unmyelinated fibers produced by applying pressure locally to the muscle.

In our recent experiments we have used the method of antidromic nerve block of Douglas and Ritchie (1962), as well as multiples of threshold stimulation (Eccles & Lundberg, 1959) to stimulate selectively specific group of muscle afferents. These experiments have been done on dogs and were designed to determine the nature of the exercise stimulus. The data obtained from these experiments have made it possible for us to define the nature of the exercise stimulus which originates from muscles. The term ergoreception has been used to describe the sensory entity in the muscle. We have chosen this general term, since neither the exact nature of transduction of the exercise stimulus into electrical afferent activity, nor the morphology of the sensory receptor has been determined so far. This ergoreception is conveyed to the central respiratory apparatus predominantly via 'C'fibers (Kalia et al, 1972; Kalia, 1973; Kao et al, 1978). The spinothalamic tract has been suggested as being possibly involved in conveying this ergoreception stimulus to the brainstem respiratory apparatus (Kao, 1963). In the brainstem, a considerable amount of processing and interaction with other afferent influences on the central respiratory mechanisms must go on.

So far, our studies have focused on determining the type of nerve fibers involved in transmitting the neurogenic stimulus from the exercising limbs. Our observations tend to support the concept that 'C' fibers in muscle nerve must have a regulatory function (Ranson & Davenport, 1931). It also provides us with a role for these 'C' fibers which are so abundant in muscle nerves. It is logical to assume that 'C' fibers must be involved in the hyperpnea of muscular exercise.

Our recent experiments have also shown that ventilatory responses of similar parameters could be obtained using a variety of 'exercise' stimulus. This includes: (1), direct electrical stimulation of the muscles, (2), using the same electrical stimulus characteristics as those used for muscle to stimulate muscle nerve, and (3), stimulation of specific group of muscle afferents using electrical stimulation in the presence of differential nerve block (Douglas & Ritchie, 1962); this stimulus was applied to the intact muscle nerve and to the central end following nerve section. The similarity in ventilatory responses observed using each of these different modes of stimulation supports the notion that the neurogenic exercise drive can be produced with or without muscle contraction. It should be emphasized that there was no significant difference in the ventilatory responses following stimulation of muscle nerve (central end or intact nerve) or stimulation of muscle directly, thus excluding the possibility of metabolic factors influencing the hyperpnea response (Kao et al, 1978; Kalia et al, 1978). A major difficulty of studying the mechanisms of exercise hyperpnea lies in the complete isolation of each individual factor causing exercise hyperpnea without actually inducing exercise (the detailed account of these observations is being published, Kalia et al, 1978).

Having established the existence of the neurogenic exercise drive and its nature, we are now in a better position to present a preliminary concept of the pathways involved in the neurogenic exercise drive together with the known chemical drive (Fig. 1.). We are aware of the difficulties involved in such an over simplification,

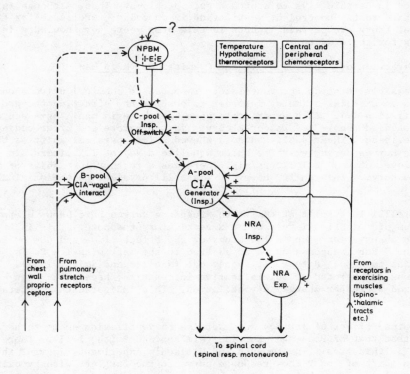

Fig.1. A diagram modified from the work of Euler and Trippenbach (1976) showing the major inputs on ventilation. CIA= Central Inspiratory Activity; NRA=Nucleus Retroambigualis; NPBM=Nucleus Parabrachialis Medialis. Exercise drive from the muscle nerves influences the CIA and possibly also the NPBM.

especially, since this represents an interpretation of a complex phenomenon. But, at least, for the present time, such a scheme will help to clarify the picture until more experimental information is made available. Even as far as the chemical drive for ventilatory control is concerned, in spite of the overwhelming amount of information is currently available to us regarding the peripheral and central chemoreceptor mechanism (Po_2, Pco_2-pH), there are still considerable gaps in our knowledge about the central processing of this chemoreceptor input. It is interesting to note that these gaps in our knowledge about chemical drive exist in areas that are identical with the neurogenic drive. There is no information currently available regarding the exact nature of the central processing of the pathways of the neurogenic exercise drive and chemical drive.

THE INTERACTION OF THE NEUROGENIC EXERCISE DRIVE AND CHEMICAL DRIVE

The matter of interpreting the mechanism underlining central responses to a single input is difficult enough, yet the problem becomes overwhelmingly complex when one attempts to interpret the responses of multiple factors and their interaction in a physiological state. It is obvious that when two or more stimuli influence a physiological response, there must be interaction. However, without knowing the complete anatomical pathways and their functional responses, how can one attack such an intricate problem? In spite of these difficulties, physiologists have attempted in certain ways to approach such problems. Thus, although information with regard to the control of ventilation in muscular exercise is far from being complete, there are certain aspects in this area where our knowledge is helpful in planning for the studies.

The Interaction of Exercise Drive and Chemical Drive in Man

It is possible to study the ventilatory response to chemical drive alone and in the presence of exercise stimulus in order to observe the effect on the gross change of ventilation ($\dot{V}$). Such experiments have been done in man. Asmussen and Nielsen (1957) studied the $\dot{V}$-Pco_2 response curves in man before and after adding various exercise loads. Their published data showed a left parallel shift of the $\dot{V}$-Pco_2 response curves during exercise which equalled a $\dot{V}o_2$ of 1.1 liters/min. With a higher level of $\dot{V}o_2$ (2.1 liters/min) there was a further left shift of the $\dot{V}$-Pco_2 response curve. This shift, however, was still parallel to the original response curve.

This parallel left shift of the $\dot{V}$-Pco_2 response curves have been interpreted as a summation of two stimuli to produce a ventilatory response. This is at variance with the observation made in the study of the effect of O_2 and CO_2 on ventilation, where the $\dot{V}$-Pco_2 response curve is shifted to the left with low Po_2's, but not in a parallel fashion. Rather, it fanned out (Nielsen and Smith, 1951). This observation was interpreted as multiplicative interaction, because at high Pco_2's, low Po_2 caused a greater change in ventilation. This indicated that interaction took place.

The combined effect of low Po_2 and exercise on ventilation seems to have a different effect than that of Pco_2 and exercise (Nielsen and Smith, 1951). There is paucity of data in this area. In Asmussen and Nielsen's experiments in man, there was a definite shift of the $\dot{V}$-Pco_2 response curve to the far left with hypoxia for the same work load. The shift of the $\dot{V}$-Pco_2 response curve during the same exercise with hypoxia also fanned out at high Pco_2. Weil et al (1972) also published data based on their observations in man. The $\dot{V}$-Po_2 plot, which they used, was shifted upwards during exercise in an unparallel fashion.

Interaction of the Exercise Stimulus with Chemical Drive in Anesthetized Dogs

In anesthetized dogs, we have done two types of experiments: (1), Subjected the dog to CO_2 inhalation and obtained the $\dot{V}$-Pco_2 response curve, then, added an exercise load. There was a left shift of the $\dot{V}$-Pco_2 response curves during exercise in a parallel fashion in intact single dogs and in cross-perfused dogs in which the head of the exercising dog was supplied by blood from a donor dog. The donor dog was given CO_2 to breathe, thus making both the donor dog and the exercising dog's head hypercapnic. In the latter arrangement, the $\dot{V}$-Pco_2 response curves of exercising dog (whose head alone received hypercapnic blood), also shifted to the left in a parallel fashion (Kao et al, 1963). (2), Subjected the dog to normoxia and hypoxia and then, induced exercise in the dog. First we established the $\dot{V}$-Po_2 response curve which was a curvilinear one. With additional induced exercise, the whole $\dot{V}$-Po_2 response curve was shifted upwards and the distance of these two curves at very low Po_2 was exaggerated. This finding was consistently obtained whether the experiments were carried out in single intact anesthetized dogs or in cross-circulated dogs in which the exercising dog's carotid apparatuses were perfused with blood from a donor dog and thus their Po_2 could be altered independent of the circulation of the dog induced to exercise (Kao et al, 1967). It seems that the ventilatory effect of Pco_2 and exercise summates and that of Po_2 and exercise interacts.

The question of the influence of the magical carotid bodies on the study of regulation of ventilation has dominated the field for the past half a century, and it is unlikely that we have seen the end of the enthusiasm shown to this minute body (Purves, 1975). Since the ventilatory response to hypoxia is so important to man's existence, that the study of the carotid body has also invaded the field of exercise physiology (Kao et al, 1967; Eisele et al, 1967; Lugliani et al, 1971; and Weil et al, 1972).

In vagotomized dogs, $\dot{V}$-Pco_2 response curve shifted to the left at both high and low Po_2's. In this connection, it is natural to raise the question whether or not the vagal afferents in different species is responsible for different effects on the $\dot{V}$-Pco_2 response curves. If this were true, then, the $\dot{V}$-Pco_2 response curves at different levels of Po_2 would produce multiple responses ranging from fanning in or fanning out or running in parallel, thus resulting in a variation of the presence or absence of the fans. For those who are skillful in doing investigations on humans, we suggest that vagal block in various degrees be done to assess the role of vagal influence on the fanning of the $\dot{V}$-Pco_2 response curves.

The Site(s) of Interaction of the Neurogenic Exercise Drive and Chemical Drive

Bhattacharyya et al (1970) also performed human experiments integrating the total response of hypoxia, CO_2, and exercise. These investigations have demonstrated the importance of the carotid body or rather its chemosensitivity in exercise hyperpnea. It can be inferred from their results that somehow there is an interaction of Po_2 and exercise at the peripheral chemoreception level. Our experiments employing cross-circulation techniques have revealed that when the carotid body's Po_2 was controlled by the second animal's circulation while its own hindlimbs were induced to exercise, the $\dot{V}$-Po_2 curves in the exercising animal changed in a similar fashion as that obtained in single intact exercising dogs during exercise with changing Po_2. The same is true where the head of one dog's Pco_2 was controlled via the arterial blood of a donor dog. The donor dog's Pco_2 was altered to influence the Pco_2 of the head of the recipient dog which was induced to exercise (Kao et al, 1963). This shows that if there is an interaction of exercise with Po_2 and a summation of exercise with Pco_2, they must be by means of a central (or intracranial) mechanism, similar to that of what we have established for the site of Po_2 and Pco_2 interaction (Kao and Mei, 1978). In a preliminary communication in this volume, Schlaefke maintains that all chemical drives and non-feed-back-afferent signals are amplified by the intermediate areas of the central chemosensitive mechanisms. It may be possible that such a relay pathway is necessary.

Muscle Nerve Stimulation and CO_2 Interaction

It is interesting to note that the stimulation of the central end of the severed muscle nerve or the intact nerve also caused a summation with the CO_2 effect on ventilation. This summation existed even when Pco_2 was at a level equal to or abov 100 mm Hg (Kao et al, 1978). The similarity of ventilatory response,when the muscle is directly stimulated to induce exercise or when the muscle nerve is stimu-lated with the same stimulation parameters,makes one feel that perhaps the stimula-tion of the muscle nerve directly can be used as a means to simulate the mode of exercise. Thus, it is possible to produce an exercise response without actual exercise, a methodology which is necessary for the neurological study of the inter-action of respiratory stimuli.

The Interaction of The Neurogenic Exercise Drive and Chemical Drive in Single Breath Studies

The interaction of various respiratory stimuli can be studied employing $\dot{V}$ as the final titration point. In addition, we can study a variety of the characteristics of $\dot{V}$, namely tidal volume (V_T), and respiratory frequency (f). These parameters can be divided into inspiratory time (T_I), expiratory time (T_E), the slope of the rise of the inspiratory tracing (S) using the recording of the electrical phenomen-on of the phrenic activity or the ordinary tidal volume, or the averaged V_T/T_T, where T_T is the total time for one complete cycle of the tidal volume, and the height of the amplitude of the tidal volume.

Since the work of Clark and Euler (1972) and Hey et al (1966), many articles have appeared using the detailed measurement of single breath characteristics. This rekindled interest in the detailed analysis of $\dot{V}$ has afforded respiratory physio-logists the possibility of studying the components of the integrated mechanisms of the central respiratory regulation apparatus (cf Bradley, 1977).

Our preliminary work on investigating the interaction of neurogenic exercise sti-mulus and chemical drive employing single breath techniques has revealed interest-ing phenomenon.

Experiments were carried out in nembutalized dogs with or without vagotomy. Single breath tracings were displayed on a Tektronix storage oscilloscope from which polaroid photographs of the oscilloscope tracing were made. Dogs were induced to exercise with or without CO_2 inhalation in order to produce hypercapnia, and with

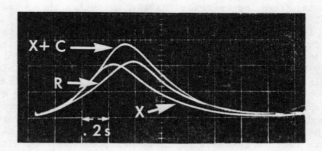

Fig.2. Single breath tracings of tidal volume in a nembutalized
dog before vagotomy. R = resting (control); X = exercise;
X+C = exercise with CO_2 inhalation. The time scale is 0.2
seconds between the arrows.

or without N_2 inhalation in order to produce hypoxia. In CO_2 inhalation and hypoxia experiments, exercise was induced after a control period during which a reasonable steady state level of ventilation was achieved. The first few breaths were
recorded for analysis so that the end-tidal CO_2 changes were minimal.

Figure 2 shows the result of such an experiment with recordings of single breath at
rest (R), during induced exercise (X), and during exercise with CO_2 inhalation (X+C)
in a dog with intact vagi. The rising slope of V_T during exercise shifted to the
left, but with exercise and CO_2 inhalation together, similar slope of V_T was obtained. CO_2 inhalation increased the amplitude of V_T and shortened T_I.

Figure 3 shows the changes in the slope of V_T at rest (R), during nitrogen administration (N) and with induced exercise during nitrogen inhalation (X+N). Similar
results regarding the rise of the slope of the tidal volume were obtained as that
with exercise and CO_2 inhalation (cf Fig.2.), namely, exercise with nitrogen inhalation followed a similar rise in the slope of V_T as that of nitrogen inhalation alone.

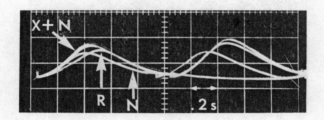

Fig. 3. Single breath tracings of tidal volume in a nembutalized
dog before vagotomy. R = resting; N = N_2 inhalation; X+N =
exercise with hypoxia. The time scale is 0.2 seconds between
the arrows.

After vagotomy, the rise of the slopes of V_T was quite different from that seen with
vagi intact. As shown in Figure 4, the rise of the slopes of V_T with CO_2 inhalation
and with exercise in the presence of CO_2 were quite separate. With CO_2 inhalation

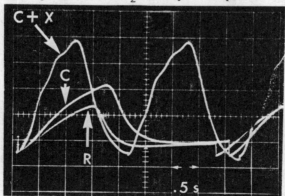

Fig. 4. Single breath tracings of V_T in a nembutalized dog after
vagotomy. R = resting; C = CO_2 inhalation; C+X = exercise
during CO_2 inhalation. The time scale is 0.5 seconds between
the arrows.

there was a shift to the left of the slope of V_T. With additional exercise, there
was a further shift of the slope of V_T to the left. CO_2 and exercise both increased the amplitude of V_T, although they are not of the same magnitude.

The same pattern was observed in nitrogen inhalation in vagotomized dogs (Fig. 5.).
First of all, nitrogen inhalation produced a shift in the slope of the V_T to the
left, CO_2 inhalation with N_2 further shifted this slope to the left, and with exercise, there was an even greater shift of the slope leftward.

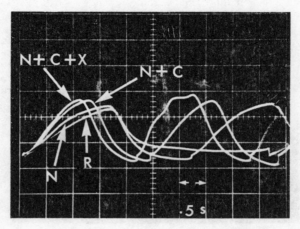

Fig. 5. Single breath tracings of V_T in a nembutalized dog after
        vagotomy. R = resting; N= N_2 administration; N+C = CO_2 in-
        halation during hypoxia; N+C+X = exercise during CO_2 inhala-
        tion and hypoxia. The time scale is 0.5 seconds between the
        arrows.

Further analyses were performed and shown in Figures 6 and 7. In Figure 6, T_I
(inspiratory time) vs S (slope of the V_T) was plotted in vagi intact (I) and in
vagotomized (Vg) dogs during exercise with and without CO_2 inhalation. The results
shown in Figure 6 is bound to pose a serious question concerning interactions of
respiratory stimuli. As shown in Figure 6, before vagotomy, exercise alone and
exercise with CO_2 showed two different slopes of the T_I-S plot, whereas, after
vagotomy the same plot showed parallel slopes (cf Agostoni & D'Angelo,1976). Con-
trarily, the $\dot{V}$-Pco_2 response curve was shifted leftward in a parallel fashion with
exercise before vagotomy. After vatogomy the $\dot{V}$-Pco_2 response curves fanned out
with exercise drive.

Recently, much work has been published concerning the T_I-T_E studies in various types
of experiments (D'Angelo & Agostoni, 1975). In Figure 7, we plotted the T_I-T_E relationship with data obtained in nembutalized dogs with high O_2, N_2 inhalation, CO_2
inhalation and with induced muscular exercise. These relationships have been shown
under two conditions: vagotomized and vagi intact. With high dose of nembutal,
vagotomy shifted the T_I-T_E lines merely upwards. Within normal range of anesthesia,
T_I-T_E lines with and without vagotomy changed almost proportionately and these lines
converged towards the origin of the graph (cf Gautier, 1976).

With deep anesthesia and oxygen inhalation,vagotomy merely pushed the T_I-T_E lines
upwards. CO_2 inhalation in animals with deep anesthesia with and without vagotomy
only changed the T_E. From the information shown in Figure 7, one is tempted to
postulate that there must be a threshold phenomenon which is indicated by the sharp

bend of the T_I-T_E plot. If this postulation were valid, then, in vagotomized dogs, the threshold for both T_I and T_E was about 1.5 seconds. For intact dogs, the values

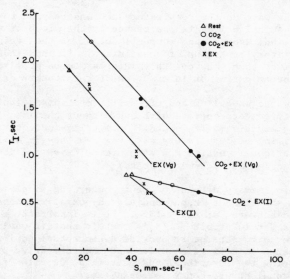

Fig. 6. Inspiratory time (T_I) is plotted against the slope (S) of
the steepest portion of the rise of the tidal volume in
nembutalized dog with intact vagi (I) and after vagotomy
(Vg) under several physiological conditions including
exercise and increased chemical drive.

of this threshold fell under 1.0 in this series of our studies. These curves also indicated that T_I response was limited, whereas T_E was responsive over a large range under various physiological (or pathological) states. Under conditions of irreversible anesthesia, T_I would be at zero and T_E would be at infinity.

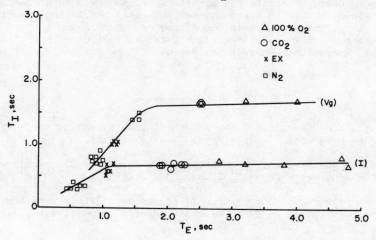

Fig. 7. Relationship between inspiratory time (T_I) and expiratory
time (T_E) in nembutalized dog with intact vagi (I) and
after vagotomy (Vg) in a variety of conditions.

The results obtained from our studies have brought out two fundamental questions concerning the interaction of neurogenic exercise drive and chemical drive:

1. In what ways do the respiratory neurons respond to exercise and chemical drive? Is the change in the slope of V_T a valid indicator of the neuronal output of the central respiratory apparatus of ventilation? If this indicator is valid, then, how can this information be utilized in our investigation of interaction of respiratory drives?

2. How do the on-switch and off-switch mechanisms in the respiratory centers operate with and without chemical drive during exercise? If T_I and T_E are valid indicators of the timing of respiratory act, how can they be utilized for further investigation of exercise drive and its interaction with chemical drive?

Since we have only preliminary data at present concerning single breath analysis during exercise with and without hypercapnia or hypoxia, we cannot be expected to provide sophisticated answers at this stage. It is important, however, to point out the intrigueness of this problem. It is certain that it would not be possible to understand,or even attempt to provide a conceptual notion regarding the interaction of the neurogenic exercise drive and chemical drive without further investigation concerning the functional and anatomical details of the total central (and peripheral) neuronal crypto-control-mechanisms.

We are fortunate, however, that some informational concepts have become available to formulate a frame work for future experimentation. We know that there is interaction at different levels between the neurogenic exercise drive and the chemical drive, but our understanding of the mechanisms is fragmentary. Is there only one type of central neuron which can respond to different drives or are there specifically designated neurons each functionally is for a specific drive? Are there central neurons capable of increasing recruitment for summation or interaction of respiratory drives so as to result in a total response in ventilation? Or a purely graded neuronal response with various inputs can explain this complex intriguing situation? During exercise,the situation becomes even more puzzling, for it requires physiological changes in systems other than that regulating ventilation. What are the effects of change in brain blood flow or other regional blood composition on the interaction of multiple respiratory drives including that of neurogenic exercise stimulus? Whatever the answer may be, we will be patiently waiting for its revelation!

REFERENCES

Agostoni,E. and D'Angelo,E. The effect of limb movements on the regulation of depth and rate of breathing. Respir.Physiol. 27,33 (1976).

Asmussen, E. and Nielsen, M. Ventilatory response to CO_2 during work and at low oxygen tension. Acta Physiol. Scand. 39,27 (1957).

Bessou,P., Dejours, P. and Laporte,Y. Effets ventilatoires réflexes de la stimulation des fibres afférentes de grand diametre, d'origine musculaire, chez le chat. C.R. Soc. Biol. Paris. 153,477 (1959).

Bhattacharyya, N.K., Cunningham, D.J.C., Goode, R.C., Howson, M.C. and Lloyd, B.B. Hypoxia, ventilation, Pco_2 and exercise. Respir. Physiol. 9,329 (1970).

Bradley, G.W. Control of the breathing pattern. In: MTP International Review of Physiology. Respiratory Physiology II. Editor, J.G. Widdicombe. University Park Press, Baltimore pp 185-217 (1977).

Clark, F.J. and Euler, C. von. On the regulation of depth and rate of breathing. J. Physiol (London). 222, 267 (1972).

Comroe, J.H. The hyperpnea of muscular exercise. Physiol. Rev. 24, 319 (1944).

Comroe, J.H. and Schmidt, C.F. Reflexes from the limbs as a factor in the hyperpnea of muscular exercise. Am. J. Physiol. 138, 536 (1943).

Cropp, G.J.A. and Comroe, J.H. Role of mixed venous blood Pco_2 in respiratory control. J. Appl. Physiol. 16, 1029 (1961).

Cunningham, D.J.C. Integrative aspects of the regulation of breathing: a personal view. In: MTP International Review of Physiology. Respiratory Physiology I. Editor J.G.Widdicombe. University Park Press, Baltimore. pp305,347 (1974).

Cunningham, D.J.C., Elliott, D.H., LLoyd,B.B., Miller, J.P. and Young, J.M. A Comparison of the effects of oscillating and steady alveolar partial pressures of oxygen and carbon dioxide on pulmonary ventilation. J. Physiol. (London) 179,498 (1965).

D'Angelo, E. and Agostoni, E. Tonic vagal influences on inspiratory duration. Respir. Physiol. 24, 287 (1975).

Douglas, W.W. and Ritchie, J.M. Mammilian nonmyelinated nerve fibers. Physiol.Rev. 42, 297 (1962).

Eccles, R.M. and Lundberg, A. Synaptic actions in motorneurons by afferents which may evoke the flexion reflex. Rev. Arch. Ital. Biol. 97, 199 (1959).

Eisele, J.H., Ritchie, B.C.,and Severinghaus, J.W. Effect of stellate ganglion blockade on the hyperpnea of exercise. J. Appl. Physiol. 22, 966 (1967).

Gautier, H. Pattern of breathing during hypoxia or hypercapnia of the awake or anesthetized cat. Respir. Physiol. 27, 193 (1976)

Geppert, J. and Zuntz, N. Ueber die Regulation der Atmung. Pflueg. Arch. ges. Physiol. 42, 189 (1888).

Gonzalez, F. Jr., Fordyce, W.E., and Grodins, F. S. Mechanisms of respiratory responses to intravenous $NaHCO_3$, HC1, and KCN. J. Appl. Physiol. 43, 1075 (1977).

Granit, R. (1955) Receptors and Sensory Perception, Yale University Press, New Haven.

Gray, J.S. (1950) Pulmonary Ventilation and its Physiological Regulation, C.C. Thomas, Springfield.

Grodins, F.S. Analysis of factors concerned in regulation of breathing in exercise. Physiol. Rev. 30,220 (1950)

Haggard, H.W. and Henderson, Y. The fallacy of asphyxial acidosis. J. Biol. Chem. 43,3 (1920).

Hey, E.N., Lloyd, B.B., Cunningham, D.J.C., Jukes, M.G.M. and Bolton, D.P.G. Effects of various respiratory stimuli on the depth and frequency of breathing in man. Respir. Physiol. 1, 193 (1966)

Heymans, C., Jacob, J. and Liljestrand, G. Regulation of respiration during muscular work, as studied on the perfused isolated head. Acta Physiol. Scand. 14, 86 (1947).

Hodgson, H.J.F. and Matthews, P.B.C. The ineffectiveness of excitation of the primary endings of the muscle spindle by vibration as a respiratory stimulant in the decerebrate cat. J. Physiol. (London). 194,555 (1968).

Iggo, A. Non-myelinated afferent fibres from mammalian skeletal muscle. J. Physiol. (London). 155, 52-53p (1960).

Kalia, M. Role of muscle receptors connected to non-medullated fibers in reflex hyperventilation. Acta Neurobiol. Exp. 33, 71 (1973).

Kalia, M., Kao, F.F., Mei, S.S., and Babich, A.M. An electrophysiological investigation of the neurogenic exercise stimulus. In preparation.

Kalia, M. Serapati, J.M., Parida, B. and Panda, A. Reflex increase in ventilation by muscle receptors with non-medullated fibers (C fibers). J. Appl. Physiol. 32, 189 (1972).

Kao, F.F. Regulation of respiration during muscular activity. Am. J. Physiol. 185,145 (1956).

Kao, F.F. An experimental study of the pathways involved in exercise hyperpnea employing cross-circulation techniques. In: The Regulation of Human Respiration, editors D.J.C.Cunningham and B.B.Lloyd, Blackwell, Oxford. pp461-502 (1963).

Kao, F.F., Lahiri, S., Wang, C. Mei, S.S. Ventilation and cardiac output in exercise: Interaction of chemical and work stimuli. Circulation Research XX-XXI, Suppl. I. pp179-191, (1967).

Kao, F.F. and Mei S.S. The central multiplicative interaction of Po_2 and Pco_2 on ventilation. In: The Regulation of Respiration During Sleep and Anesthesia, Editors R.S. Fitzgerald, H. Gautier, and S. Lahiri Pergamon Press, New York. pp 403-414 (1978).

Kao, F.F., Mei, S.S., Babich, A. and Kalia, M. Neurogenic ergoreception of exercise hyperpnea. Fed Proc. 37, 805 (1978).

Kao, F.F., Michel, C.C. and Mei, S.S. Carbon dioxide and pulmonary ventilation in muscular exercise. J. Appl. Physiol. 19, 1075 (1964).

Kao, F.F., Michel, C.C., Mei, S.S. and Li, W.K. Somatic afferent influence on respiration. Ann. New York. Acad.Sci. 109, 696 (1963)

Lugliani, R. Whipp, B.J., Seard,G., Wasserman, K. Effect of bilateral carotid body resection on ventilatory control at rest and during exercise in man. N.Engl. J. Med. 285, 1105 (1971).

Nielsen, M. and Smith, H. Studies on the regulation of respiration in acute hypoxia. Acta Physiol. Scand. 24, 293 (1951).

Perkins, J.F., Buchthal, A. Domizi, D.B., Schafer, J. and Shapiro, S. Lack of influence of changes in arterial Pco_2 on ventilatory response to a constant stimulus to the carotid bodies. Fed. Proc. 25, 389 (1966).

Ponte, J. and Purves, M.J. Carbon dioxide and venous return and their interaction as stimuli to ventilation in the cat. J. Physiol. 274, 455 (1978)

Purves, M.J. (Editor) (1975) The Peripheral Arterial Chemoreceptor, Cambridge University Press, Cambridge.

Ranson, S.W. and Davenport, H.K. Sensory unmyelinated fibers in the spinal nerve. Am. J. Anat. 48,331 (1931).

Rexed, B. and Therman, P.O. Calibre spectra of motor and sensory nerve fibers of flexor and extensor muscle. J. Neurophysiol. 11, 133 (1948).

Wasserman, K., Whipp, B.J., Casaburi, R., Huntsman, D.J., Castagna, J. and Lugliani, R. Regulation of arterial Pco_2 during intravenous CO_2 loading. J. Appl. Physiol. 38, 651 (1975).

Weil, J.V., Byrne-Quinn, E., Sodal, I.E., Kline, J.S. and McCullogh, J.S. Augmentation of chemosensitivity during mild exercise in normal man. J. Appl. Physiol. 33, 813 (1972).

Yamamoto, W.S. and Edwards, M.W. Homeostasis of carbon dioxide during intravenous infusion of carbon dioxide. J. Appl. Physiol. 15, 807 (1960).

ACKNOWLEDGEMENTS

This investigation was supported in part by USPHS, NIH grants HL-04302, HL-17800, RCDA (to M.K.) HL-00103, and an Anonymous Biomedical Research Grant. The authors wish to express their thanks to Anthony M. Babich for his invaluable technical assistance.

AN ASSESSMENT OF THE EFFECT OF THE OSCILLATORY COMPONENT OF ARTERIAL BLOOD GAS COMPOSITION ON PULMONARY VENTILATION

B. A. CROSS, B. J. B. GRANT, A. GUZ, P. W. JONES,
S. J. G. SEMPLE and R. P. STIDWILL

*Departments of Medicine, Charing Cross Hospital Medical School,
London W6 8RF and The Middlesex Hospital Medical School,
London W1N 8AA, U.K.*

There is now accumulating evidence that the oscillation of blood gas composition with breathing can affect respiration independant of mean arterial pH, PCO_2 and PO_2 (Ref 1, 2, 3, 4). The magnitude of this effect is unknown; in this paper we make an estimate of the magnitude from our experiments in anaesthetised dogs (Ref 2, 4). In these experiments the phase relationship between the respiratory and blood gas cycles were changed and the effect on the phrenic motoneurone output measured. Figure 1 is a schematic drawing showing the relationship between the cycles at the peripheral chemoreceptors. In the first part of the figure end inspiration coincides with the trough of the pH cycle whilst in the second part it coincides with the peak. The phase relationship (Φ) is described in relation to end inspiration because it is a point which can be readily and accurately determined in the respiration cycle and because the end of inspiration is thought to be the part of the respiratory cycle when chemical stimuli have their maximum effect (Ref 5, 6, 7).

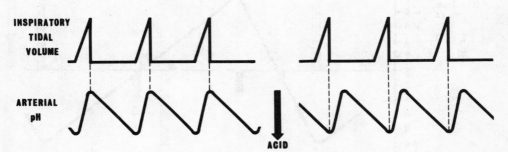

Fig 1.

In our experiments the phase relationship between respiratory and blood gas cycle was changed keeping mean blood gas composition constant. This was done by using a ventilator which was activated by the animal's own phrenic motoneurone output but in which the value of inflation was constant. Interposing a time delay between the start of phrenic discharge and activation of the ventilator was one method of changing the relationship. Another was to use the ventilator in an automatic mode independant of motoneurone output, but set at a rate which was slightly different from the animals central respiratory rhythm (as determined from the phrenic motoneurone). Because the rates were different a continually changing phase relationship was obtained and the effect of this change on each

breath could be determined. A necessary condition of these experiments however
was that the animals were paralysed and vagotomised. Vagotomy enabled the ventilator to be manipulated without inducing changes related to lung volume feedback.
From these experiments the maximum and minimum effect of changes in phase
relationship on respiratory rate, inspiratory time (T_i) expiratory time (T_e) and
the peak amplitude of phrenic motoneurone output (P) were determined. Peak
amplitude of the phrenic output was used as an index of tidal volume (Ref.8).

T_e was maximal when end inspiration coincided with the upstroke of the pH oscillation and minimal when it coincided with the downstroke- the variation between
maximum and minimum being 21% of T_e. P was maximal when end inspiration coincided with the trough of the oscillation and minimal when it coincided with the
early part of the downstroke - the variation between maximum and minimum being 7%.
T_i was the opposite to P in that it was maximal when end inspiration coincided
with the trough and minimal when it coincided with the early part of the downstroke; the variation between maximum and minimum being 7%. All these effects
were abolished by carotid body denervation.

Thus the magnitude of the effect of the phase relationship in each of the
respiratory variables was different,as was the ϕ at which they were maximal and
minimal. Allowance for these varying effects has been made when calculating the
overall effect of ϕ on respiration. For the purpose of our calculations respiratory minute volume (RMV) was assumed to be 2.60 L/min $^{-1}$, respiratory frequency
(f) 13 min $^{-1}$ and T_i 1.3 s (Figs 2 & 3). RMV was smallest when end inspiration
coincided with the trough of the oscillation and greatest when it coincided with
the middle of the downstroke. In the example shown in fig. 1 RMV varies between
2.3 and 2.8 L/min^{-1} according to the ϕ. This effect on minute volume was entirely
due to a change in f and this in turn was mainly determined by changes in T_e
(Fig. 3); indeed P was maximal when RMV was smallest.

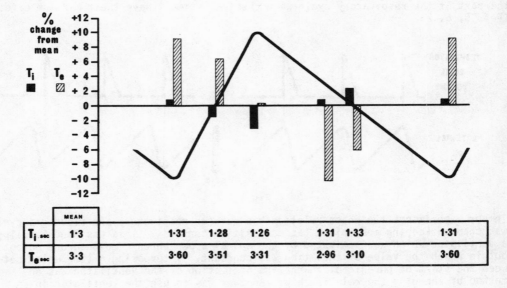

	MEAN						
T_i sec	1·3	1·31	1·28	1·26	1·31	1·33	1·31
T_e sec	3·3	3·60	3·51	3·31	2·96	3·10	3·60

Fig 2.

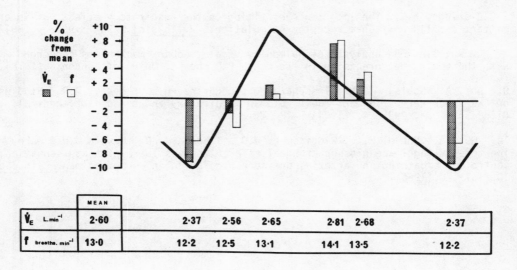

$\dot{V}_E$ L.min^{-1}	MEAN 2·60		2·37	2·56	2·65		2·81	2·68		2·37	
f breaths. min^{-1}	13·0		12·2	12·5	13·1		14·1	13·5		12·2	

Fig 3.

Our calculations predict a maximal effect of the changes in φ on respiratory minute volume of about 17%. These predictions are based on measurements on anaesthetised and vagotomised dogs so that extrapolation to the conscious intact state must be done with caution. Vagotomy however may not invalidate the extrapolation for in man, there appears to be no influence of lung volume feedback on the pattern of breathing during eupnoea (Refs. 9 & 10).

References

1. Black, A.M.S & Torrance R.W. Respiratory oscillations in chemoreceptor discharge in the control of breathing. Respir. Physiol. 13, 221-237 (1971).

2. Cross, B.A., Grant, B.J.B., Guz, A., Jones, P.W. & Semple, S.J.G. Relationship between the respiratory oscillation of arterial pH and phrenic motoneurone output. J. Physiol. 272, 79-80P. (1977).

3. Mueller, J., Plaas-Link, A., Luttman, A., Mückenhoff, K & Loeschcke, H.H. Respiratory responses to artificial arterial CO_2 oscillations in cats. Fedn. Proc. 36, 425 (1977).

4. Cross, B.A., Grant, B.J.B, Guz, A., Jones, P.W. & Semple, S.J.G. Changes of phrenic motoneurone output associated with altering its relationship to the respiratory oscillations of arterial blood gas composition. J. Physiol. 278, 12-13P. (1978).

5. Black, A.M.S. & Torrance, R.W. Chemoreceptor effects in the respiratory cycle. J. Physiol. 189, 59-61P. (1967).

6. Eldridge, F.L. The importance of timing on the respiratory effects of intermittent carotid sinus nerve stimulation. J. Physiol. 222, 297-318 (1972a).

7. Eldridge, F.L. The importance of timing on the respiratory effects of inter-mittent carotid body chemoreceptor stimulation. J. Physiol. 222, 319-333. (1972b).

8. Cross, B.A. An analysis of pulmonary vagal feedback mechanisms concerned with the control of breathing in the dog. PhD thesis, Univ. of London. (1978).

9. Guz, A., Noble, M.I.M., Trenchard, D., Cochrane, H.L. & Makey, A.R. Studies on the vagus nerves in man: their role in respiratory and circulatory control. Clin. Sci. 27, 293-304. (1964).

10. Guz, A., Noble, M.I., Widdicombe, J.G., Trenchard, D., Mushin W.W.& Makey A.R. The role of vagal and glossopharangeal afferent nerves in respiratory sensation, control of breathing and arterial pressure regulation in conscious man. Clin. Sci. 30, 161-170 (1966).

DISCUSSION

Semple was asked if he believed that the mechanisms he described would act to minimize or to enhance the oscillations in blood gas tensions and arterial pH. Widdicombe further asked Semple about how he reacted to the concept advanced by Purves in his introduction to the session that one of the roles of breathing is to minimize the potential oscillations of the chemical composition of arterial blood.

Semple replied that he regarded the pH oscillations as significant signals, and that the organism possibly by adjustments of the breathing rate might aim at diminishing the amplitude of the oscillations. He emphasized, however, that in his opinion the animal would have to breath very fast to be able to abolish them.

Torrance pointed out (in agreement with Purves) that the oscillations in afferent discharge from the innervated chemoreceptors, rather than the oscillations in arterial pH or gas tensions, constitute the significant signals to the brain mechanisms. At rest the selection of respiratory rate might be such that the oscillations in afferent discharge is hardly above the noise level. At exercise, however, the oscillations in arterial gas tensions and pH might well be increased to such an extent that they would get through and produce some oscillations also in the afferent discharge. The PCO_2 settled for in this state might then be dependent on the phase relationship between the oscillations in afferent discharge and central respiratory activity.

THE PERIPHERAL ARTERIAL CHEMORECEPTORS AS DETECTORS OF OXYGEN FLOW TO THE BRAIN

P. WILLSHAW and S. MAJCHERCZYK

Department of Physiology, The Medical School, Vincent Drive,
Birmingham B15 2TJ, England and Department of Physiology,
Warsaw Medical Academy, 26/28 Krakowskie Przedmiescie,
00-927, Warsaw, Poland

INTRODUCTION

Oxygen flow to the brain may be equated as the product of arterial oxygen content and cerebral blood flow. The object of this communication is to consider the evidence that the peripheral arterial chemoreceptors sense both parts of the oxygen flow equation.

ARTERIAL OXYGEN CONTENT AND PERIPHERAL CHEMORECEPTOR ACTIVITY

Arterial oxygen content is a function of both arterial PO_2 and blood oxygen capacity. Perhaps the best-known property of the peripheral chemoreceptors is their ability to sense arterial PO_2. The relationship between chemoreceptor activity and PO_2 is hyperbolic, increased activity becoming readily apparent below an arterial PO_2 of about 150 mm Hg (1, 2). The shape of the oxygen dissociation curve for blood converts the hyperbolic response of the chemoreceptors to oxygen partial pressure into a rectilinear response to oxygen content when this is below 15 mls O_2/100 mls blood (1, 3). The oxygen content of the blood may be varied independently of PO_2 by altering its oxygen capacity. Mills and Edwards (4) found that both carotid and aortic chemoreceptors were stimulated when the oxygen capacity of the blood was decreased by the use of carbon monoxide. The finding was confirmed in the case of the carotid body by Hornbein (1). Biscoe and co-workers (6) demonstrated that carotid chemoreceptor activity is independent of haematocrit. They used a preparation with intact sympathetic innervation. In contrast, Hatcher and co-workers (5) found that a direct reduction of haematocrit achieved by exchanging blood for dextran led to increased aortic chemoreceptor activity, but had no effect on carotid chemoreceptor activity unless the ipsilateral cervical sympathetic trunk had been sectioned. This latter finding is remarkable, in that it indicates an inhibitory role for the sympathetic innervation of the carotid body.

As a working hypothesis we must accept that the aortic bodies are directly sensitive to the oxygen content part of the oxygen flow equation, whereas the carotid bodies sense primarily oxygen partial pressure.

CEREBRAL BLOOD FLOW AND CHEMORECEPTOR ACTIVITY

The core idea of this communication is that a disturbance of cerebral blood flow can of itself engage either the sympathetic or the inhibitory sinus nerve/aortic nerve efferent neuronal pathway to the peripheral chemoreceptors and thereby engender a peripheral chemoreflex which would act to compensate for the disturbance. It is first necessary to summarise the effects of the two motor innervations of the peripheral chemoreceptors upon chemoreceptor activity.

i) The Sympathetic Innervation

The sympathetic innervation is generally considered to be an excitatory drive to the carotid body (7, 8, 9) although O'Regan (10) has shown some inhibitory effects of the sympathetic on chemoreceptor activity, and as mentioned previously the work of Hatcher (5) suggests that the sympathetic acts to inhibit carotid chemoreceptor activity during anaemia.

ii) Sinus and Aortic Nerve Efferent Activity

Biscoe and Sampson (11) found that it was possible to record neuronal activity arising from the central end of the sinus nerve. This activity persisted after section of the cervical sympathetic trunk, and has since been termed sinus nerve efferent activity. Neil and O'Regan (12) confirmed Biscoe and Sampson's finding and demonstrated a similar type of activity in the aortic nerve. Sinus and aortic nerve efferent activities are inhibitory to peripheral chemoreceptor afferent activity (12, 13, 14, 15). This inhibitory activity is tonically present in the eupnoeic anaesthetised cat to the extent that its withdrawal by section of the sinus nerve will result in an increase of chemoreceptor afferent activity by about 30% (14).

iii) Cerebral Perfusion and Motor Activity to Chemoreceptors

An important feature of the idea that peripheral chemoreceptors may be reflexly engaged by alteration of their sympathetic and non-sympathetic nerve supplies is that although the peripheral chemoreceptors must sample arterial blood it is not necessary to position them on arteries carrying a blood flow representative of cerebral blood flow. This is exemplified in the cat, an animal which does not have a patent internal carotid artery. It is sufficient for the activity of the motor nerves to the peripheral chemoreceptors to be modified as part of the brain's own reaction to altered perfusion. In the case of the sympathetic nervous system, a reduction of cerebral oxygen supply has been shown to augment sympathetic motor activity (16) despite the absence of peripheral chemoreceptors. The effects of altered cerebral perfusion on sinus nerve efferent activity are at present being studied by the authors of this communication. We found that haemorrhage produced a dramatic decrease of sinus nerve efferent activity (17). An example of this type of response is shown in Fig. 1. We have also investigated the increase in efferent activity seen during adrenaline-induced hypertension (11, 12, 17), an example of which is shown in Fig. 2. We find that β-adrenergic blockade considerably attenuates the efferent response to adrenaline-induced hypertension whilst leaving unaffected the response to haemorrhage or to an increase in arterial pressure induced by infusion of blood into the venous side of the circulation (Willshaw and Majcherczyk, in preparation). This result indicates that sinus nerve afferent activity responds not to arterial pressure per se but to some correlate of the pressure change such as a change of blood flow. Further support of such an idea is provided by the experiment of occluding a common carotid artery, which will produce a cerebral 'steal syndrome' by virtue of the anastomotic connections in the cat between the carotid rete and the cerebral vasculature. The arterial input pressure to the cerebral circulation should be essentially unaffected by this manoeuvre, and yet sinus nerve efferent activity decreases in response, as shown in Fig. 3. No baroreflex was obtained because the ipsilateral sinus nerve was cut in order to record the efferent activity. In the intact preparation, it is therefore possible that a small decrease of cerebral perfusion will result in the attenuation of sinus nerve efferent activity leading to increased chemoreceptor afferent activity.

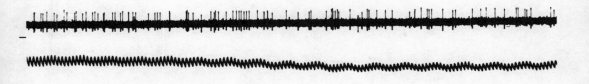

Fig. 1. Cat. Chloralose 40 mg Urethane 400 mg/kg. Artificial
ventilation. Upper trace:- efferent activity, left sinus nerve.
Lower trace:- femoral arterial pressure. Between marks, 20 mls
blood removed via femoral vein. Calibration:- horizontal, 5 secs.
Vertical - 0 and 200 mm Hg.

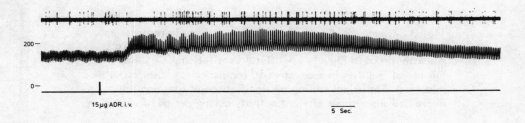

Fig. 2. Cat. Anaesthesia as in Fig. 1. Spontaneous ventilation.
Traces as in Fig. 1. Effect of intravenous injection of 15 µg
adrenaline at mark.

In summary, evidence does exist which indicates that both the sympathetic and efferent
inhibitory drives to the chemoreceptors may be modulated by altered cerebral perfusion.
Although the intrinsic response of the denervated carotid body to changed arterial pressure
is one of autoregulation of its neuronal activity if the pressure change is small (6) the motor
effects of the efferent innervations of the chemoreceptor will cause it to alter its neuronal
activity in response to those changes of cerebral perfusion which it cannot sense directly.

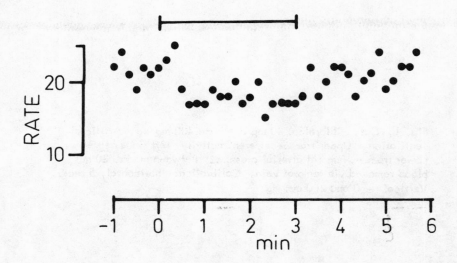

Fig. 3. Change in sinus nerve efferent activity in response to
ipsilateral common carotid occlusion, indicated by bar. Cat.
Anaesthesia as in Fig. 1. Artificial ventilation. Ordinate:-
number of impulses in successive 10 sec periods. Abscissa:- time,
minutes. Statistical testing by significance of runs confirms
decreased sinus nerve efferent activity during period of occlusion.

CONCLUSION

Evidence has been presented which indicates that the peripheral chemoreceptors may act as
oxygen flow detectors by virtue of their intrinsic sensitivity to arterial oxygen partial pressure
and content coupled with the extrinsic influences of their sympathetic and inhibitory efferent
innervations. The extrinsic innervation represents a mechanism through which chemoreceptor
activity may be modified by the response of the brain to alteration of its oxygen supply. The
teleological implication of this conclusion is that a protective chemoreflex (18, 19) may be
engaged when the brain is subject to inadequate oxygen supply due to a decreased blood flow,
a decrease in blood oxygen content, or a combination of these factors.

÷

ACKNOWLEDGEMENT

Our work in this field is supported by the Medical Research Council and the Polish Academy
of Sciences. The Royal Society provided travel expenses for P.W.

REFERENCES

(1) T. F. Hornbein, The relation between stimulus to chemoreceptors and their response, Arterial Chemoreceptors, Ed. R. W. Torrance, Blackwell, Oxford, pp. 65-68 (1968).

(2) T. J. Biscoe, M. J. Purves and S. R. Sampson, The frequency of nerve impulses in single carotid body chemoreceptor afferent fibres recorded in vivo with intact circulation, J. Physiol. (Lond.) 208, 121-131 (1970).

(3) U. S. von Euler, G. Liljestrand and Y. Zotterman, The excitation mechanism of the chemoreceptors of the carotid body, Skand. Arch. Physiol. 83, 132-152 (1939).

(4) E. Mills and W. McIver Edwards, Jr., Stimulation of aortic and carotid chemoreceptors during carbon monoxide inhalation, J. Appl. Physiol. 25 (5) 494-502 (1968).

(5) J. D. Hatcher, L. K. Chiu and D. B. Jennings, Anemia as a stimulus to aortic and carotid chemoreceptors in the cat, J. Appl. Physiol.: Respirat. Environ. Exercise Physiol. 44 (5) 696-702 (1978).

(6) T. J. Biscoe, G. W. Bradley and M. J. Purves, The relation between carotid body chemoreceptor discharge, carotid sinus pressure and carotid body venous flow, J. Physiol. (Lond.) 208, 99-120 (1970).

(7) W. F. Floyd and E. Neil, The influence of the sympathetic innervation of the carotid bifurcation on chemoreceptor and baroreceptor activity in the cat, Arch. int. pharmacodyn. 91, 230-239 (1952).

(8) C. Eyzaguirre and J. Lewin, The effect of sympathetic stimulation on carotid nerve activity, J. Physiol. (Lond.) 159, 251-267 (1961).

(9) E. Mills and S. R. Sampson, Respiratory responses to electrical stimulation of the cervical sympathetic nerves in decerebrate unanaesthetised cats, J. Physiol. (Lond.) 202, 271-282 (1969).

(10) R. G. O'Regan, Variable influences of the sympathetic nervous system upon carotid body chemoreceptor activity, Chemoreception in the Carotid Body, Ed. H. Acker and others, Springer-Verlag (Berlin) (1977) pp. 160-165.

(11) T. J. Biscoe and S. R. Sampson, Rhythmical and non-rhythmical spontaneous activity recorded from the central cut end of the sinus nerve, J. Physiol. (Lond.) 196, 327-338 (1968).

(12) E. Neil and R. G. O'Regan, Efferent and afferent impulse activity recorded from few fibre preparations of otherwise intact sinus and aortic nerves, J. Physiol. (Lond.) 215, 33-47 (1971).

(13) E. Neil and R. G. O'Regan, The effects of electrical stimulation of the distal end of the cut sinus and aortic nerves, J. Physiol. (Lond.) 215, 15-32 (1971).

(14) S. R. Sampson and T. J. Biscoe, Efferent control of the carotid body chemoreceptor, Experientia (Basel) 26, 261-262 (1970).

(15) S. J. Fidone and A. Sato, Efferent inhibition and antidromic depression of chemo-
      receptor A-fibres from the cat carotid body, Brain Res. 22, 181-193 (1970).

(16) S. E. Downing, J. H. Mitchell and A. G. Wallace, Cardiovascular responses to
      ischaemia, hypoxia, and hypercapnia of the central nervous system, Am. J. Physiol.
      204 (5) 881-887 (1963).

(17) P. Willshaw and S. Majcherczyk, The effects of changes in arterial pressure on sinus
      nerve efferent activity, Adv. Exp. Med. Biol. 99, 275-280. Edited by R. S.
      Fitzgerald and others, Plenum Press (1978).

(18) J. E. Angell-James and M. de B. Daly, Cardiovascular responses in apnoeic asphyxia:
      role of arterial chemoreceptors and the modification of their effects by a pulmonary
      vagal reflex, J. Physiol. (Lond.) 201, 87-104 (1969).

(19) Janice M. Marshall, The cardiovascular response to stimulation of carotid chemo-
      receptors, J. Physiol. (Lond.) 266, 48-49P (1977).

DISCUSSION

The discussion after the paper of Willshaw and Majcherczyk beared
out that virtually no knowledge is available, as yet, about the
neuroanatomy or the transmittor properties of the efferent, non-
sympathetic innervation of the carotid chemoreceptors.

CENTRAL NEURAL DRIVE MECHANISMS AND RESPIRATORY AFTERDISCHARGE — THE "T-POOL" CONCEPT

F. L. ELDRIDGE and P. GILL-KUMAR

Departments of Medicine and Physiology, University of North Carolina, Chapel Hill, North Carolina 27514, U.S.A.

Over the past several years, this laboratory has been reporting studies demonstrating the existence of a central neural mechanism which has the property of maintaining an increased but slowly declining respiratory activity for some minutes after cessation of a primary stimulus (1,2). A variety of stimuli, including electrical stimulation of the carotid sinus nerve and chemical stimulation of the carotid body (1), squeezing of the calf muscles (1), and voluntary hyperventilation (3,4) have been shown to activate the process. The level of CO_2-H^+ stimulus, if constant, does not appear to affect the time constant of the declining respiratory activity resulting from the process (1) but changes do interact with it (5). Anesthesia or lack of it and a number of ablative procedures, including decerebration (2), decerebellation (6), spinal cord section at C_7-T_1 (1) and carotid sinus nerve or vagal section (1) have not had obvious effects on the process. Changes in circulation do not appear to be causal (1,5).

The various findings have led to a conclusion that the mechanism is neural and located in the ponto-medullary region of the brain, and that it probably acts through the medium of neural positive-feedback circuits which produce an *afterdischarge*, or reverberation, in some neuronal network. This activity in turn, results in the continuing but slowly decaying stimulation of respiration.

Although in earlier reports we suggested the possibility that such reverberatory activity might be in the respiratory feedback loops involved in inspiratory-expiratory cycling, several pieces of evidence have suggested that it lies outside these areas. First, the reverberatory process may take some time to become fully activated, even though tidal neural activity for each breath has reached its maximum (1). Second, a large augmented breath, or sigh, occurring during the slow recovery period in vagally intact animals does not affect the process (2).

The studies reported here extend the findings on this mechanism. They support the conclusion that it lies outside the primary neuronal networks producing inspiratory-expiratory cycling and is best explained by the action of a separate network of neurons.

METHODS

The experiments were performed in cats anesthetized with chloralose and urethane. Vagi and carotid sinus nerves were usually cut. The animals were paralyzed and their end-tidal P_{CO_2} maintained at a constant level ($\pm$ 0.5 torr) by means of a servo-controlled ventilator (7). Electrical activity of a phrenic nerve root (C_5) was recorded and integrated in 0.1 sec. periods by means of an integrating digital voltmeter (8). The peak value for each breath was used as the neural equivalent of tidal output. Neural minute output was calculated as the product of this tidal value and respiratory frequency.

In each experiment base conditions were recorded after attaining a fixed end-tidal P_{CO_2} and stable respiratory output. Respiration was then increased by a facilitatory input (electrical stimulation of a carotid sinus nerve (CSN) or area M of the medulla, calf muscle squeezing or warming of a previous cooled area S of the ventral medulla). Stimulation was given usually for 1 min, following which the slow recovery respiratory pattern was recorded for another 5 min or until it approached the control level.

RESULTS

A typical experiment is shown in Fig. 1. At the onset of CSN stimulation there is a rapid increase in phrenic activity which lasts throughout the period of stimulation. The off-transient consists of two components, 1) an immediate

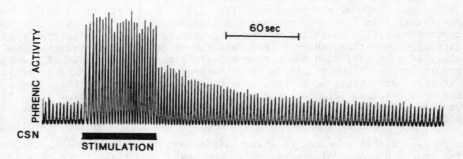

Fig. 1. Inspiratory neural (integrated phrenic) activity in
         a typical experimental run, showing baseline level
         at the left of the recording, facilitatory effect
         of 60 sec of continuous carotid sinus nerve (CSN)
         stimulation and slow recovery process (afterdischarge)
         following cessation of stimulation.

decrease in inspiratory output to about half its maximum value and 2) a slow decrease (the afterdischarge) to control level over a period of minutes. The decay of the second component usually has the form of an exponential function with time constants (TC) in the range of 50-60 sec in anesthetized animals. The TC of the recovery function in Fig. 1 is 58 sec.

Facilitation of respiration by calf muscle stimulation leads to a different respiratory response, characterized by a much higher respiratory frequency, than does the CSN. Nevertheless, the poststimulation recovery patterns are similar in form.

Effect of central chemoreceptor input

In these experiments central chemoreceptor input was facilitated in two ways. In the first, electrical stimulation of the exposed medulla was accomplished by means of a small electrode placed on chemoreceptor area M of the ventrolateral surface (9). An example is shown in Fig. 2 where the stimulation parameters were trains of pulses of 2 volts intensity and 2 msec duration, at a frequency of 25 Hz. It can be seen that phrenic activity increased in response to the stimulation in a manner similar to that of carotid sinus nerve or calf-squeezing and that a slowly decaying afterdischarge was also produced.

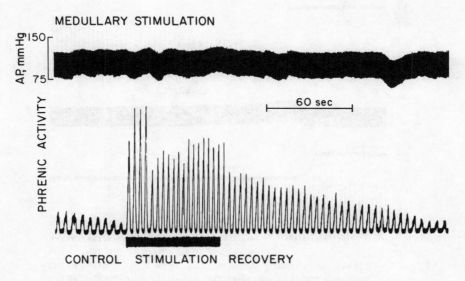

Fig. 2.   Effect of electrical stimulation of area M of the ventrolateral medulla, showing increase in phrenic activity during stimulation and activation of mechanism causing afterdischarge. AP=arterial pressure.

The second method of producing central chemoreceptor facilitation was that of Schlaefke and Loeschcke (10), where a thermode with 2x2 mm tip dimensions was placed on area S of the ventral medulla and alternately cooled and warmed to block and unblock central "chemoreceptor" input. An example of this procedure is shown in Fig. 3. The increase in phrenic activity after raising the thermode tip's temperature from 23°C to 40°C is shown in panel A. The effect of blocking input by cooling the thermode from 40°C to 21°C is shown in panel B. There is a fairly rapid drop of phrenic activity over the first 20 sec as the temperature decreases, but then with constant temperature a further slow decrease, probably representing the decaying afterdischarge, still occurs.

Although it is recognized that the thermode tip's temperature may not precisely reflect the local temperature of area S, this experiment and the findings with electrical stimulation strongly support a conclusion that, in addition to the previously shown stimuli (CSN, calf muscle squeezing, voluntary hyperventilation), central chemoreceptor input also has the ability to activate the mechanism causing afterdischarge. A poststimulation increase in the ventilation after medullary surface stimulation has also been found in spontaneously breathing cats by Loeschcke et al. (9).

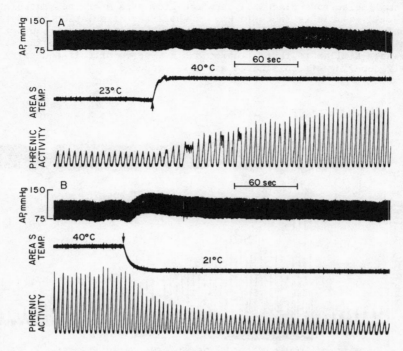

Fig. 3. Effect of warming and cooling area S of ventral surface of medulla on phrenic activity. AP=arterial
pressure.

Lack of effect of vagal afferent input on central neural respiratory afterdischarge

In these experiments the inhibitory effect of vagal nerve stimulation (100 Hz,
0.1 msec pulse duration) in vagotomized animals, or lung inflation in vagally
intact animals, on the poststimulation slow recovery process was examined. In
each animal a control experiment with CSN stimulation only, as shown in Fig. 1,
was performed first. Subsequent runs were identical except that short periods of
vagal stimulation or lung inflation were superimposed at various times during
CSN stimulation or during the afterdischarge. Vagal stimulation caused marked
inhibition of inspiratory output whenever given, but when stopped had no significant long-lasting effect on the development of the afterdischarge or on the
course of the subsequent slow recovery process. An example of this finding is
shown in Fig. 4 - the control run of the same cat is shown in Fig. 1. Despite
the inhibition, produced by vagal stimulation, there is no effect on the subsequent exponential decay of the afterdischarge.

It made no difference to the magnitude or form of the afterdischarge whether the
vagal inhibition was produced during the CSN stimulation just before onset of the
afterdischarge, during the first part of recovery or later in recovery as shown
in Fig. 4. Similar results occurred in all six of the cats studied in this manner and in the four cats in which vagal inhibition was produced by lung inflation
(11).

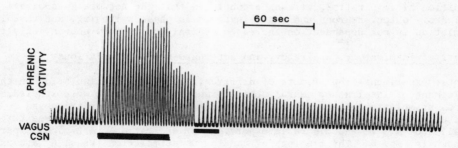

Fig. 4.   Example of lack of effect of vagal inhibition of
          inspiration on the subsequent pattern of respira-
          tory afterdischarge. The same cat's control run
          is shown in Fig. 1; all conditions are identical
          except for the 20 sec vagal stimulation given 20
          sec into the afterdischarge.

Even when the inspiratory response to carotid sinus nerve stimulation and inspiratory-expiratory cycling were totally inhibited by simultaneous stimulation of the
vagus nerve, there was development of a slowly waning afterdischarge similar to
that of the control (Fig. 5).

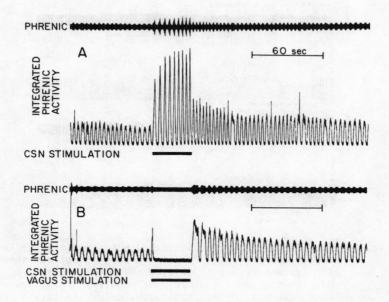

Fig. 5.   Phrenic nerve activity in two runs in one vagotomized
          cat. A: Control, showing baseline activity at left,
          effect of CSN stimulation (30 sec), and recovery;
          B: showing baseline activity, effect of combined CSN
          and vagal stimulation, and recovery.

The mechanism causing the afterdischarge is probably a buildup of activity in a
neural network in the medulla and pons. Since its activity is unaffected by vagal
inhibition of respiration, it can be concluded that the network is separate from
inspiratory output neurons and those involved in phase switching, and that its
stimulation is not dependent on increased central inspiratory neuron activity (CIA).

Effects of inspiratory, expiratory and alternate-cycle stimulations

In these experiments the effects of different modes of CSN stimulation on the
development of inspiratory neural activity and afterdischarge were studied. Continuous stimulation was as above. Inspiratory stimulation was triggered by the
onset of phrenic activity. Expiratory stimulation (0.8 to 1.0 sec) was triggered
manually to fall in the mid to late portions of expiration. A typical experiment
is shown in Fig. 6. The findings of continuous stimulation (Panel A) are as described above, a rapid increase in inspiratory output, a sharp decrease with the
first poststimulation breath and then a slowly declining afterdischarge.

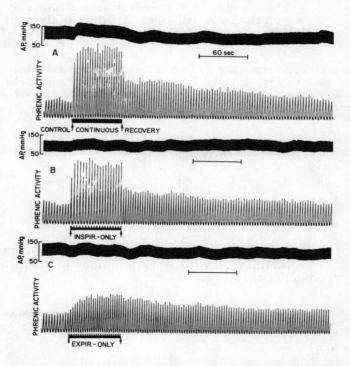

Fig. 6. Respiratory outputs (integrated phrenic activity) in
         three runs ($P_{ET_{CO_2}}$ = 30 torr in all) in one cat show-
         ing control levels at left, facilitatory effects of
         CSN stimulation for 1 min, and recovery. A: Contin-
         uous stimulation; B: inspiratory-only stimulation;
         C: expiratory-only stimultion. AP=arterial pressure.

Inspiratory stimulation (panel B) leads to a rapid rise in inspiratory activity
whose magnitude is similar to that of continuous stimulation despite the former's

smaller amount of actual stimulus time (50% of that of continuous); the after-discharge is also similar both in magnitude and time course of decay. Expiratory stimulation (panel C), on the other hand, leads to a smaller and more slowly rising (TC=25 sec) neural output during the period of stimulation. Both continuous and inspiratory stimulation runs have an immediate drop in output with the first poststimulation respiration, but this does not occur after expiratory stimulation. Nevertheless, the afterdischarge of the latter is like that of continuous and inspiratory runs in both magnitude and time course (TC=54-55 sec). All 12 cats of this study showed similar findings.

In an additional 4 cats, the effect of alternate cycle CSN stimulation was compared to that of the other modes of stimulation. It led to a dual set of patterns of increasing inspiratory neural activity (Fig. 7); the pattern of stimulated breaths resembled that of continuous or inspiratory stimulation, whereas the unstimulated breaths showed a slowly rising activity like that of expiratory stimulation. Neural activities in the first respiration after cessation of stimulation and the afterdischarge patterns (TC=51-57 sec) were similar for all stimulus modes.

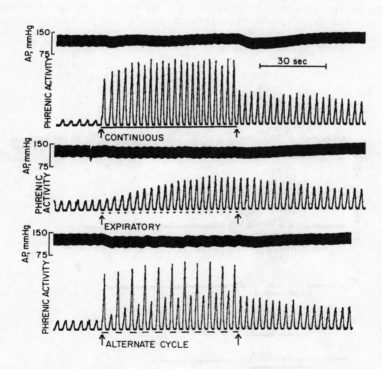

Fig. 7. Respiratory outputs in three runs (P_{CO_2}=30 torr) in one cat showing control levels at left, facilitatory effects of CSN stimulation and recovery. Top: continuous stimulation; Middle: expiratory-only stimulation; Bottom: alternate cycle stimulation. AP= arterial pressure.

The findings of this study further support the conclusion that the neural network causing the afterdischarge is separate from and does not require input from inspiratory output neurons for its activation. In addition, because inspiratory-only and expiratory-only stimulations caused similar afterdischarges despite marked differences in inspiratory output during stimulation, it can be concluded that carotid sinus nerve stimulation has dual effects, one acting relatively directly on inspiratory output neurons, the other affecting these neurons indirectly through activation of the pool of neurons causing the afterdischarge (tentatively named the "T-pool"). Stimulation during inspiration augments already activated inspiratory neurons by the more direct pathway while also increasing T-pool activity. Expiratory stimulation, on the other hand, finds inspiratory neurons below threshold or the pathway to them blocked (12) and unresponsive to the direct effect, thus allowing the indirect effect of rising T-pool activity to become apparent during succeeding inspirations. With alternate cycle stimulation, it is possible to see both responses occurring during the same period.

Effect of hypocapnia

In these experiments the effect on inspiratory activity and afterdischarge was studied (in 16 cats) during hypocapnia sufficient to stop all rhythmic respiratory activity in the absence of stimulation. An example of the findings is shown in Fig. 8. In this figure, all stimulations were given at least 5 min after the

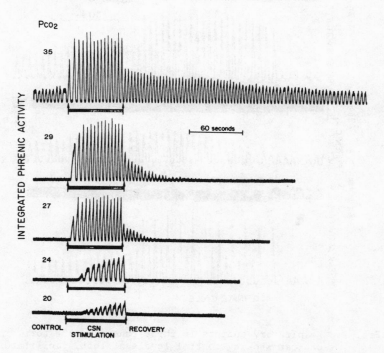

Fig. 8.   The effect of hypocapnia on phrenic response to the same CSN stimulus and on afterdischarge. Top record (P_{CO_2}=34 torr) is above CO_2 "threshold" for spontaneous respiratory activity during the control period; the remainder are progressively below the threshold.

preceding one, so previous afterdischarge activity would have had time to dissipate. The run performed at a P_{CO_2} of 34 torr is, of course, above threshold for spontaneous respiratory activity and shows the typical phrenic response to stimulation and an afterdischarge as described above. When P_{CO_2} is reduced below threshold, not only does the level of phrenic activity during stimulation become smaller, but also the afterdischarge becomes shorter, completely disappearing at P_{CO_2} levels of 24 torr and below.

The working hypothesis of this study was that gradations of central respiratory neural activity exist even when the magnitude of all input stimuli (CO_2-H^+ and others) are below the level capable of driving manifest respiratory output activity. We have termed this "concealed" activity. If such graded activity does occur, then the time from the beginning of a known input, e.g., a constant CSN stimulation, to the onset of phrenic discharge (latency) should give some indication of that activity. Consistent with the known stimulatory effects of the CO_2-H^+ input, latency was inversely related to level of end-tidal P_{CO_2} (Fig. 8). This was true in all cats studied and shows that the hypothesis is correct at least for the chemoreceptor input.

The next step was to find out if concealed activation of the T-pool occurs. The theoretical basis of this part of the experiment is shown in Fig. 9, where the minute neural activities of only the above threshold run (P_{CO_2}=35 torr) and that

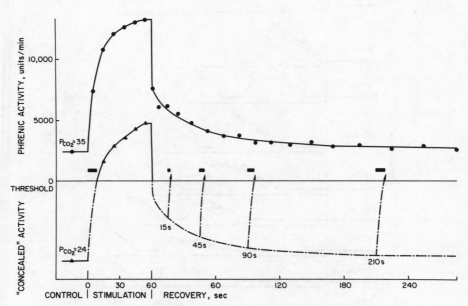

Fig. 9. Plot of mean neural (phrenic) minute activities for
         above threshold run (P_{CO_2}=35 torr) and below thresh-
         old run (P_{CO_2}=24 torr) of cat in Fig. 8. Solid curves
         above threshold represent measured values. Dashed
         curves of below threshold "concealed" activity are
         assumed. Vertical dashed curves and arrows represent
         hypothetical activity if restimulation were to occur
         at these times. Horizontal bars represent order of
         magnitude of latencies.

of the below threshold run at 24 torr are plotted. An assumption is made that
the shape of the changing concealed activity curve is the same as that of the
above threshold run. The latency (indicated by dark bars on the graph) of the
phrenic response to stimulation in the hypocapnic run should, as noted above, be
prolonged.

If a concealed afterdischarge does exist, then the level of concealed activity
(shown by the dashed curve) in central neurons should be higher shortly after a
preceding stimulation (e.g., at 15 sec) than after 5 min when the afterdischarge
will have fully decayed. A stimulation repeated at this time should therefore
produce a phrenic response after a shorter latency than one given at 5 min.
Longer delays before restimulation, e.g., at 45,90,210 sec, would allow more decay
of T-pool activity and therefore give longer latencies.

Figure 10 shows that experimentally this concept holds up. At a constant P_{CO_2},
latency of the phrenic response to a new stimulation is directly related in a
curvilinear manner to the delay from the previous stimulus. This supports a conclusion that the afterdischarge process was present even though the animal was
below threshold for manifest rhythmic respiration.

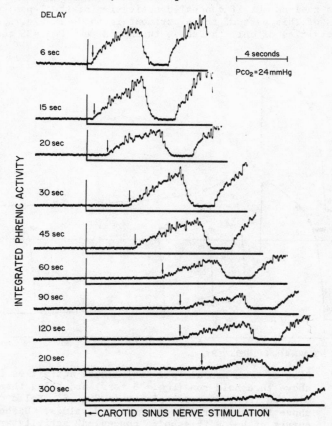

Fig. 10. Latencies of stimulus to phrenic response after various
          delays since preceding stimulation in subthreshold run
          $P_{CO_2}=24$ torr) of cat in Fig. 8. Onset of phrenic acti-
          vity in each panel indicated by vertical arrow.

DISCUSSION

On the basis of the various findings reported here we believe that the poststimu-
latory respiratory afterdischarge is due to activity in a network of neurons, the
T-pool, which when activated can maintain activity in the network of inspiratory
output neurons. Our concept of the T-pool, based on these findings, is diagrammed
in Fig. 11.

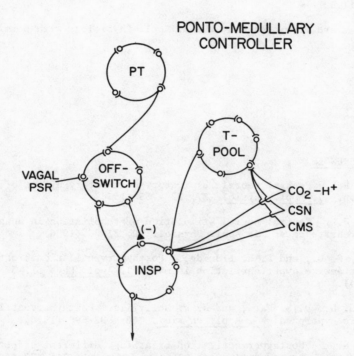

Fig. 11.   Diagram of concept of T-pool neurons. PT=pneumotaxic
           center; PSR=pulmonary sketch receptors; CO_2-H^+=central
           chemoreceptor; CSN=carotid sinus nerve; CMS=calf
           muscle squeezing. The diagram is purely schematic
           and the connections between the various pools only
           indicate the nature of the effects and not specific
           neuronal pathways.

The basic model is that of Bradley et al. (13) and von Euler and Trippenbach (14)
in which an off-switch pool of neurons, facilitated by inputs from the pneumotaxic
center (PT), vagal pulmonary stretch receptors (PSR) and inspiratory output neurons, interacts negatively with inspiratory output neurons to cause phasic cycling
of respiration. Our concern is not with the details of these interactions but
with the concept of the T-pool of neurons. The studies presented here support the
idea of the separateness of the T-pool from inspiratory output neurons and those
involved in phase switching. They show that its activiation does not depend on
increased central inspiratory activity. Facilitatory inputs appear to have dual
effects, one relatively directly on inspiratory output neurons, the other on the
T-pool itself. Further evidence for the separateness of the T-pool comes from the

finding that an afterdischarge is present even when the overall stimulus input is below that necessary to sustain rhythmic respiration. This activity, however, is "concealed" and can only be demonstrated by indirect means.

ACKNOWLEDGEMENTS

These studies were supported by U.S. Public Health Service Research Grants HL-17689 and US-11132.

Figures 5 and 7 are reprinted from the J. Appl. Physiology with permission by the publisher.

REFERENCES

1. Eldridge, F.L. Central neural respiratory stimulatory effect of active respiration. J. Appl. Physiol. 37: 723-735 (1974).

2. Eldridge, F.L. Central neural stimulation of respiration in unanesthetized decerebrate cats. J. Appl. Physiol. 40: 23-28 (1976).

3. Tawadrous, F. D., and F. L. Eldridge. Posthyperventilation breathing patterns after active hyperventilation in man. J. Appl. Physiol. 37: 353-356 (1974).

4. Swanson, G. D., D. S. Ward, and J. W. Bellville. Posthyperventilation isocapnic hyperpnea. J. Appl. Physiol. 40: 592-596 (1976).

5. Eldridge, F. L. Posthyperventilation breathing: different effects of active and passive hyperventilation. J. Appl. Physiol. 34: 422-430 (1973).

6. Eldridge, F. L. Maintenance of respiration by central neural feedback mechanisms. Federation Proc. 36: 2400-2404 (1977).

7. Smith, D. M., R. R. Mercer, and F. L. Eldridge. Servo-control of end-tidal P_{CO_2} in paralyzed animals. J. Appl. Physiol.: Respirat. Environ. Exercise Physiol. 43: 133-136 (1978).

8. Eldridge, F. L. Relationship between respiratory nerve and muscle activity and muscle force output. J. Appl. Physiol. 39: 567-574 (1975).

9. Loeschcke, H. H., J. Delattre, M. E. Schlaefke, and C. O. Trouth. Effects on respiration and circulation of electrically stimulating the ventral surface of the medulla oblongata. Respiration Physiol. 10: 184-197 (1970).

10. Schlaefke, M. E., and H. H. Loeschcke. Lokalisation eines an der Regulation von Atmung und Kneislauf beteiligten Gebietes an der ventralen Oberflache der Medulla oblongata durch Kalteblockade. Pflüg. Arch. 297: 201-220 (1967).

11. Eldridge, F. L., and P. Gill-Kumar. Lack of effect of vagal afferent input
       on central neural respiratory afterdischarge. J. Appl. Physiol.: Respirat.
       Environ. Exercise Physiol. 45: (in press), 1978.

12. Lipski, J., R. M. McAllen, and K. M. Spyer. The carotid chemoreceptor input
       to the respiratory neurones of the nucleus of tractus solitarius.
       J. Physiol. (London) 269: 797-810 (1977).

13. Bradley, G. W., C. von Euler, I. Martilla, and B. Roos. A model of the central
       and reflex inhibition of inspiration in the cat. Biol. Cybernetics
       19: 105-116 (1975).

14. Euler, C. von, and T. Trippenbach. Excitability changes of the inspiratory
       "off-switch" mechanism tested by electrical stimulation of the nucleus
       parabrachialis in the cat. Acta physiol. scand. 97: 175-188 (1976).

DISCUSSION

Richter reported that local PO_2 and pK^+ change is parallel to long-lasting peripheral chemoceptive stimulation and that these effects outlast the stimulation period. This would probably have a non-specific effect upon all neuronal structures within medullary reticular formation.

POST-STIMULUS EFFECTS AND THEIR POSSIBLE ROLE FOR STABILIZING RESPIRATORY OUTPUT

K. BUDZIŃSKA, W. A. KARCZEWSKI, E. NASLOŃSKA and
J. R. ROMANIUK

Department of Neurophysiology, P. A. S. Medical Research Centre,
00-784 Warsaw, Poland

ABSTRACT

The "inertial" behaviour of the respiratory activity during and after stimulation of the vagus nerves (VN), mesencephalic reticular formation (MRF) and rostral pons (NPB) was studied in rabbits. It was found that factors that increase the central respiratory drive reduce the time constant of post-stimulatory effects. Some anaesthetics and hypocapnia, while reducing the magnitude of the post-stimulatory effects, increase their duration. Whereas the effect of stimulation on the respiratory frequency does not depend upon the input stimulated, changes in the amplitude response are qualitatively different: vagal stimulation decreases, and NPB or MRF stimulation increases this parameter. The amplitude response is abolished or reduced by pentobarbitone. It is concluded that the reticular activating system (RAS) is not responsible for the frequency response, but may be indirectly involved in the amplitude response.
Investigations on oscillations in inspiratory discharge have shown that they depend in a similar way upon the respiratory drive. It is hypothesized that a common mechanism of leaky integration operates at various levels of respiratory control being responsible for smoothing both the inspiratory discharge and the transitions from one respiratory pattern to another.

INTRODUCTION

The attention of several authors has been recently focused upon the integrative aspects of the neural control of breathing. It became obvious that since the respiratory responses to various stimuli depend not only upon the amplitude and timing, but also upon the duration of stimulation, a mechanism of integration must be built into the system (refs 1 -- 8). This concept seems now to apply not only to the control of the parameters of a single respiratory cycle but also to the breath-by-breath regulation of the respiratory pattern. Gesell et al. (9) were the first to demonstrate a slow disappearance of changes elicited earlier by carotid sinus nerve stimulation. A similar "inertial" behaviour was later demonstrated for stimulation of the vagus nerve (refs 1, 7, 10, 11) and for stimulation of the mesencephalic reticular formation (MRF) and rostral pons (NPB) (ref. 12). Eldridge (see e.g. refs 13 and 14) re-investigated

and extended the original observations of Gesell et al. (9) and
concluded that the slow build-up and subsequent decrease of respiratory activity after CSN stimulation may be explained by reverberation (ref. 13) or afterdischarge (ref. 14) . Another Sherringto-
nian term - inertia - was used by Karczewski (10) . Swanson et al.
(15) described their observations in humans as "persistence" . We
have recently suggested that the slow transitions from one respiratory pattern to another may be interpreted in terms of short-term
memory (refs 11 and 16) . Since, however, the neuronal substrates
of both short-term memory and the inertial behaviour of the respiratory controller are equally obscure, we came to the conclusion
that a step-by-step analysis of the phenomenon may be more helpful than inventing new, even most suggestive terminology.

RESULTS AND COMMENTS

The first question we wanted to get answer to was whether the respiratory network itself or the RAS (ref. 14) or both are responsible for the slow transition phenomena. For this purpose we compared the respiratory responses elicited in anaesthetized, vagotomized, paralyzed and artificially ventilated rabbits by stimulation of the vagus nerve (VN), nucleus reticularis tegmenti (MRF)
and rostral pons (NPB). The experimental techniques were described
in detail elsewhere (refs 7, 11, 12, 16). The results can be summarized as follows:

General Characteristics of the Phenomenon
Frequency response to stimulation was qualitatively similar in all
experimental groups and consisted in a gradual decrease in the duration of the central respiratory cycle. When stimuli were applied
in late expiration, the expiratory pause was reduced immediately
(latency for precipitating a premature inspiration was between
26 and 38 msec). During stimulation in inspiration, the first inspiratory discharge was either unchanged or prolonged. The vagus-
to-phrenic and MRF-to-phrenic latency was 8 to 9 msec (see also
refs 12 and 17). With stimulation continuing, both phases of the
respiratory cycle were gradually shortened. The new steady-state
was reached after at least six respiratory cycles during which
stimulation was applied. After stimulation the duration of both
inspiratory and expiratory phases returned slowly (time constant
of "recovery" was less than 10 sec for the MRF and more than 30 sec
for the VN and NPB) to control values (Fig. 1).

Amplitude response was qualitatively different for VN stimulation
on one hand, and NPB or MRF stimulation on the other. In the former group amplitude of phrenic nerve discharge always decreased
(ref. 18). This effect, together with the increase in the respiratory frequency gave a picture equivalent to tachypnoea (see also
refs 11 and 16). The response to stimulation of the MRF or NPB was
qualitatively different: both the amplitude and rate of rise of
inspiratory discharge increased gradually during stimulation, the
final picture being similar to hyperpnoea (ref. 12). This effect
was therefore similar to that found by Eldridge (13) in his studies
on CSN stimulation. However, both in the case of stimulation of the
neuraxis and the vagus nerve, changes in the amplitude, although
opposite in direction, behaved in the same way during the post-sti-
mulation period, i.e. pre-stimulation values were gradually reached,
the time constant of the recovery period being the same as for

the frequency response (see refs 12 and 18).

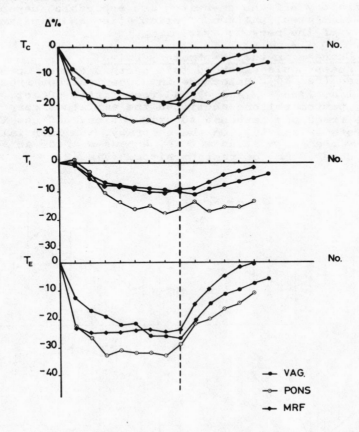

Fig. 1 Inertial behaviour of the central respiratory
cycle (Tc), inspiratory time (T_I) and expiratory pause
(T_E) during and after (vertical dashed line) stimulation of the vagus (VAG), NPB (PONS) and reticular
formation (MRF) Ordinates: change from control.
Abscissae: number of subsequent breath.

Already these results suggested that the possible involvement of RAS
varies considerably depending upon the input stimulated. It is worth
noting, that the CSN-to-phrenic nerve latencies recorded by Eldridge
(19) were approximately three times longer (25 msec in inspiration
and 75 to 100 msec in expiration) than those recorded in our experiments. This obviously implies a different pathway of response.
Moreover, changes in the amplitude of inspiratory discharge illustrate an inspiratory-facilitatory effect of CSN, MRF, and NPB stimulation and an opposite, inspiratory-inhibitory effect of VN stimulation. Nevertheless, the frequency response is similar, if not
identical, in all cases.
The above considerations led us to the conclusion that the only
component of the response that is reproducible in all experimental
groups is the slow increase in the central respiratory frequency
during, and its gradual decrease after stimulation. All other para-

meters, i.e. rate of rise and amplitude of inspiration, its duration, inspiratory off-and on-switch are separable depending upon
the input stimulated, pattern of stimulation and "instantaneous"
excitability of the nervous system.

Effects of Changes in the Respiratory Drive

Effects of anaesthesia depended to a certain degree upon the anaesthetic used (ref.16). Halothane in concentrations from 0.7 to
1.5 vol% (i.e. 1 to 2 M.A.C.) had very little effect. On the
other hand, pentobarbitone abolished the amplitude response and
reduced the frequency response to stimulation, but not its time
constant (refs 12 and 16). On the contrary, the inertial behaviour
of frequency changes was, as a rule, enhanced after an addition
of a small dose (8 mg) of pentobarbitone (Fig. 2).

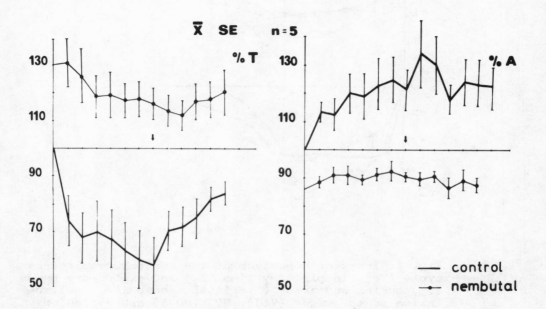

Fig. 2 Effect of pentobarbitone on the frequency
and amplitude response to NPB stimulation. T - cycle
duration (subsequent respiratory cycles marked by
a vertical bar on the abscissae) A - amplitude of
integrated phrenic n. discharges (ordinates - percent of control before Nembutal). Note that reduction of T continues after stimulation (which ends
at arrow). See text.

This is in agreement with the findings of Urabe et al. (20) who
have shown that potentials evoked by vagal stimulation in the solitary tract nucleus are suppressed or abolished by stimulation of
the MRF and enhanced by Nembutal or decortication; this would again
indicate that RAS is not the primary locus of the phenomenon. An
additional support can be found in the behaviour of EEG: stimulation of the NPB elicited, in agreement with the findings of Hugelin
and Cohen (21) an immediate EEG arousal. This response outlasted by

about a minute any change in the pattern of respiratory activity
elicited by the same stimulation.

These observations (together with the fact that arterial blood
pressure did not virtually change during VN and NPB stimulation but
rose considerably during MRF stimulation) allow the conclusion
that at least the main (i.e., frequency) component of the respiratory response to stimulation of various inputs to the "controller"
does not primarily depend upon the reticular activating system but
is specific for the neural network of the respiratory complex itself.
On the other hand, the responses of the rate of rise and amplitude
of inspiratory activity during MRF or NPB stimulation suggest that
these components may depend to some degree upon a positive feedback mechanism postulated by Hugelin and Cohen (21) and "responsible
for recruitment and increasing activity of inspiratory neurones
during the inspiratory phase; reticular input probably facilitates
discharge of neurones in this feedback loop, thus producing a more
rapid growth of the inspiratory discharge" (21).

Effects of hypocapnia were studied by Romaniuk (7) and Romaniuk et
al. (in the press). Slow changes in activity of respiratory neurones were demonstrated also in the absence of the central respiratory rhythm, i.e. during hyperventilation apnoea (Fig. 3).

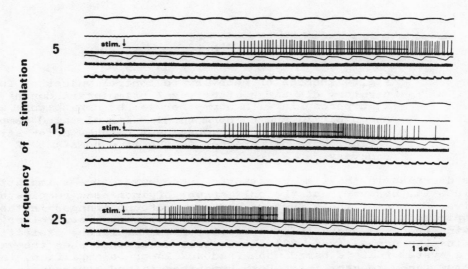

Fig. 3 Vagal stimulation during hyperventilation. Traces from top: end-tidal carbon dioxide (1.4 vol%) ,
integrated activity of the phrenic n., stimulus marker,
single phrenic motoneurone, pump stroke (33 cc), phrenic n. activity, art.blood pressure (90 torr). Frequencies of stimulation 5, 15 and 25 imps per sec.

Phrenic n.motoneurones with no activity during hyperventilation
were made to fire again by vagal stimulation, their evoked activity being roughly proportional, and the latency between the start
of stimulation and start of activity being inversely proportional
to the frequency of stimulation. After stimulation the activity
was slowly vanishing again.

<u>Effects of hypercapnia and hyperthermia</u> are summarized in Fig. 4.
It shows that an increase in the respiratory drive reduces the
time constant of the gradual return of respiratory parameters to
pre-stimulation values.

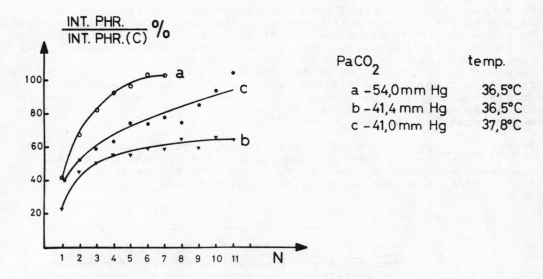

	PaCO$_2$	temp.
a	$-54,0$ mm Hg	$36,5°C$
b	$-41,4$ mm Hg	$36,5°C$
c	$-41,0$ mm Hg	$37,8°C$

Fig. 4 Process of recovery to control values of inspiratory discharge after vagal stimulation during
a) hypercapnia with normothermia; b) normocapnia with
normothermia and c) normocapnia with elevated temperature. N - number of subsequent breaths after stimulation. Note differences in the time constant of
recovery.

The decrease in the time constant of recovery to pre-stimulation
values is, however, not the only effect of increased respiratory
drive. Either of these factors induces profound changes in the
respiratory pattern. Both increase the respiratory controller´s
"gain" (ref. 3) probably as a result of an "avalanche excitation"
of insp. neurones (ref. 22). It is well known that when the gain
of a system that is based upon feedback loops is amplified, the
system tends to oscillate. Both hyperthermia and hypercapnia can
produce oscillations in the respiratory activity and although some
features of these oscillations are different, they may also have
quite a lot in common.

<u>Low-frequency oscillations.</u> With body temperature going up (and
carbon dioxide down - see ref. 23 for fuller discussion) the
phrenic nerve activity begins to disintegrate slowly into short
bursts followed by abortive expiratory pauses. The basic inspiratory discharge divides eventually into two, three or more short
volleys. The process of "fragmentation" which reflects, indeed,
the transition from hyperpnoea to panting can be regarded as a
gradual development of low-frequency oscillations in the respira-

tory system. Similar oscillations can be elicited in hypocapnic
cats by stimulation of the hypothalamus (ref.24), their neural
mechanism is, however, unclear. Increases in carbon dioxide gradually abolish these oscillations, the sequence of events being
a mirror image of their development (Fig. 5).

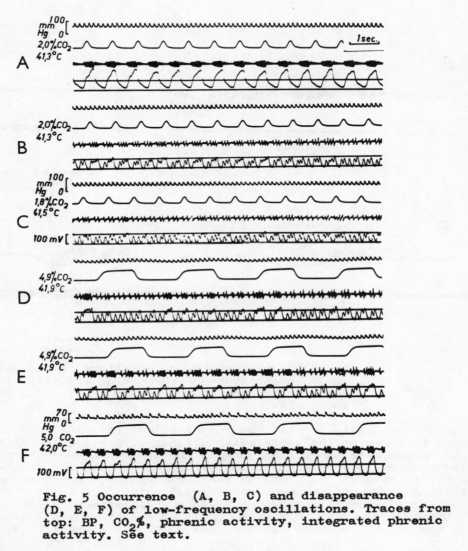

Fig. 5 Occurrence (A, B, C) and disappearance
(D, E, F) of low-frequency oscillations. Traces from
top: BP, CO_2%, phrenic activity, integrated phrenic
activity. See text.

High-frequency oscillations were first reported by Gasser (25)
and then studied in detail by several authors (refs 26-28) but
their mechanism and origin are still unknown. It has been suggested that they may arise from re-excitant connections or similar
time courses of post-spike inexcitability in different inspiratory
neurones (ref. 26) but intracellular studies of Mitchell and

Herbert (27) did not give support to either of these assumptions.
In our experiments with anaesthetized, vagotomized, paralyzed and
artificially ventilated rabbits high-frequency oscillations could
have been almost deliberately elicited by moderate hypercapnia
and gradually eliminated by normocapnic ventilation. They were
very similar to those described in the other species (Fig. 6).

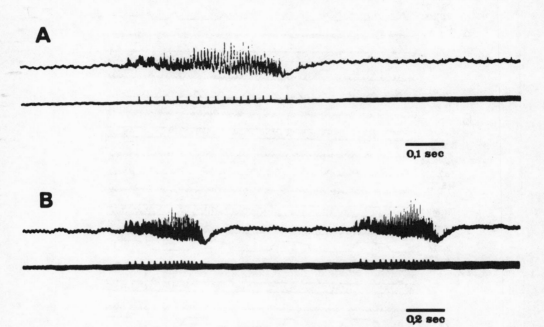

Fig. 6 High-frequency oscillations in a rabbit. In
A and B upper traces - phrenic n. activity, lower
traces - phrenic motoneurone activity. Note different
time scales.

Computer analysis of the frequency spectrum revealed some interesting features of the oscillating discharge. Non-sequential interval
histograms have shown that whereas the control frequency spectrum
seems to reflect Poisson distribution, an oscillating discharge
exhibits several peaks of "chosen" frequencies. The same applies
to single phrenic motoneurones (Figs 7 - 10).
       The hypothesis that inspiratory oscillations result from in-
hibitory influences of similar (but shifted in phase) oscillations
in expiratory neurones has been abandoned since Merrill (29) had
shown no connections from expiratory to inspiratory neurones thus
excluding the reciprocal inhibition. Although this problem is being
still discussed, one can also speculate that neurones other than
those firing in the expiratory phase might interfere with the inspiratory discharge. One possible candidate might be the group of
neurones firing in inspiration but being probably inspiratory - inhibitory (ref. 30). Although for the time being their "paradoxical"

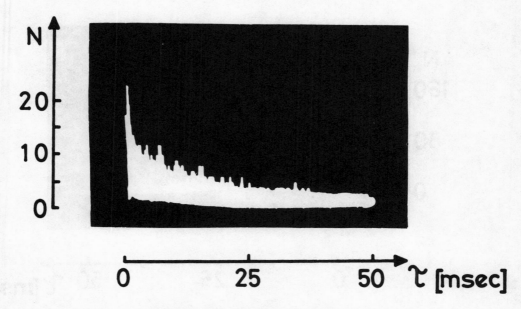

Fig. 7 Interval histogram of inspiratory discharge
(phrenic nerve) in a normocapnic (CO_2 4.4%) rabbit.
In this and next figures ordinates - number of
events, abscissae - interval duration.

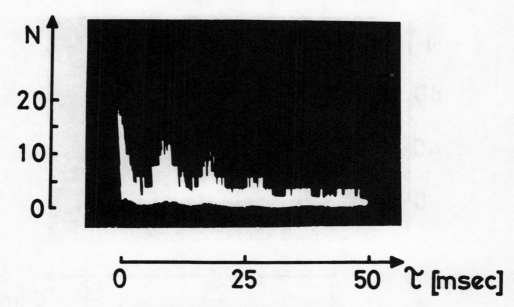

Fig. 8 Interval histogram from the same animal during hypercapnia (CO_2 6.2%). See text.

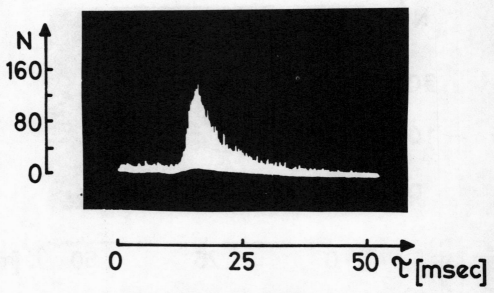

Fig. 9 Interval histogram of a single phrenic motoneurone in a normocapnic (CO_2 3%) rabbit.

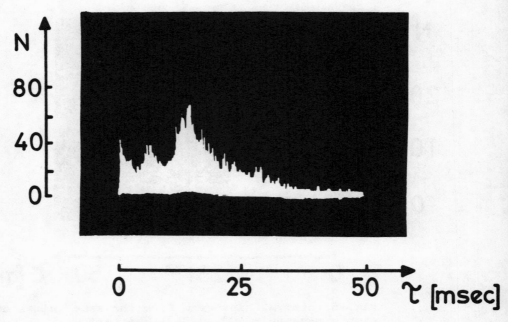

Fig. 10 Interval histogram of the same motoneurone
during hypercapnia (CO 5.4 %). See text.

response applies only to lung inflation, Mitchell and Berger (31)
believe that these units (I-beta neurones in their model) may
play the role of inhibitory interneurones also for inputs other
than vagal. Gromysz and Karczewski (17) recorded also from medullary expiratory-inspiratory neurones (VRN) that responded with excitation when stimulated in expiration, and with inhibition followed
by a post-inhibitory rebound when stimulus was applied in inspiration. The latter phenomenon deserves probably special attention
(see refs 31 and 32) . Post-inhibitory rebound is, however, only
one out of several possible mechanisms underlying oscillations in
neural networks (cf. ref. 33) and further experiments are certainly
needed.
For the time being all interpretations are rather speculative, but
some of them should perhaps be shortly discussed. The occurrence
of high-frequency oscillations may result from short-term synchronization described by Sears and Stagg (34). The problem is that
phrenic motoneurone pool is not homologous (refs 18 and 35) and,
moreover, that oscillations can be seen also in the activity of
single members of the population of phrenic neurones (Fig. 10).
Another possibility is that there is a number of oscillators whose
activity is integrated under normal conditions but which start to
play the role of "ectopic pacemakers" (similar to those observed
in lower organisms - ref. 36) when respiratory drive increases
like in hypercapnia or hyperthermia.
If a process of leaky integration discussed in many recent papers
(see Introduction) is responsible for smoothing both the inspiratory discharge and all transitions from one pattern of breathing
to another one may suppose that - at least phenomenologically -
all types of respiratory oscillations: those of "infra-low" frequency (i.e., "inertia", periodic breathing etc.) and those of
high-frequency reflect an impairment of the ability of the respiratory complex to integrate all activities into one smooth act.
In this case, not only the "millisecond-to-second gap" but also
the "second-to-minute gap" would be equally important for the
proper regulation of breathing.

(1) W. Karczewski, Vagal control of breathing (in Polish) , <u>Post. Hig. Med. Dośw.</u> 19, 507, (1965) .

(2) Brenda A. Cross and A. Guz, (1976) The effect of changing the rate of inflation of the lung on the associated phrenic moto-neurone output. In: Colloque, <u>Respiratory Centres and Afferent Systems.</u> B. Duron Editor, INSERM, vol. 59, 155

(3) C. von Euler and Teresa Trippenbach, Excitability changes of the inspiratory " off-switch " mechanism tested by electrical stimulation in Nucleus Parabrachialis in the cat, <u>Acta physiol. scand.</u> 97, 175 (1976) .

(4) J. R. Romaniuk, M. Ryba, Joanna Kulesza, The effect of volume and duration of lung inflation on the parameters of respiratory rhythm, <u>Acta physiol. pol.</u> 27, 505 (1976) .

(5) M. I. Cohen and J. L. Feldman, Models of respiratory phase-swi-tching, <u>Federation Proc.</u> 36, 2367 (1977) .

(6) A. Huszczuk, Lidia Jankowska, Joanna Kulesza and M. Ryba, Studies on reflex control of breathing in pigs and baboons, <u>Acta Neurobiol. Exp.</u> 37, 275 (1977) .

(7) J. R. Romaniuk, Central summation of respiratory information from the lungs (in Polish), Ph. D. Thesis. Warsaw 1977.

(8) M. Younes, J. P. Baker, J. Polacheck and J. E. Remmers, (1978) Termination of inspiration through graded inhibition of inspi-ratory activity. In: Advances in Experimental Medicine and <u>Biology. The Regulation of Respiration During Sleep and Anesthesia</u> (R. S. Fitzgerald, H. Gautier and S. Lahiri Eds.), Plenum Press, New York. vol. 99, 383

(9) R. Gesell, C. R. Brassfield and M. A. Hamilton, An acid-neuro-humoral mechanism of nerve cell activation, <u>Am. J. Physiol.</u> 136, 604 (1942) .

(10) W. A. Karczewski, (1963) A model of proprioceptive information from the lungs, Proc. V. Int. Conf. Med. Electronics Liége, 78

(11) W. A. Karczewski, Krystyna Budzińska, H. Gromysz, R. Herczyński and J. R. Romaniuk, (1976) Some responses of the respiratory complex to stimulation of its vagal and mesencephalic inputs. In: Colloque, <u>Respiratory Centres and Afferent Systems.</u> B. Du-ron Editor, INSERM, vol. 59, 107

(12) Krystyna Budzińska, Respiratory cycle as an index of the level of CNS excitability (in Polish) , Ph. D. Thesis. Warsaw 1978.

(13) F. L. Eldridge, Central neural respiratory stimulatory effect of active respiration, <u>J. Appl. Physiol.</u> 37, 723 (1974) .

(14) F. L. Eldridge, Maintenance of respiration by central neural feedback mechanisms, <u>Federation Proc.</u> 36, 2400 (1977) .

(15) G. D. Swanson, D. S. Ward and J. W. Bellville, Posthyperventi-lation isocapnic hyperpnea, <u>J. Appl. Physiol.</u> 40, 592 (1976) .

(16) W. A. Karczewski, Krystyna Budzińska, Elżbieta Nasłońska, Elżbieta Jazowiecka, J. R. Romaniuk and M. Ryba, (1978) Rate of rise of inspiration at various levels of CNS excitability. In: <u>Advances in Experimental Medicine and Biology. The Regula-tion of Respiration During Sleep and Anesthesia</u> (R. S. Fitzge-rald, H. Gautier and S. Lahiri Eds.), Plenum Press, New York. vol. 99, 23

(17) H. Gromysz and W. A. Karczewski, Respiratory neurons of the ventral respiratory nucleus of the rabbit and their vagal con-nections, <u>Acta Neurobiol. Exp.</u> 36, 581 (1976) .

(18) Elżbieta Nasłońska, The correlation between integrated phrenic nerve activity and discharges of single phrenic units in different experimental conditions (in Polish) , M. sc. Thesis. Warsaw 1978.

(19) F. L. Eldridge, (1978) The different respiratory effects of inspiratory and expiratory stimulations of the carotid sinus nerve and carotid body. In: Advances in Experimental Medicine and Biology. The Regulation of Respiration During Sleep and Anesthesia (R. S. Fitzgerald, H. Gautier and S. Lahiri Eds.), Plenum Press, New York. vol. 99, 325

(20) M. Urabe, T. Tsubokawa and N. Hamabe, Studies of the activities of vagal afferents in the medulla oblongata and thalamus with special reference to a central regulatory mechanism, Physiol. Behav. 3, 17 (1968) .

(21) A. Hugelin and M. I. Cohen, The reticular activating system and respiratory regulation in the cat, Ann. N. Y. Acad. Sci. 109 (2), 586 (1963) .

(22) G. L. Gebber and Susan M. Barman, (1977) Brain stem vasomotor circuits involved in the genesis and entraintment of sympathetic nervous rhythms. In: Progress in Brain Research. Hypertension and Brain Mechanisms (W. De Jong et al. Eds.), Elsevier/North-Holland Biomedical Press, Amsterdam vol. 47, 61

(23) R. Monteau, G. Hilaire and C. Ouedraogo, Contribution à l´étude de la fonction ventilatoire au cours de la polypnée thermique ou hypocapnique, J. Physiol. (Paris) 68, 97 (1974) .

(24) R. Monteau and G. Hilaire, Recyclage de l´inspiration et polypnée obtenus par stimulation électrique de l´hypothalamus, J. Physiol.(Paris) 73, 1057 (1977) .

(25) H. S. Gasser, The analysis of individual vawes in the phrenic electroneurogram, Amer. J. Physiol. 85, 569 (1928) .

(26) M. I. Cohen, Synchronization of discharge, spontaneous and evoked, between inspiratory neurons, Acta Neurobiol. Exp. 33, 189 (1973) .

(27) R. A. Mitchell and D. A. Herbert, Synchronized high frequency synaptic potentials in medullary respiratory neurons, Brain Research, 75, 350 (1974) .

(28) G. K. Suthers, D. J. Henderson-Smart and D. J. C. Read, Postnatal changes in the rate of high frequency bursts of inspiratory activity in cats and dogs, Brain Research, 132, 537 (1977).

(29) E. G. Merrill, Interactions between medullary respiratory neurones in cats, J. Physiol. 226, 72P (1972) .

(30) M. I. Cohen, Discharge patterns of brain-stem respiratory neurons during Hering-Breuer reflex evoked by lung inflation, J. Neurophysiol. 32, 356 (1969) .

(31) R. A. Mitchell and A. J. Berger, Neural regulation of respiration, Am. Rev. Resp. Dis. 111, 206 (1975) .

(32) D. H. Perkel and B. Mulloney, Motor pattern production in reciprocally inhibitory neurons exhibiting postinhibitory rebound, Science, 185, 181 (1974) .

(33) H. M. Pinsker, Aplysia bursting neurons as endogenous oscillators. II. Synchronization and entrainment by pulsed inhibitory synaptic input, J. Neurophysiol. 40, 544 (1977) .

(34) T. A. Sears and D. Stagg, Short-term synchronization of intercostal motoneurone activity, J. Physiol. 263, 357 (1976) .

(35) B. S. Nail, G. M. Sterling, J. G. Widdicombe, Some properties of single phrenic motoneurones, J. Physiol. 200, 137P (1968) .

(36) J. H. Byrne and J. Koester, Respiratory pumping: neuronal control of a centrally commanded behavior in aplysia, Brain Research, 143, 87 (1978) .

DRIVES FOR BREATHING

B. Drive Mechanisms in Fetuses and Neonates

FETAL BREATHING

G. S. DAWES

The Nuffield Institute for Medical Research, University of Oxford, U.K.

The principal aim of this paper is to describe the main features of
fetal breathing movements as a basis for discussion. The description
is complicated by the fact that only in the sheep, and only to a
limited extent in that species as yet, is information available as to
the changes in the natural history of fetal breathing movements over
a wide range of gestational age.

Fetal Breathing and Electrocortical Activity

During the last three weeks of gestation (0.15 of term) in sheep, by
which time the fetal electrocorticogram is differentiated into predominantly high voltage slow or low voltage fast components, rapid
irregular fetal breathing movements are associated with rapid eye
movement sleep. These episodic movements are normally present up to
40% of the time and have a strong diurnal variation; the incidence
(i.e. the proportion of time during which such breathing movements
are present) increases more than two-fold towards night-fall. In
addition in sheep there are occasional respiratory efforts at a
lower frequency (normally 1 - 4 per minute), not associated with the
phases of sleep. Dr. Richard Harding has recently suggested that
they may be associated with fetal rumination. They have not yet been
reported in the other species investigated (monkey, guinea pig or
man).

Observations in the rhesus monkey by direct recordings from an intratracheal catheter, and in man using either a real-time ultrasound
B-scanner or/and a continuous Doppler system (to detect either the
changes in shape of the chest wall or in the velocities of blood flow
in the great veins below the heart, respectively) have shown the same
type of rapid (30 - 100 per minute), irregular and episodic breathing
movements. There is no direct evidence in man as yet to prove that
these episodes of rapid irregular breathing are associated with rapid
eye movements sleep, as demonstrated in the sheep by direct electrocortical and eye movement records.

In both the sheep and in the human fetus <u>in utero</u> the episodic
character of the rapid irregular breathing movements is apparent

early in gestation, at 85 days in sheep and by 20 weeks in man. At
85 days gestation in sheep electrocortical activity is small and
still undifferentiated (Bernhard & Meyerson, 1973), though bursts of
positive waves and spindling activity can be seen. However destruction of the fore-brain, by tying both carotid arteries at 85 days
gestation, does not alter the normal episodic character of fetal
breathing. These observations are consistent with the hypothesis
that both associated rhythms, of breath movements and of electrocortical activity, arise from a lower centre or centres.

Physiological changes which alter the incidence of low voltage
electrocortical activity also alter the incidence of fetal breathing
movements in sheep. For example hypercapnia (induced by giving the
mother a high CO_2 mixture in which the oxygen content was reduced to
maintain maternal and hence fetal PO_2 approximately constant) caused
an increase in the incidence of low voltage electrocortical activity
by a mean value of 41%. There was a corresponding increase in the
incidence of fetal breathing (Boddy et al, 1974). Conversely,
pentobarbitone, administered in sedative doses (4 mg/kg i.v.) to the
mother causes a reduction by more than 50% in the incidence of low
voltage electrocortical activity in the lamb; fetal breathing movements are temporarily abolished (Boddy, Dawes, Fischer, Pinter &
Robinson, 1976). The effect of hypoxia also is to reduce the
incidence of low voltage electrocortical activity, also by about 50%,
and this too is associated with abolition of fetal breathing
movements.

The Systemic Chemoreceptors

The role of the systemic arterial chemoreceptors is not altogether
clear; chronic experiments have not yet been done under good
conditions after carotid denervation. There are however a number of
observations which bear on the question. Acute experiments on
anaesthetised fetal lambs wholly or partly exteriorised have shown
that the aortic chemoreceptors can readily be excited in the fetus,
either by injection of cyanide (Dawes et al, 1969a) or by manipulation
of the arterial PO_2 and PCO_2 over the physiological range (Dawes et al,
1969b). This causes changes in heart rate, blood pressure and hind
limb blood flow in the directions which were to be anticipated from
observation on adult animals. Acute experiments on anaesthetised
fetal lambs also suggest the anticipated interaction of CO_2 and
oxygen on the aortic chemoreceptors (Baillie et al, 1969).[2] At the
time that these experiments were carried out it was concluded that
the principal effect of hypoxia was to cause redistribution of
cardiac output through the aortic chemoreceptors, though actions
either centrally or locally on the adrenal medulla were also known to
be involved.

So far as carotid bodies are concerned a wide variety of experiments
have failed to produce evidence for their activity over the range of
blood gas values normally encountered in the fetus, in acute experiments on sheep. However, there is no question that in such experiments
under general anaesthesia or under maternal epidural or spinal
anaesthesia, administration of drugs such as cyanide, lobeline or
nicotine which stimulate chemoreceptors in adults also are effective
in the fetus. They induce a series of deep inspiratory movements
abolished by bilateral section of the carotid nerves. In chronic

unanaesthetised fetal lamb preparations in utero also injection of
nicotine or lobeline induces respiratory movements (e.g. Manning &
Walker, 1977). And manoeuvres, spontaneous or induced, which cause
a rapid fall of PO_2 and rise of PCO_2 also are associated with the
initiation of deep inspiratory efforts in the fetus; in this instance
it is uncertain as to whether the primary effect is central or on the
peripheral chemoreceptor mechanisms.

Afferent Stimuli from the Lungs and Respiratory Muscles

The next question concerns the possibility that fetal breathing is
modulated by afferent signals from stretch receptors in the lungs or
muscle spindles. The fact that the pulmonary stretch receptors can
be activated in the fetus was established in acute experiments on
exteriorised lambs long ago (Dawes, 1968). When the fetal lamb is
cooled to induce respiratory movements, raising tracheal pressure
will make them slower and deeper, and lowering tracheal pressure
increases their frequency. Both changes are abolished by cutting the
cervical vagi bilaterally. This response has been seen as early as
106 days gestation; its earlier development has not been pursued.

Muscle spindles are present, sparsely in the diaphragm and extensively
in the intercostal muscles of the fetal lamb near term, but the part
they play in the normal regulation of fetal breathing movements is
uncertain.

Bilateral section of the cervical vagi does not appear to cause a
gross distortion of the normal character of episodic irregular fetal
breathing movements. At the time when these experiments were carried
out (Dawes et al, 1972) we did not have the means of breath by breath
analysis of the rate and depth of fetal breathing movements. We
therefore cannot say that the detailed regulation of fetal breathing
is unaltered.

Movements of Lung Fluid and of the Fetal Chest Walls

With each fetal breathing movement in the lamb there is a small
inward and outward flow of tracheal fluid, normally less than 1 ml
and certainly much less than the dead space or the fluid capacity of
the lung. These movements are imposed upon the net outward flow of
pulmonary liquid which in the lamb is about 100 ml/kg/day, which is
reduced or abolished 36 - 48 hrs before the onset of parturition and
can be modulated by catecholamine secretion. Experiments by
T. Luther in Oxford (unpublished) in 1974 showed that the glottis was
patent in both high voltage and low voltage electrocortical activity,
as judged by the flow of fluid through a tracheal electromagnetic
flowmeter on injection of warm saline into the tracheo-bronchial
tree.

There is no doubt that fetal breathing is primarily determined by the
activity of the diaphragm as shown by direct EMG recordings. In the
past few years there has been some discussion as to whether the
intercostal muscles are normally active during fetal breathing.
Recently Poore (1978) has shown that the normal movements of the
chest wall in the fetal lamb are more complex than was thought. It
was known from observations on fetal lambs delivered under maternal

epidural anaesthesia into a warm saline bath, and also from observations on human fetuses in utero using a real-time B-scanner, that
each breathing movement is normally accompanied by an inward movement
of the chest wall in the lateral direction and dorso-ventrally, with
an outward movement of the abdomen, (so called paradoxical movements).
However, it was also known that from time to time the fetus makes
deep inspiratory efforts with inhalation of 10 - 20 ml. liquid;
observations suggested that the movements of the chest wall were then
not always in the same direction. Poore has studied this in the
fetal lamb in utero by implanting ultrasound emitters and receivers
up and down the chest wall below the skin, laterally and dorso-
ventrally. The changes in the diameter of the chest and abdomen were
measured as the transit time of ultrasound at 2 MHz. Even during
quiet breathing the lateral movements of the chest wall are not
always in the same direction. In hypercapnia they usually move
bidirectionally. In addition the hinge point or fulcrum, about which
the chest or abdomen move in opposite directions, alters its position
within a few minutes. These results are best explained by activation
of the intercostal muscles from time to time and especially in
hypercapnia, combined perhaps with flexure of the fetal body. The
correlation between changes in transthoracic pressure and diameter
was so poor as to make measurements of thoracic diameter an unacceptable index of the depth of fetal breathing.

Conclusion

There remain several problems to be tackled. We know that in the
fetal lamb the normal episodes of rapid irregular fetal breathing
contain within them periods of more regular breathing. During
hypercapnia breathing not only becomes much deeper but also more
regular; because of the large change in the frequency distribution
it is usually impossible to put a precise figure on the change in
breath interval.

This point exemplifies one of the principal methodological problems
in studying the phenomena more closely. The combination of irregularity with the episodic character of fetal breathing movements
requires studies over many hours and data reduction with a computer
to obtain valid reliable information. This has been one of the
principal difficulties in the more rapid development of the subject.

Finally we are left with some major problems. First and foremost,
why are fetal breathing movements episodic and whence is this
controlled? There are important subsidiary questions, for example,
why is there such a large diurnal variation in the incidence of
fetal breathing and in the volume of liquid ventilation? Whence is
this controlled? And why in man, but not so far as we can ascertain
in the sheep, is the incidence of fetal breathing movements so
closely dependent on the maternal plasma glucose concentration?

There are other practical aspects of the use which can be made of
fetal breathing movements in man to obtain information about fetal
health (in association with other measurements of course) which are
outside the scope of this summary.

Acknowledgements

I am most grateful to my many colleagues for permission to quote
their work and to the Medical Research Council for their generous
support.

References

Baillie, P., Dawes, G.S., Merlet, C.L. & Richards, R., Arterial CO_2
    tension and the aortic chemoreceptors in foetal lambs,
    J. Physiol. 204, 88P (1969).

Bernhard, C.G. & Meyerson, B.A., Morphological and physiological
    aspects of the development of recipient functions in the
    cerebral cortex, Foetal and Neonatal Physiology: Proceedings of
    the Sir Joseph Barcroft Centenary Symposium. Cambridge University
    Press, Cambridge. 1 (1973).

Boddy, K., Dawes, G.S., Fischer, R., Pinter, S. & Robinson, J.S.,
    Foetal respiratory movements, electrocortical and cardiovascular
    responses to hypoxaemia and hypercapnia in sheep, J. Physiol.
    243, 599 (1974).

Boddy, K., Dawes, G.S., Fischer, R.L., Pinter, S. & Robinson, J.S.,
    The effects of pentobarbitone and pethidine on foetal breathing
    movements in sheep, Br. J. Pharmac. 57, 311 (1976).

Dawes, G.S., Fetal and Neonatal Physiology, Year Book Medical
    Publishers, Chicago. (1968).

Dawes, G.S., Duncan, S.L., Lewis, B.V., Merlet, C.L., Owen-Thomas, J.B.
    & Reeves, J.T., Cyanide stimulation of the systemic arterial
    chemoreceptors in fœtal lambs, J. Physiol. 201, 117 (1969a).

Dawes, G.S., Duncan, S.L., Lewis, B.V., Merlet, C.L., Owen-Thomas, J.B.
    & Reeves, J.T., Hypoxaemia and aortic chemoreceptor function in
    foetal lambs, J. Physiol. 201, 105 (1969b).

Dawes, G.S., Fox, H.E., Leduc, B.M., Liggins, G.C. & Richards, R.T.,
    Respiratory movements and rapid eye movement sleep in the
    foetal lamb, J. Physiol. 220, 119 (1972).

Manning, F.A. & Walker, D., Nicotine and breathing movements in the
    fetal lamb, Gynecol. Invest. 8, 69 (1977).

Poore, E.R., The relationship between fetal breathing movements as
    measured by thoracic pressure changes and the movements of the
    chest measured directly in vivo, Proceedings of the Fifth
    Conference of Fetal Breathing, Nijmegen. In press (1978).

DISCUSSION

C.Bryan remarked that fetal breathing may be of importance for the development of the respiratory muscles. From the 24th week there is a substantial increase in the number of muscle fibres containing oxidative enzymes in both the diaphragm and the intercostals. These represent the endurance capacity of the respiratory muscles.

Euler raised the question as to the presence of spontaneous 'augmented' breaths or 'sighs' in fetal breathing. Recordings of fetal breathing have shown the occurrence of spontaneous deep breaths which seem to show a biphasic configuration of "a breath on top of a breath" similar to the spontaneous 'sighs' in adults. There was no information available about the effect of vagotomy on the occurrence of 'augmented' breaths or 'sighs' in fetal lamb.

A CRITICAL ANALYSIS OF THE DEVELOPMENT OF PERIPHERAL AND CENTRAL RESPIRATORY CHEMOSENSITIVITY DURING THE NEONATAL PERIOD

H. RIGATTO

Department of Pediatrics, University of Manitoba, Winnipeg, Manitoba, Canada

The notion that the fetus breathes in utero brought a new dimension to birth (Ref. 1). We now say that birth does not initiate respiration but modifies it. During this unique moment in life, which Henderson so poetically labelled "the most dangerous event in life," there is a general arousal of all sensors affecting respiration. The peripheral and central chemoreceptors, somehow dormant in utero, become more active. The fact that morphologically the peripheral chemoreceptors are well developed in utero and the observation that CO_2 enhances fetal breathing, suggests that the chemoreceptors are "alive and well" in utero (Ref. 2,3). The functional arousal of these structures after birth must be related, at least teleologically, to the new role of the lungs, now solely responsible for the process of gas exchange. It is interesting however, that the arousal does not lead to maximal chemoreceptor activity instantaneously after birth. There is a gradual progress in this activity which reaches peak levels after the first two days of postnatal age. This must be part of an adaptation process which we know little about.

How do we know that the peripheral and central chemoreceptors are active and that this activity changes during the postnatal life? Our studies have been done in human neonates mostly, and I shall restrict myself to them. In such infants, the presence and importance of the peripheral chemoreceptors activity is assessed by measuring the change in ventilatory output in response to a change in inspired O_2; that of the central chemoreceptors is assessed by measuring the change in ventilatory output in response to an increase in inspired CO_2.

THE PERIPHERAL CHEMORECEPTORS

It is now well accepted that peripheral chemoreceptor activity is present during the immediate neonatal period in humans. This notion comes from numerous observations showing that high O_2 (100%) causes an immediate decrease and hypoxia an immediate increase in ventilation (Ref. 4,5,6,15,16). Because the response to high O_2 is independent of respiratory impedance, it may be slightly superior than hypoxia to judge the performance of these receptors. Numerous studies have also shown that the decrease in ventilation in response to 100% O_2 is frequently associated with apnea (Ref. 6,15). The length of apnea per se may be used as an index of peripheral chemoreceptor activity (Ref. 11). We have measured this response to high O_2 in neonates and adult subjects using similar methods. The immediate decrease in ventilation when 100% was substituted for 21% O_2 was less in adults than in infants but this was probably due to higher resting arterial PO_2 in adult subjects (Ref. 14). When we matched the resting PaO_2, the decrease in ventilation was of the same magnitude (Fig. 1). These findings suggest that peripheral chemoreceptor activity is present and, generally speaking of the same magnitude in neonates and adult subjects.

After the immediate decrease in ventilation, there is a rebound, ventilation increasing by approximately 20% above control levels both in infants and adult
subjects (Ref. 5,6,14,15,16). This late response is believed to be centrally
mediated but the intimate mechanism is not known. The identical response to
hyperoxia observed in neonates and adult subjects is contrary to the traditional
teaching which claims that the responses are different (Ref. 5,6,12,15).

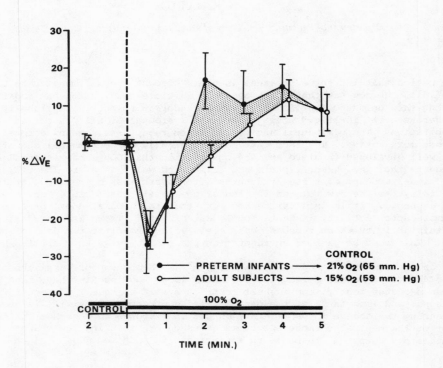

Fig. 1 Percentage of change in ventilation when 100% O_2
was substituted for 21% O_2 in preterm infants (closed circles)
and 15% O_2 in adult subjects (open circles). Note that
when the control resting PaO_2 were matched, the response to
100% O_2 was essentially the same in infants and adult subjects.
(Reproduced by permission of Critical Care Medicine.)

The explanation for our findings lies in the use of similar methods probably. In
addition, if the response is stratified longitudinally, it appears that the decrease in ventilation is less in the first two days of life, suggesting that immediately after birth there is a gradual increase in peripheral chemoreceptor
activity which peaks after two days of postnatal life (Fig. 2).

The assessment of peripheral chemoreceptors using hypoxia is made by measuring the percent increase in $\dot{V}_E$ when 15% O_2 is substituted for 21% O_2. Our observations suggest that this increase is similar in neonates and adult subjects, confirming the idea that the peripheral chemoreceptors are not only present after birth but

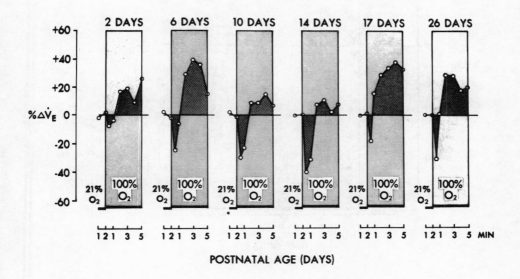

POSTNATAL AGE (DAYS)

Fig. 2 Ventilatory response to inhalation of 100% O_2 in preterm infants according to postnatal age. The immediate decrease in ventilation, reflecting peripheral chemoreceptor activity becomes more pronounced after 2 days of age.

their peak activity matches that in adult man (Ref. 14). After this initial increase in ventilation, however, there is progressive decrease in breathing towards the fifth minute of hypoxia in infants (Ref. 4,6,14,16). Adult subjects sustain their hyperventilation with hypoxia (Fig. 3).

Others and ourselves have suggested that this late paradoxical response in infants
is due to direct central depressant effects of hypoxia (Ref. 6,16). In recent
observations, however, expressing the output of the respiratory system in terms of
mean inspiratory flow and "effective" timing, we discovered that the depression in

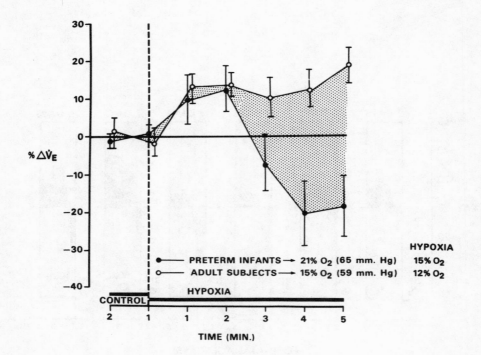

Fig. 3 Percentage of change in ventilation when 15% O_2 was
substituted for 21% O_2 in preterm infants (closed circles)
and 12% O_2 substituted for 15% O_2 in adult subjects (open
circles). Preterm infants do not sustain hyperventilation
and ventilation decreases towards the end of 5 minutes on
15% O_2. (Reproduced by permission of Critical Care Medicine)

ventilation with 15% O_2 is due mostly to a change in the timing mechanism, via
prolongation in expiratory time (Te) (Fig. 4) (Ref. 20). There was little or no
change in mean inspiratory flow. This raises some doubts about the notion that
the paradoxical response to hypoxia in preterm infants is solely centrally mediated.
Factors determining Te, such as vagal modulation of breathing, upper airway resistance and diaphragmatic contraction may conceivably be affected by hypoxia and
therefore, be responsible for hypoventilation observed with hypoxia. The other
possibility is that the neurotransmitter reserves at the peripheral or central
chemoreceptor levels are rapidly exhausted during the hypoxic challenge and hyperventilation cannot be sustained. This would agree with the observation that
chemodenervated animals tend to depress their ventilation with hypoxia (Ref. 13).

Again if we stratified the immediate response longitudinally, we would notice that this response is less pronounced during the first two days of postnatal life (Fig. 5). This reinforces the thought that it takes awhile after birth for the

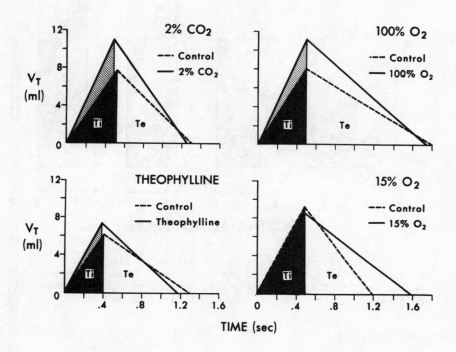

Fig. 4 Relationship between tidal volume (V_T) and duration of inspiration (Ti) and expiration (Te), during control (---) and while preterm infants were subjected to 2% CO_2, 100% O_2, theophylline and 15% O_2 (——). Respiratory stimulants (2% CO_2, 100% O_2, theophylline) increased mean inspiratory flow (V_T/Ti) but did not affect the "effective" timing (Ti/Ti+Te). A respiratory depressant (15% O_2) however, did not change V_T/Ti but significantly decreased the inspiratory time "on duty", (Ti/Ti+Te) via an increase in Te.

peripheral chemoreceptors to respond maximally. One fascinating aspect of the development of the peripheral chemoreceptors is the fact that hyperventilation in response to hypoxia becomes sustained after the third week of postnatal life in preterm infants, mimicking the mature response to adult subjects (Ref. 17). The reason for this "switch" at three weeks of age is unknown.

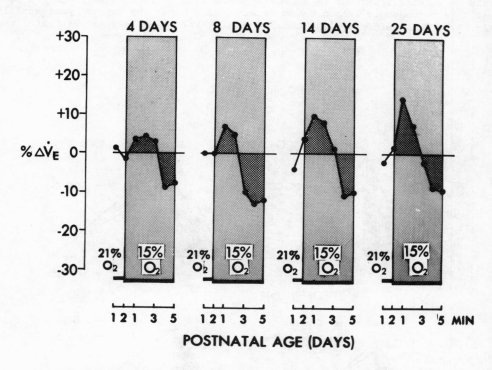

Fig. 5 Ventilatory response to inhalation of 15% O_2 in
preterm infants according to postnatal age. The immediate
increase in ventilation, reflecting peripheral chemoreceptor
activity, becomes more pronounced with increasing age.

THE CENTRAL CHEMORECEPTORS

The responsiveness of the ventilatory apparatus to inhaled CO_2 has been used as an
index of the integrity of the central chemoreceptors in patients with normal lungs
and respiratory "pump." The pressure generated after airway occlusion seems to be
a "purer" index of the central output, but in neonates the presence of chest
distortion and changes in sleep states makes the results obtained with airway
occlusion difficult to interpret (Ref. 14).

The ventilatory response to CO_2 is similar in neonates and adult subjects. The
only difference is that the intercept is shifted to the left in neonates, a finding
probably related to their lower bicarbonate levels (Ref. 15). These observations
imply that the central chemoreceptors are intact in human neonates. When we assessed the change in response to CO_2 with progressive gestational and postnatal age, it
was obvious that the ventilatory response to CO_2 increased with gestation (Ref. 18).
The consensus at the present time is that this is both due to changes at the
central chemoreceptor level and possibly at the peripheral level, i.e. lungs and
respiratory "pump" (Ref. 9,18). Also, when this response was stratified longitudinally with postnatal age, the response during the first two days of life was decreased (Ref. 18) (Fig. 6). This may suggest that the central mechanism also takes
some time to respond maximally after birth.

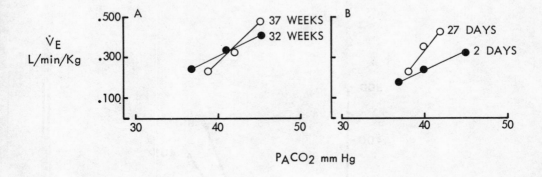

Fig. 6 The ventilatory response to inhaled carbon dioxide
increases with increasing gestational age (A) and increasing
postnatal age (B). (Reproduced by permission of Pediatrics).

In attempting to elucidate the effect of CO_2 on ventilation under various background concentrations of O_2, we found that this response was the opposite of that
in adult subjects (Ref. 19) (Fig. 7). In other words, the lower the inspired O_2
concentration, the flatter was the response to CO_2 in neonates. This finding
became provocative when we observed that the interaction of CO_2/O_2 at the peripheral chemoreceptor level was the same in infants and adults (Fig. 8). Thus the
paradoxical response to CO_2/O_2 is likely mediated at the central chemoreceptor
level. This in itself creates controversy, as the CO_2/O_2 interaction has been
entirely attributed to its effect at the peripheral chemoreceptor level (Ref. 10).
This brings up the question of whether we have not been overestimating the role of
the peripheral chemoreceptor in modulating the ventilatory response to various
CO_2/O_2 combinations. In any event, the peripheral chemoreceptors in neonates are
doing what they should, if judged on the basis of adult behaviour. The late
response, which is likely central seems to be unique however. Because the ventilatory response to CO_2 is the same in infants and adults, we thought that this late
paradoxical response to CO_2 under various background concentrations of O_2 might be
due to the peculiar responses of these infants to high and low O_2. This turned
out not to be the case, as our findings have shown that the response of neonates
to high O_2 does not differ from that in adult subjects. Hypoxia per se may have
something to do with the depressed ventilation on CO_2 but we still are left with

the question of why 100% O_2 enhances the response to CO_2 in these infants.   It is possible that changes in cerebral blood flow have a key role in this sequence of events but this is speculation.

Of interest are studies showing that the control of respiration may be affected by the state of sleep.   An hypothesis might be raised, therefore, that some of the responses we are seeing are peculiar to certain sleep states.   To investigate this

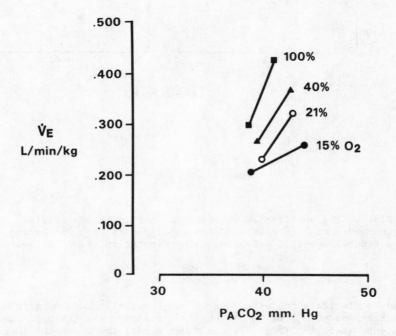

Fig. 7 Steady state CO_2 response curves at different
inspired O_2 concentrations. The lower the inspired O_2,
the flatter the response to CO_2. (Reproduced by permission
of the Journal of Applied Physiology.)

possibility we studied a few babies during wakefulness and sleep. One interesting observation made was that periodic breathing and/or apnea is not triggered by sleep.   Secondly, the response to low and high O_2, does not seem to be affected by sleep in a major way. These findings suggest that if sleep alters the control of breathing in neonates, it does so in a mildly quantitative rather than qualitative way.

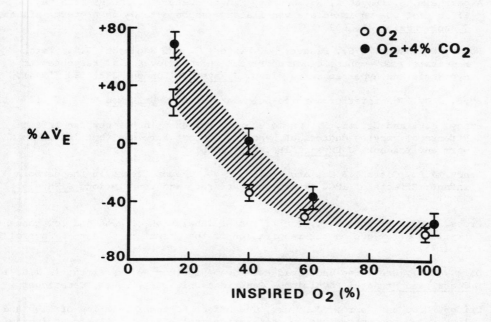

Fig. 8 Adding 4% CO_2 to the inspired gas enhanced the
immediate response to 15% O_2, reduced the response to 40%
O_2, and did not affect the response to 60% and 100% O_2.
This response is similar to that in adult subjects.
(Reproduced by permission of the Journal of Applied Physiology.)

CONCLUSION

In conclusion, our studies tend to support the idea that central and peripheral
chemoreceptors, somewhat dormant in utero, become active at birth and reach
maximal activity after two days of postnatal age. The paradoxical response to CO_2
under various background concentrations of O_2 remains unexplained and the likelihood that it is centrally mediated makes the subject of CO_2/O_2 interaction at
the central chemoreceptor level provocative. This fact plus the unique decrease
in ventilation with hypoxia point out qualitative differences on the behaviour of
the respiratory chemoreceptors in neonates and adult subjects.

H. Rigatto

REFERENCES

1. Albersheim, S., Boychuk, R., Seshia, M.M.K., Cates, D. and Rigatto, H.,
    Effects of CO_2 on immediate ventilatory response to O_2 in preterm infants,
    J Appl Physiol 41, 609 (1976).

2. Boddy, K., Dawes, G.S., Fisher, R., Pinter, S. and Robinson, J.S., Fetal
    respiratory movements, electrocortical and cardiovascular responses to
    hypoxemia and hypercapnea in sleep, J Physiol (London) 243, 599 (1974).

3. Boyd, J.D., The inferior aortico-pulmonary glumos, Brit Med Bull 17, 127 (1961).

4. Brady, J.P. and Ceruti, E., Chemoreceptor reflexes in the newborn infant:
    Effects of varying degrees of hypoxia on heart rate and ventilation in a
    warm environment, J Physiol 184, 631 (1966).

5. Brady, J.P., Cotton, E.C., and Tooley, W.H., Chemoreflexes in the newborn
    infant: Effects of 100% oxygen on heart rate and ventilation, J Physiol 172,
    332 (1964).

6. Cross, K.W. and Oppé, T.E., The effect of inhalation of high and low concen-
    trations of oxygen on the respiration of the premature infant, J Physiol 117,
    38 (1952).

7. Dawes, G.S., Breathing and Rapid-Eye-Movement Sleep Before Birth, in (1973)
    Foetal and Neonatal Physiology, Cambridge University Press, Cambridge.

8. Dripps, R.D. and Comroe, J.H. Jr., The effect of the inhalation of high and
    low oxygen concentrations on respiration, pulse rate, ballistocardiogram
    and arterial oxygen saturation (oximeter) of normal individuals, Am J Physiol
    149, 277 (1947).

9. Frantz, I.D. III, Adler, S.M., Thach, B.T. and Taeusch, H.W. Jr., Maturational
    effects on respiratory responses to carbon dioxide in premature infants,
    J Appl Physiol 41, 41 (1976).

10. Horbein, T.F., Griffo, L.J. and Roos, A., Quantitations of chemoreceptor
    activity: interrelation of hypoxia and hypercapnea, J Neurophysiol 24, 561
    (1961).

11. Krauss, A.N., Tori, C.A., Brown, J., Soodalter, J. and Auld, P.A.M., Oxygen
    chemoreceptors in low birth weight infants, Pediatric Res 7, 569 (1973).

12. Purves, M.J., Respiratory and circulatory effects of breathing 100% O_2 in the
    newborn lamb before and after denervation of the carotid chemoreceptors,
    J Physiol 185, 60 (1966).

13. Purves, M.J., The effects of hypoxia in the newborn lambs before and after
    denervation of the carotid chemoreceptors, J Physiol 185, 60 (1966).

14. Rigatto, H., Respiratory control and apnea in the newborn infant, Critical Care
    Medicine 5, 2 (1977).

15. Rigatto, H. and Brady, J.P., Periodic breathing and apnea in preterm infants.
    I. Evidence of hypoventilation possibly due to central respiratory depression,
    Pediatrics 50, 202 (1972).

16. Rigatto, H. and Brady, J.P., Periodic breathing and apnea in preterm infants. II. Hypoxia as a primary event, Pediatrics 50, 219 (1972).

17. Rigatto, H., Brady, J.P. and de la Torre Verduzco, R., Chemoreceptor reflexes in preterm infants. I. The effect of gestational and postnatal age on the ventilatory response to inhalation of 100% and 15% oxygen, Pediatrics 55, 604 (1975).

18. Rigatto, H., Brady, J.P. and de la Torre Verduzco, R., Chemoreceptor reflexes in preterm infants. II. The effect of gestational and postnatal age on the ventilatory response to inhaled carbon dioxide, Pediatrics 55, 614 (1975).

19. Rigatto, H., de la Torre Verduzco, R. and Cates, D.B., Effects of O_2 on the ventilatory response to CO_2 in preterm infants, J Appl Physiol 39, 896 (1975).

20. Rigatto, H., Desai, U., Cates, D. and MacCallum, M., The effect of 2% CO_2, 100% O_2, theophylline and 15% O_2 on "respiratory drive" and "effective" timing in preterm infants, (Submitted to Clinical Research).

DISCUSSION

Purves made the following written contribution to the discussion:

The paper by Rigatto raises a number of questions as to the suitability of using traditional methods for assessing the respiratory 'sensitivity' to hypoxia and hypercapnia in the newborn infant – especially if it is premature. Indeed, it may be the right moment to consider how useful these methods are in the adult.

Under clearly defined conditions – which usually means the physiological laboratory – the so-called 'CO_2 – response curve' has proved to be a very valuable method of assessing the steady-state respiratory response to hypoxia and hypercapnia, the way in which these stimuli interact and the way in which the response is affected by such factors as noradrenaline, temperature etc. The drawbacks of this approach are fairly obvious. Thus the inhalation of varying concentrations of CO_2 for many minutes must be regarded as a completely unphysiological procedure and with respect to the newborn baby this may impose such a powerful stimulus that the respiratory musculature is incapable of sustaining an adequate response. Further, it is becoming clear that it is the respiratory response to small transient changes in CO_2 which is of importance. Finally it is equally clear from what we have heard today that the steady state CO_2 response can be enormously varied by non-chemical factors so that unless the conditions are rigidly controlled, virtually any answer can be obtained.

There is an additional problem, as I see it, in the newborn infant since it is occasionally uncertain whether the signal that is applied is in fact the signal which is affecting respiration. For example, the persistance of foetal vascular channels for hours or days after birth can markedly affect the imposition of hyperoxic or hypoxic stimuli. The effect of inhaling a few breaths of pure oxygen can be

markedly attenuated if there is a significant level of venous admix-
ture so that the absence of a fall in ventilation in these circumstances does not necessarily mean that the peripheral arterial chemoreceptors are not functioning. Similarly if the newborn in the first
hours or days of life is made hypoxic at a constant level of end-
tidal CO_2, the action of hypoxia which constricts pulmonary vessels
and dilates the ductus arteriosus will mean that an increasing proportion of right ventricular output is diverted away from the lungs
into the aorta and it then remains quite uncertain what is the true
chemical stimulus to possible CO_2 sensitive receptors in the lungs,
the peripheral arterial and central chemoreceptors. Thus, as I see
it, it is not only very difficult to apply the traditional tests to
the newborn especially in quantitative terms and this is particularly
difficult if longitudinal studies are attempted. However, it is
equally clear from Rigatto and the other contributors to this symposium that it is of the first importance that we should have an accurate idea about the development of chemosensitivity in the newborn
period if, for no other reason, that there is a strong suspicion
that many newborn infants may have delayed maturity of chemosensitivity and may come to grief some weeks after birth.

Johnson pointed out that the dogs in REM sleep arose when they were
tested for their responses to elevated PCO_2 levels and to hypoxia as
found by Phillipson et al. (J.Appl.Physiol. 40, 895, 1976; Am.Rev.
resp.Dis. 115, 251, 1977). The question was raised concerning the
possibility that immaturity of the arousal mechanisms might permit
profound hypoxia to occur in the preterm infant and that this, in
turn, might be an important causal factor for the Sudden Infant
Death Syndrom.

Lahiri drew attention to the fact that newborns at high altitude do
breathe and live, although they are exposed often to environmental
hypoxia greater than 15 per cent O_2 breathing at sea level. They
should not do that according to the effect of acute hypoxia on newborns at sea level presented by Rigatto.

APNEA AND HYPOVENTILATION IN INFANTS: RELATIONSHIPS TO THE DEVELOPMENT OF RESPIRATORY CONTROL REFLEXES

D. C. SHANNON

Pediatric Intensive Care Unit, Massachusetts General Hospital, Boston, Massachusetts 02114, U.S.A.

Broadly, two types of faulty regulatory mechanisms have been invoked to explain life-threatening apnea or hypoventilation in various infants. One type involves deficiency, the other, exaggeration of normal reflex responses. Deficiency of activity of mechanisms which normally sustain ventilation by their tonic activity would be expected to cause hypoventilation whereas exaggeration of the latter group would cause episodic apnea.

TABLE I   Deficiency or Absence Causes Hypoventilation

1. Medullary chemoreceptors
2. Carotid body chemoreceptors
3. Central nervous system induced gasping

Stimulation Causes Apnea

1. Laryngeal chemoreceptors
2. Vagal reflexes
3. Diving reflex
4. Central nervous system hypoxic depression

Criteria which permit assigning a cause-effect relationship between a mechanism and an observed abnormal respiratory pattern in a patient have not been established. I propose to outline such criteria and then compare them to observed clinical syndromes and physiologic investigations in infants in order to explore such cause-and-effect relationships.

TABLE 2   Criteria for Determining that Deficiency or
             Absence of a Reflex Causes Apnea

1. Quantify apnea-hypoventilation
2. Quantify abnormal reflex response and determine that other respiratory control reflexes are normally active
3. Quantify resolution of apnea with normalization of reflex: with development -- with pharmacology

CLINICAL SYNDROMES OF PROLONGED APNEA

In this discussion, prolonged apnea is defined as any episode of apnea longer than 20 seconds duration. Hypoventilation is defined as an elevated arterial or alveolar P_{CO2} compared to expected values for age and development. These are seen in several distinct syndromes which affect infants either in the neonatal period or at home and are frequently life-threatening. I am assuming that apnea related to identifiable disease has been excluded, e.g. hypoglycemia, seizures, etc.

Apnea During Sleep in the Neonate

Prolonged apnea is identified with increasing frequency in newborns of shorter gestational age and is generally considered to be the result of delayed development of regulatory reflexes. It is often accompanied by increased frequency and duration of periodic short apnea in the same infant. Although Daily et al (1) stated that prolonged "apnea occurred only in conjunction with periodic breathing", neither these investigators nor others have published data to support this statement.

Variations in the balance of activity of regulatory reflexes which determine alveolar ventilation in one state compared to another might be important in permitting or promoting prolonged apnea. Deuel, (2), in a study of 13 infants, 32-58 weeks post-conceptional age, observed that apnea of less than 5 seconds occurred in non-REM state. Gabriel et al (3), on the other hand, conducted a study of 8 infants 31-35 weeks post-conception using similar techniques and found that 59% of all apneas including those 10-20 sec. and over 20 sec. duration occurred in REM which accounted for 65% of sleep time. They suggest that this apparent relationship to the REM state may be due to inhibition of respiratory motor neurons similar to that seen in other mono-synaptic pathways. Such discrepancies in determining the relation of apnea to state are in part due to differences in an investigator's definition of one state compared to another. This is particularly true in defining what percent of sleep will be allotted to an indeterminate or transitional state. For example, Krauss et al (4), in conducting a polygraphic study of 15 pre-term infants at 30-33 weeks, defined 44% of sleep time as REM compared to 65% in Gabriel's study. Perhaps as a result, Krauss et al concluded that a disproportionate number of prolonged apneas were seen in quiet sleep when compared to the % time in that state, i.e. what Gabriel defined as transitional, Krauss designated quiet sleep. While it is clear that prolonged apnea is sleep-related, a sleep-state relationship has not been fully clarified.

Among the possible defects in regulation of ventilation that might explain apnea in the neonate, numerous investigations have focused on the development of medullary and carotid body chemoreceptor control and on the Hering-Breuer vagally-mediated inflation reflex in human infants. Others, such as the laryngeal chemoreflex are currently the subject of animal investigations.

a. Medullary chemoreflex activity. A small group of infants develop life-threatening apnea in the first few days of life and continues to need ventilatory support during sleep for an indefinite duration.

Physiologic studies confirm profound <u>sleep hypoventilation</u> proceeding
to apnea during quiet sleep; after the first few months, ventilation
can be sustained at a subnormal level during sleep and is characterized by reduction in tidal volume rather than frequency (5). Without ventilatory support at this stage, episodic apnea and
biventricular cardiac respiratory failure develop in 2-4 weeks.
These infants also manifest a paucity of REM sleep, about 90% of
sleep time showing the characteristics of the quiet state. Ventilation in the awake state is normally reflected in tidal volumes
averaging 7.1 ml/kg and $PaCO_2$ within the normal range.

TABLE 3   Characteristics of Breathing in the
                     Congenital Hypoventilation Syndrome

(N = 5 infants) Condition	$\dot{V}_E$ (ml/kg/min)	f	VT (ml/kg)	$PACO_2$ (mmHg)
Awake	235	33	7.1	34-39
REM	196	37	5.3	43-51
Quiet Sleep	75	31	2.4	63-76
Exercise	300	38	8	32
Fever-awake	177	34	5.2	55

The response to cycle-pedaling exercise was qualitatively
normal in two children at 2 1/2 and 6 yrs. respectively.
In all infants, fever was not well tolerated even when it
didn't reflect a respiratory infection and required ventilatory support when they were awake.

Given 5% CO_2 in air to breathe, there is little or no increase
in ventilation and progressive hypercapnea progresses to narcosis
fig. 1.

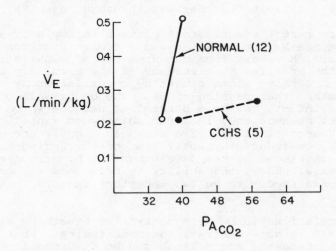

Fig. 1. Steady state ventilatory response to CO_2 in air
         breathing in congenital central hypoventilation
         syndrome

During hyperoxic ventilation, there is sustained depression to
40-60% of resting $\dot{V}_E$ even at six years of age fig. 2. During 15%
O_2 breathing, hyperventilation (up to 30 sec.) is followed by depression fig. 2.

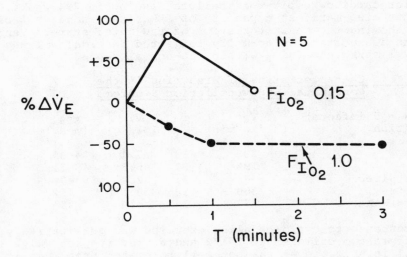

Fig. 2. Transient responses to altered F_{IO_2} in congenital
         central hypoventilation syndrome

Administration of theophylline is without effect while administration
of doxapram increases ventilation in these infants; tachyphyllaxis
and serious side effects limit its therapeutic usefulness (6).

    These infants represent the clearest clinical example of a re-
lationship between apnea-hypoventilation and chemoreceptor control of
breathing. It appears, however, from measurements of ventilation beyond the first months of life, that absence of the medullary chemoreceptor control of breathing alone causes hypoventilation by reducing tidal volumes rather than causing apnea. The occurrence of
sleep apnea in these infants may be a natural occurrence which is
unnaturally prolonged because they lack the ability to sense increasing acidity. Younes et al (7) have shown in lightly anesthetized dogs that apnea induced by activation of the Hering-Breuer
inflation reflex is shortened by the development of hypercapnea and
lengthened by hyperoxia. Thus, the ability to sense and respond to
hypoxia and hypercapnea appear to be two important factors in terminating apnea.

    A tantalizing relationship between control of breathing and
state is seen in these infants. First, the data indicate that control of breathing in the awake state is or can be divorced from
medullary chemoreceptor control. What then regulates ventilation in
the awake state? What accounts for the near absence of REM in these
infants? How are the pathways which regulate state related to those
which regulate breathing?

A much larger number of pre-term and even term infants manifest episodic prolonged apnea; for example, infants of younger gestational ages experience an increasing number of such episodes particularly during the first weeks of life. Over 50% of infants under 34 weeks must be treated for this problem which can occasionally be related to a specific disease but is frequently a manifestation of immaturity (8). Investigators have naturally looked for pathogenic clues in studies of medullary chemoreceptor control because this mechanism is so important in the regulation of ventilation during sleep.

Cross et al (9) and Miller (10) independently demonstrated that term and even pre-term infants were able to increase ventilation in response to CO_2 breathing. In fact, the magnitude of change measured with the plethysmograph and Krogh spirometer was comparable to that found by investigators during the past few years. Using the Read rebreathing method via a mask, Avery (11) observed a slope of 45 ml/kg/min/mm Hg PCO_2 in term newborns, and a comparable level in adults. Chernick (12) then attempted to determine whether pre-term infants with periodic breathing (which can be associated with prolonged apnea) responded less well to CO_2 breathing than those who breathed regularly. Probably because of inadequate control of post-natal age, and excessive withdrawal of expired air through the CO_2 analyzer, the slopes of CO_2 responses were similar and end-tidal PCO_2 values were very low. In a study which overcame the latter problem, Rigatto et al (13) found that end-tidal CO_2 values were not different on the average in pre-term infants with periodic breathing from those with regular breathing and that the slope of the CO_2 response in 31 week gestation infants was 22% less than 34 week infants, a difference which only approached statistical significance. When these studies were repeated, Rigatto et al (14), Krauss et al (15) and Frantz et al (16), with careful control for post-natal as well as gestational ages, a significant increase in slope was found with increased gestational as well as post-natal age. These investigators used the nasal pneumotachygraph steady state, face-mask pneumotachygraph rebreathing and face-mask pneumotachygraph steady state methods respectively. Because of variations in dead space, the absolute levels of ventilation in each study varied but the relative changes in minute ventilation during CO_2 breathing were similar. Krauss et al (17) also measured total respiratory resistance and compliance while measuring ventilatory responses to CO_2 and concluded that in some infants, responses were reduced because of impaired respiratory impedance, others because of insensitivity to CO_2. The possibility that respiratory muscles could not sustain the required workload was not considered.

The weight of recent evidence, therefore, indicates that CO_2 responsiveness is less well-developed the lower the gestational age at birth. Infants with blunted responses also manifest periodic breathing and prolonged apnea. Since these respiratory pattern abnormalities are evanescent in individual infants, it may not be pertinent to know whether responsiveness differs when they breathe regularly or periodically.

Although CO_2 responsiveness increases with post-natal age it is common experience that periodic breathing and prolonged apnea both decrease at this time, the comparative time courses of these changes in physiology and breathing pattern simultaneous with development of normal CO_2 responsiveness would strengthen the association but not prove a cause-and-effect relationship. Restoration of a normal breathing pattern is frequently possible by administration of theophylline (18-20). Davi et al (21) suggest that this is related to potentiation of the ventilatory response to CO_2 while Gerhardt et al (22) find increased alveolar ventilation and a parallel shift in slope of the response in treated infants.

While these studies strongly suggest a relationship between abnormal breathing patterns and abnormal ventilatory response to CO_2 in the neonate, they lead to further questions. Do other respiratory control reflexes mature in parallel to the CO_2 response? Is the problem one of increased promotion of apnea, inadequate termination or both? What are the biochemical influences on the CO_2 response in infants? Are they related to resolution of apnea during theophylline administration? For example, Shannon (23) observed a significant increase in steady state glucose concentration during theophylline administration in pre-term infants with apnea. Shaefer (24) has suggested that adrenal medullary response to CO_2 may influence the ventilatory response to CO_2 in adult subjects. An unidentified effect of thyroid hormone is also important (25).

b. Carotid body chemoreceptors. Although experimental evidence supports the conclusion that PaO_2, $PaCO_2$ and pH, each exert independent effects on the carotid body chemoreceptors, studies on infants have been limited to evaluation of responsiveness to variations in PaO_2. Several assumptions are made: first, that the steady state ventilatory response to CO_2 may have a carotid body component but that the measured response is due to the effects of H+ ion on the medulla; second, that the first 30 seconds of the ventilatory response to altered PaO_2 are related primarily to carotid body effects while the steady state response is also influenced by central effects.

Our studies of chemoreceptor activity in infants with congenital central hypoventilation and sleep apnea show the importance of considering the role of interaction between various respiratory reflexes. Given 100% O_2 to breathe, these infants depress ventilation to lower levels than do normal infants and maintain that depression until the stimulus is removed. It appears, therefore, that responsiveness to CO_2 limits the transient ventilatory depression during oxygen breathing and restores ventilation to resting or even higher levels in the steady state.

The search for differences in ventilatory responses to altered FIO_2 between term and pre-term infants began with the studies of Cross et al (26,27) which first identified the shapes of the curves now considered characteristic for the responses to high and low inspired oxygen respectively. Furthermore, they noted that periodic apnea in the pre-term infant was abolished by 100% and enhanced by 15% O_2 breathing. Miller (10) observed that hypoxia failed to potentiate the ventilatory response to hypercapnea characteristic of the adult response. More recent studies have confirmed these observations but have added little further information. Fenner et al (28), Rigatto et al (29), and Krauss et al (30) have confirmed the course of the ventilatory response to hyperoxia in pre-term infants but disagree over the magnitude of depression and the degree of difference in smaller pre-term infants. For example, Krauss observed a

greater depression in infants less than 34 weeks than in those more
than 34 weeks gestation but Rigatto found no difference. Because
infants of lower gestational ages respond less well to CO_2 breathing,
the observations of Krauss seem more likely, i.e., impaired recovery
from hyperoxic ventilatory depression would be expected. Rigatto
et al (31) have conducted the only satisfactory reported study of
development in response to 15% O_2 breathing and found a biphasic
response in 32 compared with 37 weeks gestation infants at 2 days
but a sustained response in both at 18 days post-natal age. Both
Rigatto et al (31) and Krauss et al (30) agree that hypoxia precipi-
tates periodic breathing and prolonged apnea. In a study designed
to evaluate the interaction between oxygen and CO_2 receptors,
Rigatto (32) found that in the steady state hypoxia blunted and
hyperoxia potentiated the ventilatory response to CO_2. It is not
possible to assess the relative contributions of carotid body and
central nervous system to these effects.

Hypoxia, then, can account for periodic breathing and prolonged apnea in pre-term infants. But what accounts for this? Is
it an unusual susceptibility to the central depressant effects of
hypoxia? Is it mediated indirectly through interaction with hydrogen ion effects at the medulla? None of the reported studies have
controlled for PaO_2. Perhaps the explanation for apparent development in the response to hypoxia lies not in the sensor itself but in
the level of oxygen tasted by carotid body and brain. Prospective
studies of post-natal development which will control for gestational
and post-natal age as well as arterial oxygenation and relate
responsiveness to respiratory pattern are needed before these questions can be answered.

c. Central nervous system-induced gasping. From animal (33) as well
as human studies (34), it appears that gasping respirations following
prolonged apnea serve as an emergency self-resuscitating mechanism.
This role is generally attributed to the central nervous system but
its neuro-anatomic site and pathways are unknown. It may be related
to the gasping respirations which characterize the first few breaths
of the newborn following the asphyxial birth process. This is
probably a sub-cortical influence because Bystrzycka (35) found that
umbilical cord occlusion in fetal sheep, which exhibit breathing
movements in utero, caused apnea along with an isoelectric ECoG
followed by gasping respirations while the ECoG remained flat.

Investigations in infants of the four reflex mechanisms which,
when stimulated, can induce apnea (see above) are sparce.

a. Laryngeal chemoreceptors. No investigations have been found
which report the importance of these intriguing receptors for infants.
In animals of numerous species (36), stimulation with a variety of
chemical agents, e.g., water, glucose, HCl and heterologous milk,
causes apnea and even death. In piglets, the apneic response to
water didn't change with age while the response to cow's milk
diminished in both the percent of animals affected as well as the
intensity of the response. It appears that this reflex is designed
to protect the lung against foreign material especially at a critical
period of development.

Before we understand the role of this reflex relative to other
controlling influences, its independent development must be fully

understood. At a neuro-anatomic-chemical level we need to know how
it over-rides other controlling mechanisms sufficient to result in
ventilatory failure and death.

b. Vagal reflexes. Activation of vagal inhibition by inflating the
lungs of infants from 30 weeks gestation was demonstrated by Bodegard and Schweiler (37). Developmental changes in activity of this
reflex have been observed by Kirkpatrick et al (38). They examined
the time course of the pressure change developed against end-
expiratory occlusion in pre-term and term infants studied sequentially and found that inspiratory inhibition was more prominent in
an infant at any age if birth was premature. They suggested that
this represents reliance on a more primitive mechanism of control
in infants with incomplete neurologic maturation because of
premature birth.

c. Diving reflex. Developmental changes in this reflex have not
been recorded.

d. Central nervous system hypoxic depression. Hypoxia depresses
the central nervous system at some critical level of delivery of
aerobic substrate and apnea of increasing duration causes progressive hypoxia. However, the role of this mechanism in initiating
or perpetuating apnea has not been examined.

    There are then a number of chemoreflexes which modulate
respiratiory output from the ponto-medullary controller in response
to need. Failure or deficiency in their activity results in
inadequate pulmonary gas exchange and may encourage perpetuation of
apnea. Both CO_2 ventilatory responsiveness and sustained hypoxic
hyperventilation are inadequately developed in the pre-term infant
who is prone to irregularities of respiratory pattern including
life-threatening apnea. Other reflexes modify ventilation in
response to feeding and mechanical impedance. Our understanding of
the interaction between these controlling influences, their respective developmental patterns, neuro-anatomic and chemical interrelationships and their role(s) in accounting for periodic breathing
and apnea in the newborn is primitive.

Apnea in Infants at Home

    As in the neonate, apnea in the infant can accompany a variety
of readily identifiable diseases, but it is also identified with
increasing frequency as an isolated sign.

    The onset of congenital central hypoventilation can be delayed
for several months. The respiratory pattern both awake and asleep
as well as the ventilatory responses to carbon dioxide and oxygen
are the same as those in the neonate. The usual patient, however,
manifests a more subtle alteration in respiratory pattern and control reflexes. Several investigators have now identified infants,
nearly all in the first year of life, who sustain repeated episodes
of life-threatening apnea (39-42), manifest a higher than normal
prevalence of periodic breathing (43) and exhibit modest alveolar
hypoventilation and blunting of the ventilatory response to CO_2
during quiet sleep (44). The abnormal respiratory pattern matures
over the first year of life so that neither prolonged apnea nor
periodic breathing can be identified by 10-12 months of age in over

90% of affected infants (45,46).

It is tempting because of the resemblance to consider that the pathophysiology of respiratory control in these infants is the same as that in pre-term infants. However, this is almost certainly too simple an explanation. The respiratory system has a limited number of ways it can manifest diseases which can affect a variety of reflex mechanisms. Because this syndrome can cause sudden death in infants (42), it is imperative that techniques be developed which can quantitate ventilation and various reflex responses in sleeping infants. Although the other reflexes described above (Apnea in the Newborn) may also be involved in the abnormal respiratory patterns identified in these infants, no studies of their activity even in normal infants have appeared.

In conclusion, we understand even less about the development of respiratory control, interaction of reflexes and their relationships to abnormal breathing patterns in infants than we do in neonates. Studies of neuro-anatomic, physiologic and chemical features of respiratory control mechanisms must be extended through the first year of life.

References

(1) W.J.R. Daily, M. Klaus, and H B.P. Meyer, Apnea in premature infants: monitoring, incidence, heart rate changes, and an effect of environmental temperature, Ped. 43,510 (1969).

(2) R.K. Deuel, Polygraphic monitoring of apneic spells, Arch. Neurol. 28,71 (1973).

(3) M. Gabriel, M. Albani, and F.J. Schulte, Apneic spells and sleep states in pre-term infants, Ped. 57, 142 (1976).

(4) A.N. Krauss, G.E. Solomon, and P.A.M. Auld, Sleep state, apnea and bradycardia in pre-term infants, Develop. Med. Child. Neurol. 19, 160 (1977).

(5) D.C. Shannon, D.W. Marsland, J.B. Gould, B. Callahan, I.D. Todres, and J. Dennis, Central hypoventilation during quiet sleep in two infants, Ped. 57, 342 (1976).

(6) C. Hunt, and D.C. Shannon, Respiratory and non-respiratory effects of doxapram in congenital central hypoventilation, Am. Rev. Resp. Dis. In press.

(7) M. Younes, P. Vaillancourt, and J. Milic-Emili, Interaction between chemical factors and duration of apnea following lung inflation, J. Appl. Physiol. 36, 190 (1976).

(8) F. Miller, H. Behrle, and N. Smull, Severe apnea and irregular respiratory rhythms among premature infants, Ped. 23, 676 (1959).

(9)   K.W. Cross, J.M.D. Hooper, and T.E. Oppe, The effect of inhalation of carbon dioxide in air on the respiration of the full-term and premature infant, J. Physiol. 122, 264 (1953).

(10) H.C. Miller, Effect of high concentrations of carbon dioxide and oxygen on the respiration of full-term infants, Ped. 14, 104 (1954).

(11) M.E. Avery, V. Chernick, R.E. Dutton, and S. Permutt, Ventilatory response to inspired carbon dioxide in infants and adults, J. Appl. Physiol. 18, 895 (1963).

(12) V. Chernick, and M.E. Avery, Response of premature infants with periodic breathing to ventilatory stimuli, J. Appl. Physiol. 21, 434 (1966).

(13) H. Rigatto, J.P. Brady, Periodic breathing and apnea in preterm infants: evidence for hypoventilation possibly due to central respiratory depression, Ped. 50,2 202-18 (Aug. 1972).

(14) H. Rigatto, J.P. Brady, and R. De La Torre Verduzco, Chemoreceptor reflexes in pre-term infants: the effect of gestational and post-natal age on the ventilatory response to inhaled carbon dioxide, Ped. 55,5, 614-20 (May 1975).

(15) A.N. Krauss, D.B. Klain, S. Waldman, and P.A.M. Auld, Ventilatory response to carbon dioxide in newborn infants, Pediatr. Res. 9, 46 (1975).

(16) I.D. Frantz, S.M. Adler, B.T. Thach, H.W. Taeusch, Jr., Maturational effects on respiratory responses to carbon dioxide in premature infants, J. Appl. Physiol. 41, 41-5 (July 1976).

(17) A.N. Krauss, S. Waldman, and P.A.M. Auld, Diminished response to carbon dioxide in premature infants, Biol. Neonate. 30, 216 (1976).

(18) D.C. Shannon, F. Gotay, I.M. Stein, M.C. Rogers, I.D. Todres and F.M.B. Moylan, Prevention of apnea and bradycardia in low birthweight infants, Ped. 55, 589 (1975).

(19) R. Uauy, D.L. Shapiro, B. Smith, and J.B. Warshaw, Treatment of apnea in prematures with orally administered theophylline, Ped. 55, 595 (1975).

(20) F. Bednarek, and D.W. Roloff, Treatment of apnea of prematurity with aminophylline, Ped. 58, 335 (1976).

(21) M.V. Davi, K. Sankaran, K.J. Simons, et al, Physiologic changes induced by theophylline in the treatment of apnea in preterm infants, J. Ped. 92, 91 (1978).

(22) T. Gerhardt, and E. Bancalari, Personal communication.

(23) D.C. Shannon, Apnea or prematurity, Ross Conference on Pediatric Research (1975).

(24) K.E. Schaefer, Respiratory pattern and respiratory response to CO_2, J. Appl. Physiol. 13, 1 (1958).

(25) C.W. Zwillich, D.J. Pierson, F.D. Hofeldt, E.G. Lufkin, and J.V. Weil, Ventilatory control in myxedema and hypothyroidism, New Eng J Med. 292, 662 (1975).

(26) K.W. Cross, and P. Warner, The effect of inhalation of high and low oxygen concentrations on the respiration of the newborn infant, J. Physiol. 114, 283 (1951).

(27) K.W. Cross, and T.E. Oppe, The effect of inhalation of high and low oxygen concentrations on the respiration of the premature infant, J. Physiol. 117, 38 (1952).

(28) A. Fenner, U. Schalk, and H. Hoenicke, et al, Periodic breathing in premature and neonatal babies: incidence, breathing pattern, respiratory gas tensions, response to changes in gas composition of ambient air, Pediatr. Res. 7, 174 (1973).

(29) H. Rigatto, and J.P. Brady, Periodic breathing and apnea in pre-term infants, II. Hypoxia as a primary event, Ped. 50, 219 (1972).

(30) A.N. Krauss, C.A. Tori, J. Brown, J. Soodalter, and P.A.M. Auld, Oxygen chemoreceptors in low birth weight infants, Pediatr. Res. 7, 569 (1973).

(31) H. Rigatto, J.P. Brady, and R. De La Torre Verduzco, Chemoreceptor reflexes in pre-term infants: the effect of gestational and post natal age on the ventilatory response to inhalation of 100% and 15% oxygen, Ped. 55, 604 (1975).

(32) H. Rigatto, Respiratory control and apnea in the newborn infant, Crit. Care Med. 5, 2-9 (Jan.-Feb. 1977).

(33) J.A. Davis, The effect of anoxia in newborn rabbits, J. Physiol. 155, 56P (1961).

(34) J.M. Gupta, and J.P.M. Tizard, The sequence of events in neonatal apnea, Lancet 55 (1967).

(35) E. Bystrzycka, B.S. Nail, and M.J. Purves, Central and peripheral neural respiratory activity in the mature sheep foetus and newborn lamb, Resp. Physiol. 25, 199 (1975).

(36) S.E. Downing, and J.C. Lee, Laryngeal chemosensitivity: a possible mechanism for sudden infant death, Ped. 55, 640 (1975).

(37) G. Bodegard, and G. Schwieler, Control of respiration in newborn babies, Acta Paediat. Scand. 60, 181 (1971).

(38) S.M.L. Kirkpatrick, A. Olinski, M.H. Bryan, and A.C. Bryan, Effect of premature delivery on the maturation of the Hering-Breuer inspiratory inhibitory reflex in human infants, J. Ped. 88, 1010 (1976).

(39)   A. Steinschneider, Prolonged apnea and the sudden infant
death syndrome: clinical and laboratory observations, Ped. 50,
646 (1972).

(40)   A. Steinschneider, Nasopharyngitis and prolonged sleep apnea,
Ped. 56, 967 (1975).

(41)   C. Guilleminault, R. Peraita, M. Sonquet, and W.C. Dement,
Apnea during sleep in infants: possible relationship with sudden
infant death syndrome, Science 190, 677 (1975).

(42)   D.C. Shannon, and D.H. Kelly, Impaired regulation of alveolar ventilation and the sudden infant death syndrome, Science 197,
367-368 (July 22, 1977).

(43)   D.H. Kelly, and D.C. Shannon, Periodic breathing: a market
of impaired control of ventilation, Ped. (In press).

(44)   D.C. Shannon, D.H. Kelly, and K. O'Connell, Abnormal
regulation of ventilation in infants at risk for sudden infant
death syndrome, New Eng J Med. 297, 747-50 (1977).

(45)   D.H. Kelly, D.C. Shannon, and K. O'Connell, Care of infants
with near-miss sudden infant death syndrome,   Ped. 61, 511
(1978).

(46)   D.H. Kelly, and D.C. Shannon, Management of apnea in infants,
Perinat. (In press).

DISCUSSION

Söderberg reported on observations which might be of great relevance
in this connection. Calling attention to the well known fact that
temporal lobe epilepsia often is accompanied by respiratory depression during seizure episodes he told about his own close experience
of a few cases (adults) in whom epileptic attacks coincided with
complete apnoea. During recovery from the seizure attack, when partial consciousness returned, these patients were still apnoeic or
had insufficient ventilation. On command they could voluntarily
maintain adequate respiration. However, if not repeatedly told to
breath they turned cyanotic again and it even happened that the
respiratory deficit precipitated a new grand mal-like seizure attack.

A CRITICAL OXYGEN LEVEL BELOW WHICH IRREGULAR BREATHING OCCURS IN PRETERM INFANTS

H. LAGERCRANTZ, H. AHLSTRÖM, B. JONSON,
M. LINDROTH and N. SVENNINGSEN

Karolinska Institute, Stockholm, and University of Lund, Lund, Sweden

ABSTRACT

Very preterm infants (gestational age < 32 weeks) may develop respiratory depression and irregular breathing at a too low ambient and arterial PO_2. This is a study of the relationship between oxygenation (transcutaneous PO_2) and ventilation. A critical level of PO_2 at 10—13 kPa was found below which irregular breathing with apnea and bradycardia occurred. This level is higher than that generally supposed safe with regard to tissue hypoxia and not far from the risk zone for retrolental fibroplasia. A meticulous monitoring of oxygenation in very preterm infants is warranted.

INTRODUCTION

If preterm infants are subjected to hypoxia they react with transient hyperventilation followed by respiratory depression (Cross & Oppé, 1952; Brady & Ceruti, 1966; Rigatto & Brady, 1972). Already in 1923 Bakwin reported that irregular breathing could be induced by hypoxia, a fact that has been taken into consideration in clinical practise. Too high concentrations of inspired oxygen often used in the past commonly led to retrolental fibroplasia (James & Lanman, 1976). Our aim was to study if there is a level of PO_2 that is optimal with regard to stable ventilation but lower than levels leading to retrolental fibroplasia.

METHODS

Seven very preterm infants with a tendency of irregular breathing were studied (Table 1). They had no other sign of lung disease. During treatment in incubators they were given parenteral nutrition, in four cases together with human milk given via a nasogastric tube. Respiration was monitored by impedance plethysmography and the heart rate beat to beat on the basis of R–R intervals in ECG (Hewlett-Packard). Apnea was defined as cessation of breathing accompanied by a drop of heart rate below 100 beats/min.

Transcutaneous PO_2 ($tcPO_2$) was monitored in five infants (Radiometer TCM1). The electrodes on the chest were heated to 43.5°C. Electrode site was changed every 3—6 hours. Arterial blood for analysis of PaO_2 was sampled via umbilical catheters. Ambient oxygen concentration was determined with an O_2-monitor. The oxygen concentration was varied so as to find the lowest level with stable respiration. When this was not achieved at safe levels with regard to eye damage, treatment was supplemented with continuous positive airways pressure (CPAP, 2—4 cm H_2O) or theophylline.

H. Lagercrantz *et al.*

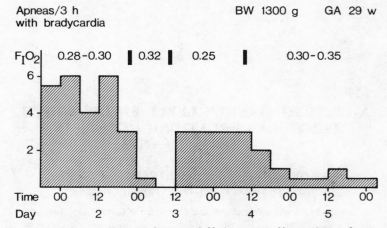

Fig. 1. The incidence of apnea fell dramatically in this infant at a slight increase of FIO_2.

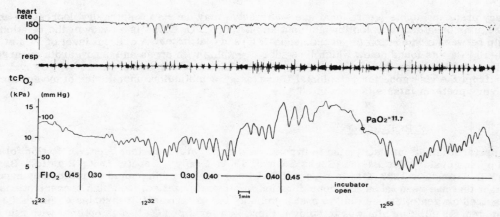

Fig. 2. The heart rate (beat-to-beat), the respiration and the $tcPO_2$ of infant no. 7.

RESULTS

All studied infants had episodes of apnea during the study. It was possible to decrease the number of attacks in each infant by elevating the oxygen concentration in the inspired air (FIO_2). In some infants it was found that even a quite small increase of oxygen could near-ly completely abolish the apneas (Fig. 1).

Figure 2 shows a recording in infant no. 7. At a decrease of oxygen concentration from 45 % to 30 % $tcPO_2$ fell from 12 to 9–6 kPa. An irregular breathing pattern started and apneas occurred. When the ambient oxygen was increased the breathing became more regular and the incidence of apnea decreased. Opening of the incubator for care caused hypoxia and apnea.

Figure 3 illustrates the relationship between apnea and $tcPO_2$. A critical level below which apnea frequently occurs was found at about 10–13 kPa (75–97 mg Hg). $tcPO_2$ was close to arterial PO_2 in each case, Table 1. The critical level for inspired oxygen concentration was between 30 and 45 %. Arterial PCO_2 was essentially normal.

TABLE 1 Birth Weight, Gestational Age, Postnatal Age at Study Procedures and Critical Levels of FIO_2, PaO_2, and $tcPO_2$

Case no.	Sex	Body weight g	Gestational age weeks	Postnatal age days	Critical levels			
					FIO_2 %	PaO_2, kPa	$tcPO_2$, kPa	$PaCO_2$, kPa
1	F	960	29	14	0.35	-	-	-
					0.32	-	-	-
					0.30	-	-	-
2	M	1100	29	7	0.32	10.5-12.5	-	5.7-5.6
				12	0.32	9.5-12.0		6.5-5.0
3	F	840	28	6	0.35	11.0-12.5	11-12.5	6.0-5.2
				12	0.32		11-13.5	
4	F	1200	30	7	0.35	11.0-13.0	11-13	5.8-4.9
				9	0.35	11.5-12.5	10-11.5	
5	F	1230	30	6	0.30	12.0-13.5	10-12	
6	F	1305	29	2	0.45	12.4-13.3	10-11	5.1
7	F	1375	30	2	0.40	10.0-12.3	11-12	4.6-5.0

DISCUSSION

The critical level below which frequent apnea occurs was as high as 10—13 kPa (75—97 mm Hg). To maintain such levels oxygen concentrations as high as 45 % were sometimes needed although the infants were considered free from lung disease and in some cases on supplementary treatment (CPAP, theophylline). These oxygen levels are not far from the range of increased risks for eye damage. The use of moderately high oxygen concentrations must be weighed against the risks and problems associated with artifical ventilation. A prerequisite for the use of oxygen at optimum levels is meticulous monitoring of PO_2.

Our unpublished data and the present study are in agreement with those of Löfgren (1978) that $tcPO_2$ is very close to arterial PO_2 when an electrode heated to 43.5°C is used. This temperature is high enough for very preterm infants with thin skin and more or less preserved cardiopulmonary function. Others have used a temperature of 44°C (Severinghaus et al. 1978). We conclude that transcutaneous PO_2 measurements offer a mean for control of oxygen administration. One advantage with this continuous recording is increased awareness of how opening of the incubator for care adversely affects the status of the infant.

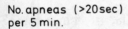

No. apneas (>20 sec) per 5 min.

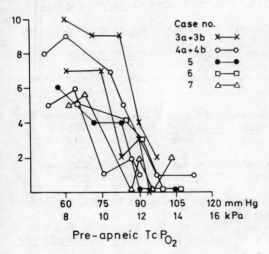

Case no.
3a+3b ×—×
4a+4b o—o
5 ●—●
6 □—□
7 △—△

Fig. 3. The number of apneas related to $tcPO_2$ recorded immediately before the apnea. Cases no. 3 and 4 were investigated twice.

Our study was not designed to illustrate reasons for instability of ventilation. However, the data offer some basis for a discussion of these matters. Three theoretical situations causing instability of ventilation control were discussed in the previous session by Cherniack, von Euler, Homma and Kao (see this volume): predominant control of breathing by hypoxia; overall increase in controller gain or prolonged circulation time. Irregular breathing occurs as a rule without signs of circulatory disturbances, and our infants showed no evidence of cerebrovascular disease. Therefore these explanations seem to be less likely. Prolonged circulation time has also not been observed in apneic infants (Rigatto and Brady, 1972). However, once bradycardia has occurred circulatory factors may modify the further course of an apneic spell.

The somewhat poor CO_2 response in some preterm infants (Rigatto and Brady, 1972) may be the basis for instability of ventilation. If such instability leads to a fall of PO_2 a further depression of ventilation may ensue as even moderate hypoxia has such effects in infants (Albersheim et al., 1976). When a respiratory pause has been long enough peripheral receptors may be activated and cause a series of augmented breaths (Bartlett, 1971) often recorded in our series.

The factor that stabilizes ventilation at high FIO_2 must not necessarily be arterial PO_2. A greater storage of O_2 in the lungs is one result of high FIO_2. At high FIO_2 the risks for hypoxia at a slight instability of ventilation is reduced and this may eliminate a further respiratory depression. A higher FRC caused by CPAP may have a similar effect.

A factor that appears to be of importance for apnea is the sleep state of infants. This state was not systematically assessed, but we got the impressione that irregular breathing occurred mainly at slow wave silent sleep.

(This study has been supported by the Swedish Medical Research Council 05234 and 04732 and by the Swedish National Association against Heart and Chest Diseases.)

REFERENCES

Albersheim, S., Boychuk, R., Seshia, M.M.K., Cates, D. and Rigatto, H., Effects of CO_2 on immediate ventilatory response to O_2 in preterm infants, J. Appl. Physiol.41, 609–611 (1976).

Bakwin, H., Oxygen therapy in premature babies with anoxemia, Am. J. Dis. Child. 25, 157 (1923).

Bartlett, P., Origin and regulation of spontaneous deep breaths, Respir. Physiol. 12, 230–238 (1971).

Brady, J. and Ceruti, E., Chemoreceptor reflexes in the newborn infant: Effects of varying degrees of hypoxia on heart rate and ventilation in a warm environment, J. Physiol. 184, 631–645 (1966).

Cross, K.W. and Oppé, T.E., The effect of inhalation of high and low concentrations of oxygen on the respiration of the premature infant, J. Physiol. 117, 38–55 (1952).

James, L.S. and Lanman, J.T. (Eds.), History of oxygen thearpy and retrolental fibroplasia, Pediatrics 57, suppl. (1976).

Löfgren, O., On transcutaneous PO_2 measurements in humans. Some methodological, physiological and clinical studies. Dissertation. Litos Reprotryck, Malmö (1978), pp. 26–46.

Rigatto, H. and Brady, J.P., Periodic breathing and apnea in preterm infants. II. Hypoxia as a primary event, Pediatrics 50, 219–228 (1972).

Severinghaus, J.W., Peabody, J., Thunström, A., Eberhard, P. and Zappia, E., Workshop on methodological aspects of transcutaneous blood gas analysis, Acta Anaesthesiol. Scand. 68, suppl. 69 (1978).

A COMMENT OF HYPOXIC RESPONSES IN INFANTS — A CONTRIBUTION TO THE DISCUSSION

A. C. BRYAN

Research Institute, Hospital for Sick Children, Toronto, Canada

The failure of infants to respond to hypoxia is a critical issue. It not only emerges from ventilatory responses to hypoxia such as Dr. Rigatto has described, it is a common clinical observation, particularly in preterm infants, that hypoxia is more likely to lead to apnea than hyperpnea. It is a problem that neonatologists need help with as we are hemmed in by ethical considerations in infants and the lack of a suitable animal model.

Perhaps the clue is provided by the work of Tenney and Ou (1) who showed that decortication markedly enhanced the ventilatory response to hypoxia and produced intense arousal. They suggested that there were balanced facilitatory and inhibitory pathways to the medulla and the inhibitory pathway was abolished by decortication. They suggested that the facilitatory pathway was mediated by a diencephalic neurotransmitter. By analogy, hypoxia is a direct myocardial depressant but by causing reflex release of catecholamine, hypoxia increases myocardial contractility.

Many neurotransmitters have an oxygen dependant step in their production (2, 3) and the fetus is in a low oxygen environment. Neurotransmitter stores in the brain are known to be low at birth (4, 5) and re-uptake mechanisms slow (6). Thus the newborn infant may have low stores of facilitatory neurotransmitters in the diencephalon, which could be rapidly depleted. Such a mechanism could account for the biphasic ventilatory response to hypoxia -- an initial hyperpnea mediated by neurotransmitter followed by hypoxic depression of the medulla.

REFERENCES

(1) S.M. Tenney & L.C. Ou, Ventilatory response of decorticate and decerebrate cats to hypoxia and CO_2. <u>Resp.Physiol.</u> 29, 81 (1977).

(2) J.N.Davis & A. Carlsson, The effect of hypoxia on mono-amine synthesis, levels and metabolism in rat brain. <u>J.Neurochem.</u>

21, 783 (1973).

(3) R.M. Brown, W. Kehr & A. Carlsson, Functional and biochemical aspects of catecholamine metabolism in brain under hypoxia. Brain Res. 85, 491 (1975).

(4) H.C. Agarwal, S.N. Glisson & W.A. Himwitch, Changes in mono-amines of rat brain during post natal ontogeny. Biochim. et Biosphys. Acta 130, 511 (1966).

(5) L. Loizon & P. Salt, Regional changes in mono-amines during post-natal development. Brain Res. 20, 467 (1970).

(6) J.T. Coyle, in: Brazier, M. & Coceani, E. (1976) Brain Dys-function in Infantile Febrile Convulsions, Raven Press, New York.

DISCUSSION

Lagercrantz raised the objection to Bryan's comment that the neuro-transmitter stores cannot be depleted after such a short period of moderate hypoxia. Even after severe hypoxia preterm infants release considerable high amounts of catecholamines at least from the peri-pheral system (Lagercrantz & Bistoletti, Pediatr.Res. 11, 889, 1977). Other have shown that long-lasting hypoxia affects the neurotrans-mitter stores and the neuroenzyme activities such as tyrosen hydroxylase in the brain surprisingly little (Hedner, Lundborg & Engel, Biol.Neonate 32, 229, 1977).

GENERATION AND REGULATION OF PATTERN OF BREATHING

A. Basic Mechanisms in the Adult Organism

WHAT IS THE PATTERN OF BREATHING
REGULATED FOR?

F. S. GRODINS and S. M. YAMASHIRO

*University of Southern California, Department of Biomedical Engineering,
Los Angeles, California 90007, U.S.A.*

Professor Purves broadened our horizons yesterday morning when he told us "What we breath for". Clearly there are many reasons, and to follow Professor Purves' lead, we can say that we think that the pattern of breathing is regulated to accomplish these tasks in some "optimal manner". To make this statement something more than a trivial tautology, we must identify and define what we mean by "some optimal manner".

I don't think we should be embarrassed because we have long concentrated on the gas exchange function of breathing as opposed to its other roles in speaking, singing, oboe playing, eating, postural adjustments and temperature regulation. After all, in any system serving multiple functions there must be a priority scheme and it is certainly clear that if we don't satisfy the requirements for gas exchange, we would not have to worry about any of the others!

But even when we concentrate on the gas exchange function, the extremely complex control task which the respiratory controller must accomplish is abundantly clear. Figure 1 shows our overall concept of the "metabolic servomechanism" whose job it is to meet metabolic demand for gas exchange while simultaneously keeping arterial P_{CO_2}, pH, and P_{O_2} constant. It could do this provided that: 1) the controller is furnished with information on $\dot{V}_{CO_2}$ (we don't know how this is accomplished!), and 2) the controller sends out a neural motor pattern which, having allowed for the dead space and the mechanics of the ventilatory apparatus, will be appropriately mapped on the respiratory muscle grid in space and time to produce a $\dot{V}_A$ proportional to $\dot{V}_{CO_2}$ (we don't know how this is done either). To this already complex task let us now add another, which though apparently not necessary for the servomechanism operation just described (but maybe it is!), will suggest one answer to the question posed at the beginning, i.e., what is the pattern of breathing regulated for? Let us say that our controller, given a specific demand for $\dot{V}_A$, as defined by $\dot{V}_{CO_2}$ and arterial composition, will pattern its output in such a way as to minimize the force or work of the respiratory muscles.

Concepts of optimality or economy in one form or another are among the oldest principles of theoretical science (e.g. Fermat, Maupertius, Hamilton) and their application to respiratory physiology dates at least from the time of Rohrer (1925). In recent years, my colleague, Dr. Yamashiro, has extended the pioneering work of Rohrer (1925), Otis (1950), and Mead (1960) and shown that a criterion function

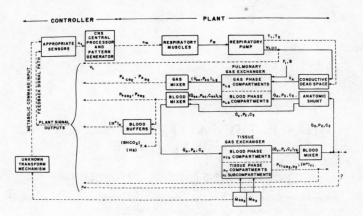

Fig. 1.   The respiratory metabolic servomechanism.

based on energetics and gas exchange efficiency can successfully predict not only res
piratory frequency but also airflow pattern shape, FRC and relative durations of T_I
and T_E, although the predictions are much closer to observation during exercise than
at rest.   Experimental measurements of all these variables show random and systemati
fluctuations which may be manifestations of some kind of goal directed search procedu
To know when the criterion function has been minimized, the system must be able to
detect some output variables related to it.   What are some possibilities?

We know that skeletal muscles in general contain both length (spindles) and tension
(Golgi) sensitive sensors, and as pointed out by Granit (1972) some old psychophysical experiments by v. Frey (1913, 1914) and Renquist (1926) demonstrated that
both force and work can be precisely estimated by human subjects during work involving the arm muscles.   Figure 2 shows an expanded version of the respiratory
pattern control system with the various proprioceptive feedback pathwys indicated.

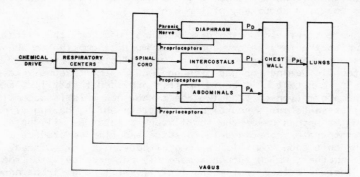

Fig. 2.   The respiratory pattern control system.

We know that the intercostal and abdominal muscles have both length (spindles) and
tension (Golgi) receptors, the diaphragm has tension receptors, and the pulmonary
stretch receptors provide information on lung volume so that feedback information
related to muscle force and work are potentially available.   In the early 1960's,
Campbell and associates showed that normal human subjects could detect both added
elastic and resistive loads to breathing provided they exceeded a certain thresh-

old, and more recently that such subjects could detect an absolute increase of 700 ml in tidal volume when ventilation was increased, Table 1. Of special interest

TABLE 1   Thresholds of Load Detection

Load	Threshold	Reference
Elastic	2.55 cm H_2O/l	Campbell et al (1960)
Resistive	0.59 cm H_2O/lps	Bennett et al (1962)
Volume	700 ml	West et al (1975)

to us is the fact that consideration of minimum detectable levels of respiratory force or work changes leads to theoretical predictions of variability in breathing pattern variables which are largest at rest and decrease during exercise and mechanical loading, which is in agreement with observation. Let us examine this point further.

Table 2 shows data recently obtained in our laboratory by Perumal Natarajan which illustrates that the variances of respiratory frequency, tidal volume, and inspiratory duration all decrease during an experimental state involving a combination of treadmill exercise (6 mph, 0 grade) and an added inspiratory resistance (11 cm H_2O/LPS).

TABLE 2   Effect of Exercise and Inspiratory Resistance Load on Respiratory Pattern Variables

	CONTROL	EXERCISE + R_I
f (BPM)	17.3 (6.0)*	21.7 (4.7)
V_T (1)	.65 (9.2)	1.45 (5.1)
T_I (sec)	1.93 (8.3)	1.73 (5.0)

*Coef. of variation for 10 breaths

The subject was a normal young man (25 years old) and the values given are the means and coefficients of variation for 10 breaths. You see that the latter are decreased by about 22% (f), 45% (V_T), and 40% (T_I) respectively during combined exercise and inspiratory resistive loading. How does this observed behavior compare with that predicted by optimization theory?

If the neural pathways for conscious and unconscious detection partly share a common circuitry, similar, although probably quantitatively different, thresholds may be involved in the automatic adjustment of respiratory pattern to external loads. By substituting the threshold values for detection of elastic and resistive loads from Table 1 into Mead's minimum force amplitude optimization criterion, we can convert them into the equivalent pressure thresholds as shown below:

Mead minimum force amplitude criterion:

$$\Delta \hat{P} = \left(\frac{V_T \sqrt{(2\pi fRC)^2+1}}{C} \right)_{LOAD} - \left(\frac{V_T \sqrt{(2\pi fRC)^2+1}}{C} \right)_{CONTROL}$$

Pressure equivalent load detection thresholds:

Elastic: ΔE of 2.55 cm $H_2O|1$ = $\Delta \hat{P}$ of 1.38 cm H_2O

Resistive: ΔR of 0.59 cm $H_2O|1ps$ = $\Delta \hat{P}$ of 0.49 cm H_2O

The fact that the equivalent pressure thresholds are so different for the two speaks against their detection through a common force or pressure pathway. The same sort of differences persist if we calculate a work equivalent threshold. Thus, some kind of mismatch between the input pressure and the output geometry as first proposed by Campbell seems a more likely sensing mechanism. However, as many people have emphasized, the mechanical consequences of internal and external loads may be quite different and a simpler detection method may work for them (or a more complex one may be needed!). Also, the thresholds for the unconscious detection of load information for use in automatic pattern optimization may be much lower than those described above.

Whatever the ultimate sensing mechanism, however, any threshold at all will set a minimum bound on the variance of the manipulated variable in any search or optimization procedure which may be involved in pattern optimization. We can illustrate this with Fig. 3 in which Mead's minimum force amplitude criterion is plotted against frequency at two levels of $\dot{V}_A$. The optimum frequency is 20 cpm at $\dot{V}_A$ = 6 1/m

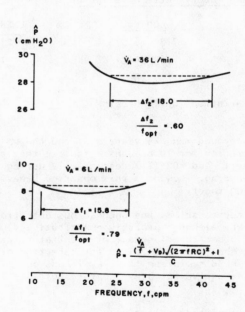

Fig. 3.   Pressure amplitude versus respiratory frequency at two levels of alveolar ventilation. The horizontal dashed lines indicate the threshold levels for detection of an added resistive load.

and 30 cpm at $\dot{V}_A$ = 36 1/min. The dashed horizontal lines represent the addition
of Campbell's resistive load detection threshold in pressure equivalents to the
minimum pressure defining the optimum frequency. The intersection of these dashed
lines with the solid curves defines the minimum frequency range within which f can
move without detecting any change in P. This both sets a limit to the precision
of optimal frequency selection and defines the minimum range of any useful search
procedure. For present purposes, we note that this range is 79% of the optimal
frequency at $\dot{V}_A$ = 6 1/min and decreases to 60% of the optimal frequency at $\dot{V}_A$ = 36 1/min,
a prediction which is qualitatively consistent with Natarajan's experimental data.

How might such an optimal frequency selection system work? We don't really know
of course, but we can describe at least two general classes of possibilities.
Figure 4 describes a search optimization procedure in which a criterion function

SEARCH OPTIMIZATION

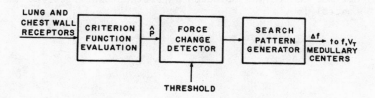

Fig. 4. Optimum controller based on criterion function evaluation and
         variable search pattern generator.

such as Mead's is calculated from appropriate sensed information, changes of at
least threshold magnitude are detected and sent to a search pattern generator
which initiates a wider Δf search. Figure 5 shows an optimization procedure based
on an initial parameter estimation procedure. As noted before, this might be
based on sensory information about input (pressure) - output (length) inappropriate-
ness, and only changes above a particular threshold value are detected. The new
values are fed into a fixed control law which calculates the change in f required
to maintain desired behavior with the new values of R and K. Both of these methods
are used in engineering systems, but we can only speculate about their possible
use here.

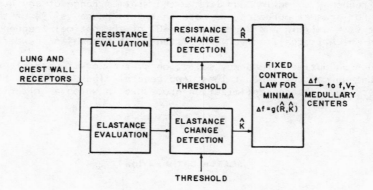

PARAMETER ESTIMATION OPTIMIZATION
"LENGTH – TENSION APPROPRIATENESS"

Fig. 5.   Optimum controller based on parameter identification and fixed
control law.

SUMMARY

In the overall metabolic servomechanism of respiration we have assumed that alveolar
ventilation is set by metabolic and chemical drive and asked what determines the
choice of cycle pattern for any such alveolar ventilation. Formulations which
assume the choice is based on minimization of a force or energy criterion have had
some success in predicting respiratory frequency, flow trajectory, FRC, and T_I/T_E
ratio particularly during exercise where the work of breathing becomes significant.
Sensory mechanisms used to detect loads, evaluate parameters, and calculate
criterion functions were briefly discussed but the details remain largely unknown.
The effect of sensory thresholds on the variance of pattern measurements was discussed, and two possible optimization mechanisms were outlined.

REFERENCES

E.D. Bennett, M.I.V. Jayson, D. Rubenstein, and E.J.M. Campbell, The ability of
man to detect added non-elastic loads to breathing, Clin. Sci. 23, 155-162 (1962).

E.J.M. Campbell, S. Freedman, P.S. Smith and M.E. Taylor, The ability of man to
detect added elastic loads to breathing, Clin. Sci. 20, 223-231 (1961).

M. Von Frey, Studien über den Kraftsinn, Zt. Biol. 63, 129 (1913).

M. Von Frey, Die Vergleichung von Gewichten mit Hilfe des Kraftsinns. Zt. Biol. 65, 203 (1914).

R. Granit, Constant errors in the execution and appreciation of movement, Brain 95, 649 (1972).

J. Mead, Control of respiratory frequency, J. Appl. Physiol. 15, 325-336 (1960).

A.B. Otis, W.O. Fenn, and H. Rahn, Mechanics of breathing in man, J. Appl. Physiol. 2, 592-607 (1950).

Y. Renqvist, Über den Bewegungswahrnehmungen zugrunde liegenden Reize. Skad. Arch. Physiol. 50, 52 (1926).

F. Rohrer, Physiologie der atembewegung. In: Handbuch der Normalen and Pathologischen Physiologie, edited by A. Bethe et al. Berlin: Springer, Springer, 1925, vol. 2, p. 70-127.

David W.M. West, Christopher G. Ellis and E.J. Moran Campbell, Ability of man to detect increases in his breathing, J. Appl. Physiol. 39, 372-376 (1975).

S.M. Yamashiro and F.S. Grodins, Optimal regulation of respiratory airflow, J. Appl. Physiol. 30, 597 (1971).

S.M. Yamashiro and F.S. Grodins, Respiratory cycle optimization in exercise, J. Appl. Physiol. 35, 522 (1973).

S.M. Yamashiro, J.A. Daubenspeck, T.N. Lauritsen and F.S. Grodins, Total work rate of breathing optimization in CO_2 inhalation and exercise, J. Appl. Physiol. 38, 702 (1975).

DISCUSSION

In the discussion following Grodin's presentation Euler drew attention to the fact that for a certain ventilation the selection by the organism of tidal volumes and respiratory rate is not unique but depends partly on the body temperature. This is the case both in man (Hey et al., Respir.Physiol. 1, 193, 1966) and in cat (Euler et al., Respir.Physiol. 10, 93, 1970). In latter species, at least, there is no concomitant change in FRC. This could mean that strive after minimization of work does not always have highest priority in determining the pattern, but that there may be other factors which are 'allowed' also to exert an influence on the variables constituting the breathing pattern.

Guz raised the question about optimization in disease. He remarked that patients with asthma breath more rapidly and are doing more work on their ventilation than they would 'need' to do if energetic optimization had been the main determinant of their pattern of breathing.

In his reply Grodins emphasized that the calculations for minimal work should include not only tidal volume and rate of breathing but also such variables as FRC and T_I to T_E ratio. At relative rest when the level of inspiratory work is fairly trivial the behaviour of these variables are not very close to predictions but in exercise when work of breathing becomes a considerable fraction of the total the behaviour of these variables becomes quite close to the predictions.

Euler mentioned the possibility that the diseased organism may have quite different priorities and different objectives for its pattern regulation than the healthy one. In the case of such a complex and multifactorial disease as asthma it might be pertinent to consider the possibility that a malfunction of the mechanisms for optimization might be of importance in this disease.

REFLEX AND CENTRAL CHEMOCEPTIVE CONTROL OF THE TIME COURSE OF INSPIRATORY ACTIVITY

E. N. BRUCE, C. VON EULER and S. M. YAMASHIRO

Nobel Institute for Neurophysiology, Karolinska Institutet,
S-104 01 Stockholm, Sweden

Recent work has provided evidence suggesting that the basic, automatic regulation of the respiratory pattern can be examined in terms of three different functions: 1) the generation and shaping of the trajectory of central inspiratory activity, CIA, 2) the 'off-switch' of the inspiratory activity including the production of graded inhibition and the final termination of the inspiratory activity along with the setting of the thresholds at which these events occur, and 3) the control of the duration of the expiratory phase. Both the time course of the increment of CIA in each inspiration and the duration of the inspiratory activity determined, as it is, by the inspiratory 'off-switch' mechanisms and their threshold functions, are drive dependent (see Fig. 1A). This is the case also when variations in drive are accomplished by direct manipulation of the afferent input from the intracranial chemoceptive structures by focal cooling of the 'intermediate' chemoceptive areas on the ventral surface of medulla (Ref. 1; see also p. 35).

The trajectory of the increase in phrenic activity as measured by the time course of the phrenic 'moving average' often bears a close relationship to the time course of the volume increase in inspiration although this mechanical aspect represents a highly smoothed version of its driving neural activity. However, in conditions of disparity between intercostal and diaphragmatic activity (some of which will be discussed later on pp 443 and 457) and in conditions when the expiratory muscles contribute substantially to the work of breathing, the phrenic activity is not representative of the variations in volume. Although several papers (e.g. Refs. 2, 3) have shown that integration of various spinal and supraspinal inputs take place in the phrenic motoneuron pools and influence the transfer of the respiratory drive signals to the motor command for the diaphragm, the shape of the trajectory of the 'moving average' of the efferent phrenic activity can under certain conditions, but certainly not always, be used as an approximation also of the initial increase in excitability of the inspiratory 'off-switch' mechanisms caused by the postulated recurrent aspect of CIA (Ref. 4).

It thus appears that under certain experimental conditions the trajectory of the 'moving average' of the efferent phrenic activity may serve as a valuable index of the CIA and of the neural and mechanical output parameters of breathing. The time course of the trajectories of the phrenic 'moving average' and the volume curve usually appear to be roughly linear up to the threshold for the graded inhibition of CIA although either convexities or concavities are often present. The dynamics of the increment of the inspiratory activity, however, have only seldomly been subject to a close study. Under conditions of experimentally induced

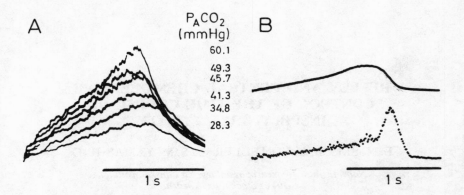

Fig. 1.   Records of 'moving average' of inspiratory phrenic
activity in the absence of cyclic vagal volume related feedback.   A. Six superimposed records of inspiratory trajectories at different P_ACO_2 levels showing that the rate of rise
of inspiratory activity increases with increasing P_ACO_2.
B. Upper trace shows the average of 30 phrenic trajectories
at a PCO_2 of 46 mm Hg. Lower trace shows the corresponding standard deviations magnified 10 times.

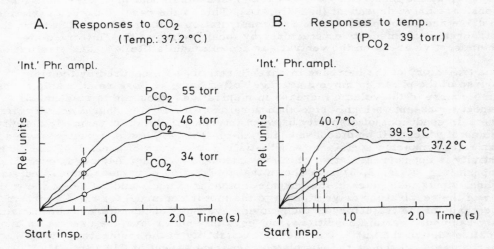

Fig. 2.   From a cat made apneustic by bilateral parabrachial
lesions and surgical vagotomy to show the effects of changes
in P_ACO_2 (A) and body temperature (B) on the initial rate of
rise of inspiratory activity ('integrated' phrenic activity).
The points on the curves (small circles) and the dashed lines
mark the 'half times' for the 'integrated' phrenic activity to
reach its apneustic plateaus. Note the 'half time' stays
almost constant in A but is markedly shortened with increased
temperature in B. (Redrawn from Ref. 5).

apneusis it has been suggested that the mechanisms determining the shape of the inspiratory trajectory may not be altered and that the main difference from 'normal' breathing may depend on an elevated threshold for the inspiratory 'off-switch' mechanisms allowing the inspiratory activity to be followed uninterrupted for longer periods of time than with 'normal' operation of the 'off-switch' (Ref. 6). Both the initial rate of rise and the final apneustic level depend on PCO_2 in the same way as does the inspiratory growth rate in the normal, intact animal. An increase in body (or hypothalamic) temperature also causes an increase in the rate of CIA increment. As is evident from Fig. 2 the mechanisms of action of these two stimuli are quite different however. In response to changes in PCO_2 the <u>fractional</u> increment in CIA per unit time did not change (Fig. 2A), whereas an elevation in body (or hypothalamic) temperature caused a very marked increase also in the relative rate of rise of CIA (Fig. 2B).

It is of interest to observe that under conditions of constant drive inputs the shape of the trajectory is subject to much less variations than is the duration of the inspiratory phase as shown in Fig. 1B (Refs. 6, 7). This strongly suggests that there are separate mechanisms for the generation and control of the shape of the inspiratory trajectory on the one hand and for the 'off-switch' of inspiration on the other. Its strong dependence on drive and its small degree of scatter, which usually exhibits a fairly linear relation to the level of activity, indicate that the rate of increment of CIA may be subject to a continuous short term regulation. It has been suggested that this regulation is accomplished by some balance between excitatory and inhibitory activities which, in turn, depends on the various 'tonic' and transient drive inputs and reflexes (Refs. 8, 9).

Although it is tempting to speculate that the high frequency oscillations which have been found at various levels of the output from the CIA generator may be signs of the operation of the controller regulating the time course of CIA (see e.g. Ref. 10) we have to admit that our knowledge about those fundamental neural mechanisms which are responsible for the generation and the control of the time course of CIA is virtually nil. We do not even know whether the so-called R_α neurons (of the solitary tract complex) which transmit the centrally generated inspiratory activity to the spinal inspiratory motoneuron pools form a part of the CIA generator or whether they merely serve as relays and projection neurons.

With the aim of giving guidance to future experimental approaches to the problems on the CIA generator mechanisms, it may be of value to consider some theoretical grounds for evaluating trajectory shapes and to create realistic models which fit experimental data.

Several mathematical models of the generation of respiratory rhythmicity have been developed e.g. Camerer (11), Feldman and Cowan (12), and Geman and Miller (13) but in general these were not aimed at predicting the shape of the inspiratory trajectory. Previous models all include non-linearities which together with the multitude of parameters involved would make a direct application of these models to interpret experimental data extremely difficult if not impossible. Close inspection of these models reveal that for the values of parameters chosen to correspond to the activity of inspiratory neurons, essentially linear responses were obtained over a significant range of activities. That is, above threshold and below saturation, most response characteristics could be predicted with a linear model. Available evidence, briefly mentioned above, indicate that different neural mechanisms are employed for 1) the generation of the inspiratory activity and 2) for the termination of this activity. It further appears that the termination of inspiration and the inspiratory-expiratory phase transition involve non-linearities such as threshold functions. In contrast, the shape of the CIA, following the start and prior to the termination of inspiration, does not appear to be critically dependent on non-linear characteristics. Thus, for the purpose of analysing those mechanisms which generate and control the growth rate of CIA in each inspiration a linearized model would seem to be adequate.

In order to begin developing a linear model which should ultimately summarize current knowledge about the mechanisms which generate CIA, and which therefore should be helpful for evaluating working hypotheses and for designing future experiments, we have first studied a simple model with two interacting components. This model has been found to reproduce adequately the changing CIA trajectory as a function of end-tidal PCO_2.

The model shown in Fig. 3 is consistent with the hypothesis mentioned above that the control of the growth of CIA may be based on a balance between self-excitatory and self-inhibitory processes, and assumes that the CIA generating pool contains neurons of two basic types; one with excitatory outputs and another with

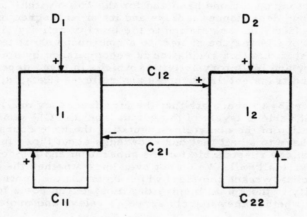

Fig. 3. Model of the generator of inspiratory trajectory. For explanation see text.

inhibitory outputs which are in balance with each other. Models with self reexcitation and -inhibition have been previously proposed by Camerer (11), Feldman and Cowan (12), and Geman and Miller (13) to explain the generation of respiratory rhythm, but for reasons given above we will only discuss the details of the shape of the inspiratory trajectory. Following the approach of Wilson and Cowan (14), the variables of our model will be defined as follows:

I_1 = The instantaneous average activity of the population of excitatory cells;

I_2 = The instantaneous average activity of the population of inhibitory cells.

In the present model which is concerned only with CIA trajectory during inspiration we have restricted our attention to neural activity levels where saturation or other non-linearities are not encountered. The following linear set of differential equations can be used to describe the model of Fig. 1:

$$\tau_1 \frac{dI}{dt} 1 = -I_1 + C_{11}I_1 - C_{21}I_2 + D_1, \tag{1}$$

$$\tau_2 \frac{dI}{dt} 2 = -I_2 + C_{12}I_1 - C_{22}I_2 + D_2 \tag{2}$$

Parameters τ_1 and τ_2 correspond to effective neural time constants; D_1 and D_2 represent constant tonic (chemical) drive inputs; C_{11}, C_{21}, C_{12}, and C_{22} refer to interaction parameters corresponding to interconnections as shown in Fig. 3. Effective neural time constants relate to build-up and decay of post-synaptic potentials (Ref. 12). The solutions of interest here are activities I_1 and I_2 as a function of time starting from zero initial conditions and driven by the tonic drive inputs D_1 and D_2. By applying the Laplace Transform, the solutions are obtained as:

$$I_1 = \frac{As + B}{S\left[\left(\frac{s}{\omega_n}\right)^2 + 2\xi\left(\frac{s}{\omega_n}\right) + 1\right]} \tag{3}$$

$$I_2 = \frac{C_{12}\, S\, I_1 + D_2}{1 + C_{22}\, S\left(\frac{\tau_2}{1 + C_{22}}\, S + 1\right)} \tag{4}$$

where

$$\omega_n^2 \equiv \frac{C_{21}C_{12} - (C_{11} - 1)(1 + C_{22})}{\tau_1 \tau_2}$$

$$\xi \equiv \frac{\left[\tau_1(1 + C_{22}) - \tau_2(C_{11} - 1)\right]\omega_n}{2}$$

$$A \equiv \frac{D_1\, \tau_2}{C_{21}C_{12} - (C_{11} - 1)(1 + C_{22})}$$

and

$$B \equiv \frac{D_1(1 + C_{22}) - C_{21}D_2}{C_{21}C_{12} - (C_{11} - 1)(1 + C_{22})}$$

Note that parameters ω_n and ξ correspond to the natural resonance frequency and the damping co-efficient, respectively, of a second order transfer function. Neural time constants τ_1 and τ_2 should be of the order of several milliseconds, but the slow dynamics of I_1 and I_2 should be primarily determined by ω_n and ξ. This also means that trajectories of I_1 and I_2 will have roughly the same shape with respect to slow dynamics and be indistinguishable when measured on a time scale of seconds. For this reason, only the I_1 trajectory need to be considered as long as, in a first approximation, the high frequency components are ignored. This trajectory is determined by the parameters A, B, ω_n, and ξ. Parameters A and B will change as a function of the tonic drive inputs (D_1 and D_2) while ω_n and ξ are independent of drive.

We will now compare model predictions with experimental results. The best available estimate of the CIA trajectory may be obtained during apneustic breaths (such as those measured by Euler <u>et al</u>. (4) assuming that in apneusis the 'off-switch' thresholds are raised above the level at which significant inhibitory effects are encountered. Figure 4 shows apneustic data at three different levels of end-tidal CO_2 tension. Also shown in this figure are the theoretical curves obtained by fitting the data with the inverse Laplace Transformed (time domain) version of Equation (3). For the three curves shown, values of ω_n = 0.8 rad/sec

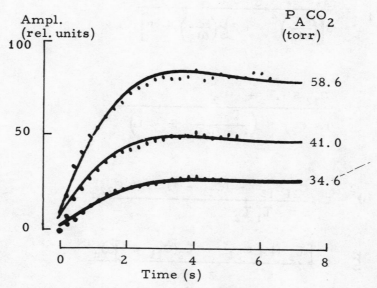

Fig. 4. Comparison of model predictions (lines) and experimental data (dots) during apneusis at three levels of end-tidal CO_2. Data from Ref. 5.

and ξ = 0.65 led to the best visual fit. Parameters A and B were chosen to best fit the individual curves assuming that CO_2 changed the tonic drive inputs D_1 and D_2 (parameters A and B) proportionally and without affecting other parameter values. It thus appears that the predictions fit data over several levels of chemical drive during apneusis (as shown in Fig. 4).

This model appears helpful in interpreting changes in trajectory in response to variations in drive inputs and to various transient reflexes as well as to such general shape characteristics as concavity and convexity obtained in different experiments and conditions (cf. Milic-Emili, p. 185). It would seem useful in trying to design key experiments to elucidate the influences on CIA generation by different reflexes and drives as well as the mechanisms for graded and final inhibition of CIA by the 'off-switch' mechanisms.

The model draws attention to the possibility that the CIA generator may not necessarily depend on the presumption that its neuronal elements interact with each other by means of action potentials. It does not seem unlikely that it is build up by populations of 'silent' neurons exciting and inhibiting each other electrotonically. In such a case only the output would be encoded to be transmitted in terms of discharge rate of action potentials.

ACKNOWLEDGEMENT

This work was supported by the Swedish Medical Research Council (project no. 14X-544) and Knut och Alice Wallenbergs Stiftelse.

REFERENCES

(1) N. S. Cherniack, C. von Euler, I. Homma & F. F. Kao, Graded changes in central chemoceptor input by local temperature changes on the ventral surface of medulla, J. Physiol. 287, 191 (1979).

(2) P. K. Gill & M. Kuno, Excitatory and inhibitory actions on phrenic motoneurones, J. Physiol. 168, 274 (1963).

(3) E. E. Decima & C. von Euler, Intercostal and cerebellar influences on efferent phrenic activity in the decerebrate cat, Acta physiol. scand. 76, 148 (1969).

(4) C. von Euler & T. Trippenbach, Excitability changes of the inspiratory 'off-switch' mechanism tested by electrical stimulation in nucleus parabrachialis in the cat, Acta physiol. scand. 97, 175 (1976).

(5) C. von Euler, I. Marttila, J. E. Remmers & T. Trippenbach, Effects of lesions in the parabrachial nucleus on the mechanisms for central and reflex termination of inspiration in the cat, Acta physiol. scand. 96, 324 (1976).

(6) G. W. Bradley, C. von Euler, I. Marttila & B. Roos, Steady state effects of CO_2 and temperature on the relationship between lung volume and inspiratory duration (Hering-Breuer threshold curve), Acta physiol. scand. 92, 351 (1974).

(7) J. Newsom Davis, L. Loh & M. Casson, The effects of diaphragm paralysis on the volume and time components of individual breaths in man, In: Duron, B. (1976) Respiratory Centres and Afferent Systems, INSERM, Paris, pp 199-202.

(8) C. von Euler, J. N. Hayward, I. Marttila & R. J. Wyman, The spinal connections of the inspiratory neurones of the ventrolateral nucleus of the cat's tractus solitarius, Brain Res. 61, 23 (1973).

(9) J. L. Feldman & J. D. Cowan, Large-scale activity in neural nets II: A model for the brainstem respiratory oscillator, Biol. Cybernetics 17, 39 (1975).

(10) M. I. Cohen, Synaptic relations between inspiratory neurons, in: Duron, B. (1976) Respiratory Centres and Afferent Systems, INSERM, Paris, pp 19-29.

(11) H. Camerer, A model of a rhythmic active neuronal network, in: Umbach, W. & Koepchen, H. P. (1974) Central Rhythmic and Regulation, Hippokrates Verlag, Stuttgart, pp 78-81.

(12) J. L. Feldman & J. D. Cowan, Large-scale activity in neural nets I: Theory with application to motoneuron pool responses. Biol. Cybernetics 17, 29 (1975).

(13) S. Geman & M. Miller, Computer simulation of brainstem respiratory activity. J. Appl. Physiol. 41, 931 (1976).

SPIROMETRIC AND AIRWAY OCCLUSION WAVEFORM

J. MILIC-EMILI

Department of Physiology, McGill University, Montreal, Canada

Since the pioneering work of Haldane and Priestley (1), in studies of control of breathing the most commonly used output variable has been pulmonary ventilation ($\dot{V}_E$). The limitations of ventilation and its two classical components, tidal volume (V_T) and breathing frequency (f) as measures of the output of the respiratory system were recognized in 1931 by Barcroft and Margaria (2). In a study on the effects of CO_2 on ventilation in man they stressed that understanding of control of breathing requires knowledge of "(a) the duration of the phases of respiration, namely inspiration, expiration and the pause (if any), (b) upon the rates at which air is taken in and given out during the various phases." Indeed, as shown schematically in Fig. 1 (C and D), a given ventilation can be obtained with the same frequency and tidal volume but with different airflows and phase durations. In C the inspiratory flow is much greater than in D, while in D duration of inspiration is much longer than in C. The behaviour of the central respiratory controller is quite different in these two examples, although $\dot{V}_E$, V_T and f are the same. Figure 1 also shows that ventilation can basically be varied as a result of changes (a) in rate of lung filling and (b) in the proportion of inspiratory time to total breath duration (T_I/T_{TOT}). The latter can be varied by changing expiratory duration (T_E) and/or T_I, such that the T_E/T_I ratio changes. Indeed :

$$T_I/T_{TOT} = T_I/(T_I + T_E) = 1/(1 + T_E/T_I) \tag{1}$$

The relationship between $\dot{V}_E$ and T_I/T_{TOT} is given by (3) :

$$\dot{V}_E = (V_T/T_I) \times (T_I/T_{TOT}) \tag{2}$$

where V_T/T_I is mean inspiratory flow per breath (overall mean inspiratory flow) and T_I/T_{TOT} is a dimentionless number, recently termed "inspiratory duty cycle"(4).

If during inspiration lung volume increases linearly with time, i.e. inspiratory flow is constant (as in Fig. 1), changes in T_I will *per se* have no effect on V_T/T_I. Under such conditions, analysis of ventilation by equation 2 is particularly advantageous because it partitions $\dot{V}_E$ into two components : one (V_T/T_I) which is a mechanical transform of the rate of rise of spinal motoneuron output and is independent of respiratory "timing" ; and the other (T_I/T_{TOT}) providing the contribution of "timing" to $\dot{V}_E$. This is not the case for the conventional relationship :

$$\dot{V}_E = V_T \times f \tag{3}$$

because both V_T and f are always time-dependent. In fact, f is inversely proportional to T_{TOT}, and V_T clearly depends on T_I as well as on rate of lung filling (Fig. 1 C and D).

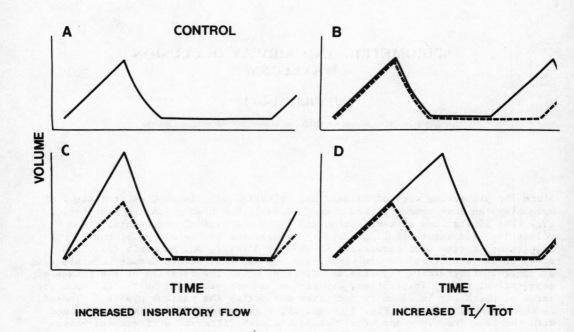

Fig. 1.   Schematic spirograms illustrating ways in which ventilation can be increased. A : control spirogram. It is reproduced as broken line in panels B-D. B : inspiratory phase as in A, but duration of expiration is shortened. C : duration of respiratory phases as in A, but inspiratory flow is increased. D : inspiratory flow and total cycle duration as in A, but inspiratory duration is increased while the opposite is true for expiratory duration. In B and D, ventilation is increased as a result of increased fraction of inspiratory time to total cycle duration , i.e. increased T_I/T_{TOT} ; in C, ventilation is increased by increased inspiratory flow. The contribution of inspiratory flow and T_I/T_{TOT} on ventilation can conveniently be assessed by equation 2.

On the other hand, if the inspiratory volume-time profile is not linear, V_T/T_I becomes T_I-dependent, as shown schematically in Fig. 2. Under such conditions, a shortening of T_I will *per se* either decrease (panel B) or increase (panel C) the overall mean inspiratory flow (i.e. V_T/T_I). Prolongation of T_I will, of course, have the opposite effect.

INSPIRED VOLUME

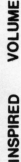
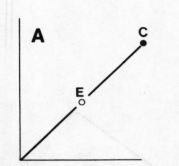
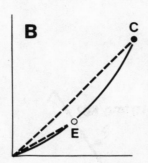
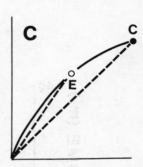

INSPIRATORY   DURATION

Fig. 2. Schematic diagram illustrating the effect of changes in inspiratory
duration on overall mean inspiratory flow (V_T/T_I) for different
inspiratory volume-time profiles. In each panel, the solid curves
depict the inspiratory limb of spirograms ; points C indicate control
V_T and T_I ; points E indicate the end-inspiratory volume when T_I is
shortened from C to E. In panel A, inspiratory flow (dV/dt) is
constant, and hence a change in T_I has no effect on mean inspiratory
flow. In panel B, rate of lung filling increases progressively with
inspiratory time. Here a shortening of T_I causes decreased V_T/T_I, as
shown by the slopes of the broken lines radiating from the onset of
inspiration to the respective end-inspiratory points (E and C).
In panel C, where the rate of rise of volume decreases progressively
with increasing T_I, a shortening of T_I causes increased overall mean
inspiratory flow. Note that the slope of the broken lines is equal to
V_T/T_I (= overall mean inspiratory flow).

The above considerations imply that in studies of control of breathing the shape
of the spirogram must be taken into account. Although in recent years there has
been considerable interest in the study of the breathing pattern, so far little
attention has been paid to detailed analysis of the configuration of the
spirogram.

In recent studies on adult cats we have found that the shape of the inspiratory
limb of the spirogram varies markedly with the type of anesthetic used, ranging
from nearly linear for sodium pentobarbital to markedly curvilinear (convex
upward) for both enflurane and ketamine. As a result, when the dose of sodium
pentobarbital is increased, the ensuing reduction in V_T/T_I is due almost entirely

to decreased slope of the inspiratory limb of the spirogram (Fig. 3). Since in this case the inspiratory volume-time relationship is linear, the prolongation of T_I caused by increased anesthetic depth is inconsequential in terms of V_T/T_I.

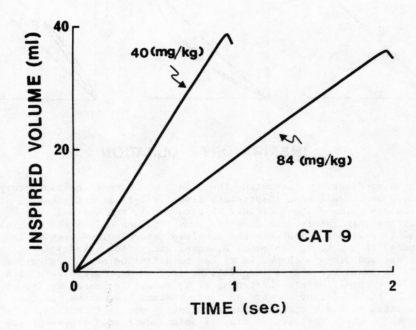

Fig. 3. Inspiratory limbs of spirograms in a cat anesthetized with 40 and 84 mg/kg of sodium pentobarbital (i.p.) breathing 100 % O_2. Increased depth of anesthesia causes reduction in rate of rise of volume and prolongation of T_I. Since the inspiratory volume-time profile is essentially linear, the prolongation of T_I at the higher anesthetic dose has not contributed to the observed reduction in V_T/T_I. This has decreased solely as a result of decreased rate of filling of the lungs (L. Murphy and J. Milic-Emili, unpublished observations).

On the other hand, an increased depth of enflurane anesthesia results in a drop in V_T/T_I due partly to reduced rate of rise of volume, and partly to prolongation of T_I (5). This is shown in Fig. 4 A which depicts inspiratory spirograms in a cat inhaling 2.4 and 3.6 % enflurane. The contribution of decreased rate of rise of volume and prolongation of T_I to the fall in V_T/T_I observed between 2.4 and 3.6 % enflurane can be quantitated as shown in Fig. 4 B, where overall mean inspiratory flow (V_T/T_I) is plotted against the mean inspiratory flow achieved up to a fixed time (0.5 sec) after the onset of inspiration ($\dot{V}_{0.5}$). The isopleth

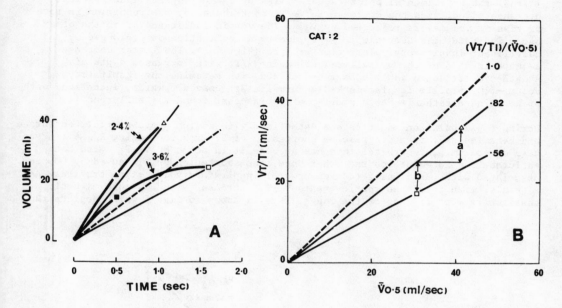

Fig. 4. A. Inspiratory limbs of spirograms (heavy lines) obtained in a cat at
2.4 % (triangles) and 3.6 % (squares) enflurane during 50 % oxygen
breathing. Filled symbols indicate volume inspired by 0.5 sec after the
onset of inspiration ($V_{0.5}$) ; open symbols indicate V_T and T_I. The
slope of the thin solid lines radiating from the onset to the end of
the inspiratory spirograms indicate overall mean inspiratory flows
(V_T/T_I) ; the slope of the broken line indicates the mean inspiratory
flow that would be obtained at 3.6 % enflurane if T_I has remained the
same as at 2.4 %. The reduction in V_T/T_I from 2.4 to 3.6 % enflurane
is thus due in part to decreased amplitude of the spirogram and in part
to prolongation of T_I. Note that the shape of the spirogram is not
affected by depth of anesthesia, i.e. with 3.6 % enflurane the fractional
decrease in volume per unit time is constant (5).

B. Relationship between overall mean inspiratory flow (V_T/T_I) and
mean inspiratory flow up to 0.5 sec from onset of inspiration ($\bar{V}_{0.5}$)
in same cat as in A with 2.4 % (△) and 3.6 % (□) enflurane concentration
during 50 % oxygen breathing. Broken line indicates a (V_T/T_I)/$\bar{V}_{0.5}$
isopleth of 1.0. Solid lines represent the isopleths pertaining to the
two experimental points. For further explanation see text.

labelled 1.0 in Fig. 4 B indicates the relationship between V_T/T_I and $\bar{V}_{0.5}$ that
is obtained when the inspiratory volume-time profile is linear. Under such
conditions $\bar{V}_{0.5}$ is of course the same as the overall mean inspiratory flow. Since
during enflurane anesthesia the inspiratory volume-time profile was convex upward
(Fig. 4 A), the experimental points lie below the 1.0 isopleth. During 2.4 %
enflurane inhalation, the experimental point (triangle) lies on a V_T/T_I vs.
$\bar{V}_{0.5}$ isopleth amounting to 0.82, whereas at the higher enflurane concentration

(3.6 %) the experimental point (square) lies on a 0.56 isopleth. The vertical
distance a indicates the decrease in V_T/T_I contributed by the reduction in rate
of rise of volume, as reflected by $\bar{V}_{0.5}$. The vertical distance b, on the other
hand, indicates the decrease in V_T/T_I due to a combination of prolonged T_I and
curvilinear inspiratory volume-time profile (Fig. 4 A). The latter decrease
amounts to 48 % of the overall reduction in V_T/T_I with increased depth of
anesthesia. Since in adult cats anesthetized with ketamine the inspiratory
volume-time profile is also markedly curvilinear (convex upward), increased depth
of ketamine anesthesia has a similar effect as that found for enflurane.

During CO_2 inhalation adult cats anesthetized with sodium pentobarbital, enflurane
and ketamine exhibit a progressive shortening of T_I with increasing P_{ACO_2}. In the
case of sodium pentobarbital this has no benefit in terms of V_T/T_I. With both
enflurane and ketamine, on the other hand, the shortening of T_I caused by CO_2 is
associated with curvilinear (convex upward) inspiratory volume-time profiles. As
a result, with these anesthetic agents V_T/T_I increases with CO_2 more markedly
than the rate of filling of the lungs. This is shown in Fig. 5 which depicts the

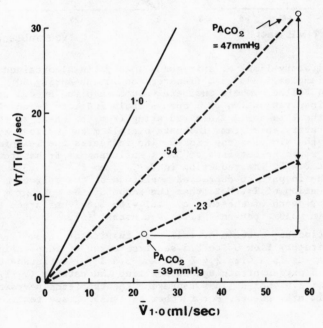

Fig. 5. Relationship between V_T/T_I and $\bar{V}_{1.0}$ obtained in a cat anesthetized
with 40 mg/kg of ketamine for P_{ACO_2} values of 39 (lower circle) and
47 (upper circle) mm Hg. Lines passing through the origin of the graph
indicate various ratios of V_T/T_I to $\bar{V}_{1.0}$. For further information see
text. (N. Jaspar, C. Tessier, M. Mazzarelli and J. Milic-Emili,
unpublished observations).

relationship between V_T/T_I and mean inspiratory flow up to 1 sec from the onset of inspiration ($\dot{V}_{1.0}$) in a cat anesthetized with 40 mg/kg of ketamine at P_{ACO2} values of 39 (lower circle) and 47 (upper circle) mm Hg. The lines passing through the origin of the graph depict various ratios of V_T/T_I to $\bar{\dot{V}}_{1.0}$. The isopleth labelled 1.0 (line of identity) indicates the relationship between V_T/T_I and $\bar{\dot{V}}_{1.0}$ which is obtained when the inspiratory spirogram is linear. Under such conditions $\bar{\dot{V}}_{1.0}$ is identical to the overall mean inspiratory flow. Since in the cat of Fig. 5 the inspiratory volume-time profile was convex upward, the experimental points lie below the 1.0 isopleth. At P_{ACO2} = 39 mm Hg, the experimental point lies on a V_T/T_I vs. $\bar{\dot{V}}_{1.0}$ isopleth amounting to 0.23, whereas at P_{ACO2} = 47 mm Hg the experimental point lies on a .54 isopleth, indicating that in these instances the overall mean inspiratory flow amounted to 23 and 54 %, respectively of the corresponding flow achieved up to 1 sec after the onset of inspiration. If at the higher P_{ACO2} the inspiratory duration has remained the same as at the lower P_{ACO2}, V_T/T_I would have increased along the .23 isopleth, and hence the vertical distance a indicates the increase in V_T/T_I due solely to increased rate of lung filling with CO_2. The vertical distance b (corresponding to 66 % of the overall increase in V_T/T_I) thus represents the gain in V_T/T_I due to a combination of decreased T_I with CO_2 and curvilinear (convex upward) inspiratory volume-time profile.

The above data indicate that the V_T/T_I (and hence $\dot{V}_E$) response to CO_2 depends in part on the shape of the inspiratory spirogram. The latter reflected the airway occlusion pressure waveform in all of our cats. Indeed, in cats anesthetized with sodium pentobarbital we found that during airway occlusion at end-expiration (6), the pressure developed by the inspiratory muscles increased approximately linearly with time, i.e. dP/dt was nearly constant. On the other hand, with both enflurane and ketamine the airway occlusion pressure profile was curvilinear (convex upward).

In adult anesthetized cats the rising limb of the airway (tracheal) occlusion pressure waves can (as a useful approximation) be described by a power function :

$$p = at^b \qquad\qquad (4)$$

where P is tracheal occlusion pressure, t is time from the onset of occluded inspiration (sec) and a and b are constants. The constant a represents the occlusion pressure at 1 sec, while b is a dimentionless index of the shape of rising limb of the occlusion pressure wave. For a linear pressure-time profile b is equal to 1, whereas $b < 1$ represents a profile with upward convexity, and $b > 1$ downward convexity. In our adult cats anesthetized with sodium pentobarbital b averaged about 1, whereas with enflurane and ketamine the corresponding values were 0.7 and 0.5, respectively. In each case, b was virtually independent of anesthetic dose and alveolar P_{CO2}.

It appears therefore, that in adult cats the airway occlusion pressure waveform changes markedly with different anesthetics. Whether this reflects changes in waveform of intrinsically generated central inspiratory activity (7-10) or changes at a more peripheral level (e.g. spinal cord and inspiratory muscles) remains as yet to be elucidated. It is clear, however, that in adult cats the temporal pattern of inspiratory driving pressure, as reflected by the airway occlusion pressure wave, determines the shape of the inspiratory spirogram. Thus, when dP/dt is nearly constant (as for sodium pentobarbital) also dV/dt is nearly constant ; whereas with both enflurane and ketamine both dP/dt and dV/dt decrease progressively during inspiration. Since in the latter case the flow is higher at the beginning than during the later course of inspiration, a reduction of T_I will be clearly advantageous for achieving high overall inspiratory flows (and hence high $\dot{V}_E$'s). No such advantage will obtain by shortening T_I for a linear inspiratory volume-time profile. In this connection it should be noted that in some newborn (1 day old) rabbits the inspiratory spirogram is markedly convex downward (11). Since in this instance dV/dt increases progressively with T_I, a longer T_I will of course result in a higher overall mean inspiratory flow.

In conclusion, ventilation depends on both T_I/T_{TOT} and V_T/T_I (equation 2). For curvilinear inspiratory volume-time profiles, V_T/T_I depends on both T_I and shape of the inspiratory spirogram. The latter, as well as the airway occlusion pressure waveform, differ with different anesthetics.

REFERENCES

(1) J.S. Haldane and J.G. Priestley, The regulation of the lung-ventilation, J. Physiol. (London) 32, 225 (1905).

(2) J. Barcroft and R. Margaria, Some effects of carbonic acid on the character of human respiration, J. Physiol. (London) 72, 175 (1931).

(3) J.-P. Derenne, J. Couture, S. Iscoe, W.A. Whitelaw and J. Milic-Emili, Occlusion pressures in men rebreathing CO_2 under methoxyflurane anesthesia, J. Appl. Physiol. 40, 805 (1976).

(4) I. Wyszogrodski, B.T. Thach and J. Milic-Emili, Maturation of respiratory control in unanesthetized newborn rabbits, J. Appl. Physiol. : Respirat. Environ. Exercise Physiol. 44, 304 (1978).

(5) M. Mazzarelli, R. Chiolero and J. Milic-Emili, Effect of enflurane on control of breathing in cats, J. Appl. Physiol. : Respirat. Environ. Exercise Physiol. (Accepted for publication).

(6) M.M. Grunstein, M. Younes and J. Milic-Emili, Control of tidal volume and respiratory frequency in anesthetized cats, J. Appl. Physiol. 35, 463 (1973).

(7) C. von Euler, I. Martilla, J.E. Remmers and T. Trippenbach, Effects of lesions in the parabrachial nucleus on the mechanisms for central and reflex termination of inspiration in the cat, Acta Physiol. Scand. 96, 324 (1976).

(8) C. von Euler and T. Trippenbach, Excitability changes of the inspiratory "off-switch" mechanism tested by electrical stimulation in nucleus parabrachialis in the cat, Acta Physiol. Scand. 97, 175 (1976).

(9) M.M. Grunstein and J. Milic-Emili, Analysis of interactions between central and vagal respiratory control mechanisms in cats, IEEE Trans. Biomedical Eng. 25, 225 (1978).

(10) T. Trippenbach and J. Milic-Emili, Temperature and CO_2 effect on phrenic activity and tracheal occlusion pressure, J. Appl. Physiol. : Respirat. Environ. Exercise Physiol. 43, 449 (1977).

(11) M.S. Goldberg, and J. Milic-Emili, Effect of pentobarbital sodium on respiratory control in newborn rabbits, J. Appl. Physiol. : Respirat. Environ. Exercise Physiol. 42, 845 (1977).

DISCUSSION

It was pointed out by Widdicombe that the shape of the inspiratory trajectory can be drastically changed by various inspiration-facilitating reflexes e.g. from the larynx.

Euler drew attention to earlier work showing that changes in chemical drive (PCO_2) does not change the relative time course ($\frac{1}{2}$ time) of the phrenic trajectory (see Bruce et al. in this volume) whereas changes in body temperature, presumably by effects mediated from the anterior hypothalamus, causes very pronounced effects on the shape of the phrenic trajectory both in relative and absolute terms. This suggests that the different inputs from central chemoreceptors, anterior hypothalamus and vagal defence reflex afferents are affecting the CIA generator in different ways. Milic-Emili's results seem to show that with respect to its effect on CIA pentobarbitone mimic specifically the effects of reductions in the input from the chemoreceptors.

Attention was further drawn to work suggesting that one action of pentobarbitone is to enhance the GABA-mechanisms for inhibition (e.g. Nicoll et al., Nature, 258, 625, 1975; Nicoll, Science 199, 451, 1978) and that topical applications of pentobarbitone and of GABA (Dr. G.Wennergren, personal communication) on the chemoceptive areas on the ventral surface of medulla causes depression of respiration similar to hypocapnia.

GRADED INSPIRATORY INHIBITION: THE FIRST STAGE OF INSPIRATORY "OFF-SWITCHING"

J. E. REMMERS, J. P. BAKER, JR. and M. K. YOUNES

Departments of Medicine and Physiology and Biophysics,
The University of Texas Medical Branch, Galveston, Texas, U.S.A.

The mammalian respiratory rhythm consists of two repetitively alternating motions, and for each mechanical phase a characteristic central neural counterpart has been identified. Investigators have questioned the neuronal basis of this rhythm, but no single mechanistic explanation has been established. One approach is to treat separately the two respiratory phases and examine the initiation and termination of each phase. We have focused on one such question, namely: what neuronal mechanisms terminate the inspiratory phase? The present communication reports our results derived from the barbiturate anesthetized, paralyzed cat, ventilated with 100% O_2 by a servorespirator.

INSPIRATORY OFF-SWITCHING IN TWO STAGES

In this preparation, inspiratory neuronal activity, once initiated, develops in a pre-programmed way appropriate to the particular level of chemical stimulus (1,2). Ultimately, it is terminated either by vagally mediated feedback or by the action of the so-called pneumotaxic area (3,4). If neither is effective, inspiratory activity reaches a limiting value and continues for a prolonged period. Recent results (5) demonstrate that volume feedback switches off the inspiratory phase in two distinct stages:

> Stage 1 - graded, reversible suppression of inspiratory activity.
> Stage 2 - complete and irreversible cessation of inspiration.

These two stages appear to constitute a necessary sequence, since inspiratory termination (Stage 2) ensues only after the suppression of phrenic discharge has reached adequate proportions during Stage 1 (6). In other words, engagement of the neuronal process responsible for termination appears to be contingent upon prior establishment of a critical level of reversible inhibition.

GLOBAL CHARACTERISTICS OF STAGE 1 INHIBITION

Stage 1 inhibition can be viewed as the output component of a reflex loop initiated by vagal afferent information. Two features characterize Stage 1 inhibition:

Gradation

The degree of suppression of phrenic efferent discharge during Stage 1 depends upon lung volume (or some related variable) and inspiratory time (5). Using constant flow, volume ramps introduced after varying delays allows systematic investigation of this dependence as shown in Fig. 1. The lung volume (above FRC) associated with first detectable inhibition (inhibitory threshold) declines during

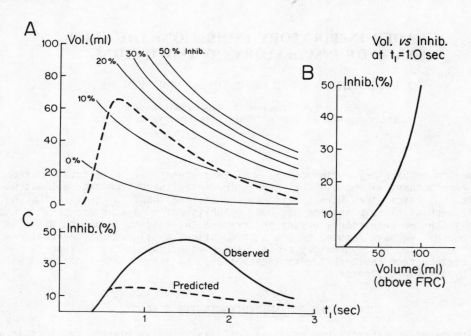

Fig. 1. Average results from a typical experiment. Panel A: Iso-inhibition curves for various values of constant fractional reduction in phrenic neurogram constructed from average phrenic inhibition during constant flow, volume ramps. Dashed curve: time course of volume during controlled volume withdrawal test. Panel B: Exponential relationship between volume and fractional inhibition derived from iso-inhibition curves in A at inspiratory time (T$_I$) = 1.0 sec. Panel C: Predicted (---) and observed (——) time course of averaged phrenic inhibition during controlled volume withdrawal test.

inspiration (bottom curve, Fig. 1). Similar relationships hold for other particular values of fractional reduction in phrenic neurogram, e.g., 10%, 20%, 30%, etc. Each hyperbolic iso-inhibition curve resembles the volume versus time relationship reported by Clark and Euler using peak phrenic as an index of inspiratory termination (1). This family of iso-inhibition curves constitutes an inhibitory band or zone which quantitates the magnitude of phrenic inhibition associated with any particular volume at any particular inspiratory time.

Reversibility

Withdrawal of the inhibitory input (e.g., decrease in lung volume or cessation of

a vagal stimulus) at the appropriate time leads to a resurgence of phrenic activity and, ultimately, the phrenic neurogram returns toward the uninhibited level
(5). The limiting or maximal value of reversible inhibition is difficult to
determine experimentally, but values as high as 90% have been reversed. Latency
between stimulus withdrawal and reversal is substantial (100-400 msec), suggesting
that the vagal input possesses delays of considerable magnitude.

INPUT-OUTPUT RELATIONSHIP FOR STAGE 1 INHIBITION

Inhibition of phrenic efferent discharge appears to serve as a useful index of
reflex response. What variable represents the input, or stimulus? Presuming that
vagally innervated receptor activity initiates Stage 1 inhibition in our preparation, airflow as well as volume should be important (7); most pulmonary stretch
receptors respond to flow rate because they transduce large airway transmural
pressure (8,9) and because they possess inherent dynamic responsiveness (10).
Moreover, if "irritant" receptors contribute to the reflex action, airflow should
determine, to some extent, inhibitory output. However, experiments designed to
identify a specific contribution of flow rate to Stage 1 inhibition failed to bear
out our expectations; we compared families of iso-inhibition curves generated with
high and low flow rates and found them to be superimposible (11). In other words,
lung volume above FRC sufficed to predict the magnitude of inhibition at any time.
The specificity of lung volume is probably more apparent than real. We propose
that the substantial central delays, mentioned above, probably manifest integrative processing of vagal input. In other words, processing delays might offset
the flow sensitivity of pulmonary stretch receptor activity, so that inhibition
correlates with volume, independent of flow.

One can examine the overall input-output characteristics of Stage 1 inhibition at
any particular time, as shown in Fig. 1B. Inhibition bears a characteristic relation to volume - successive increments in volume above the inhibitory threshold
produce progressively greater increments in inhibition (Fig. 1B). This non-
linearity has functional implications for the dynamics of inspiratory off-switching. For instance, a constant flow volume trajectory within the inhibitory band
will produce accelerating inhibition until a critical value can be achieved,
whereupon Stage 2 ensues. Also noteworthy in this regard, mechanical or neural
feedback delays can be expected to increase the probability that inhibition will
progress up to the value required for triggering irreversible inhibition. These
two effects promote inspiratory termination and lessen the possibility that Stage
1 will be protracted.

The exponential nature of the volume-inhibition relationship suggests a central
integrative process. Results obtained by manipulating the volume trajectory
within the family of iso-inhibition curves supports this speculation (12).
Single breath tests were performed wherein inspiration was not terminated during
inflation, and the subsequent time course of volume withdrawal was adjusted to
approximate the 10-15% iso-inhibition lines (dashed curve, Fig. 1A). Accordingly,
this procedure should produce a nearly constant, low level of phrenic inhibition
for a protracted period (dashed curve, Fig. 1C). However, the observed inhibition
consistently rose to unexpectedly high levels over a 1 sec interval (solid curve,
Fig. 1C) and then declined to the predicted value over a similar interval. This
"overshoot" in inhibitory output seems to reflect central neural integration of
volume information during Stage 1 inhibition. These results may underestimate the
magnitude of this behavior inasmuch as the activity of pulmonary stretch receptors
is less, for any particular volume, during expiratory than inspiratory flow.

NEURONAL CORRELATES OF OFF-SWITCHING

The two stages of inspiratory off-switching presumably derive from distinct but closely related actions of brain stem respiratory neurons. Since the general characteristics of switching persist after bilateral "pneumotaxic area" lesions, we suspect that medullary structures are responsible for switching in our preparation. We have, therefore, explored the nucleus of the solitary tract (NTS) with metal microelectrodes seeking neurons whose discharge relates to phrenic inhibition under control conditions and during a variety of single inspiration tests.

We have identified single units that discharge only in association with Stage 1 inhibition during control breathing as shown in Fig. 2b. Similar neuronal behavior has been described by Feldman and Cohen (12). Single breath tests were introduced by changing respirator gain, thereby changing the interrelationship between time, volume and phrenic amplitude during <u>Stage 1</u>. In all cases, the timing of neuronal firing shifted and maintained a close association with Stage 1 inhibition (Figs. 2a and 2c). The onset of discharge preceded the onset of inhibition by 100-500 msec, and firing frequency roughly paralleled the magnitude of

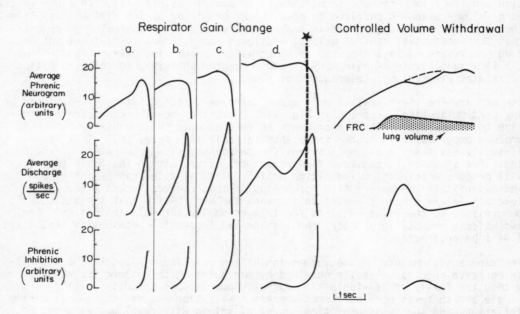

Fig. 2. Average phrenic neurograms and average discharge of a possible "switch" neuron during various single breath tests. Left panel: change in gain of servorespirator; right panel: controlled volume withdrawal test. Segment b: control gain; segments a and c: 2 fold increase and decrease in gain, respectively; segment d: respirator off (lung volume held at FRC). Only the terminal portions of the phrenic neurogram are shown in b, c and d. Shaded area shows the time course of volume during controlled volume withdrawal test. Bottom row gives average phrenic inhibition for each test.

inhibition (Figs. 2a, b and c, second row). That this type of neuron is specifically linked to inspiratory off-switching is also evidenced by its augmenting
pattern coincident with spontaneous termination of an apneustic inspiration when
lung volume is held at FRC. Finally, the controlled volume withdrawal maneuver,
described above, produced a burst of firing that preceded and paralleled the inhibitory wave (Fig. 2, right panel). We, therefore, speculate that this type of
neuron qualifies as a putative "switch" neuron, mediating Stage 1 inhibition.
Overall, average phrenic inhibition in these various tests correlates closely with
the square of average firing frequency. Discharge versus inhibition plots for the
various test maneuvers are curvilinear, reminiscent of the exponential volume
versus inhibition plot (Fig. 1B). This suggests that "integrative" processing of
volume related information occurs closer to the ultimate site of inspiratory inhibition.

A remarkable feature of this putative off-switch neuron is that during an apneustic inspiration its firing appears just prior to the onset of the plateau in the

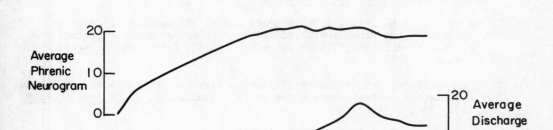

Fig. 3. Average phrenic neurogram and average discharge
rate, for cell shown in Fig. 2, during respirator off tests
(lung volume held at FRC). Note that single unit activity
appears shortly before onset of apneustic plateau.

phrenic neurogram (Fig. 3). During the plateau phase, the neuron discharges at a
low level. This observation raises the possibility that the apneustic plateau
represents, to some extent, an inhibitory process related to Stage 1 inhibition.

SUMMARY

In the barbiturate anesthetized cat, inspiration is switched off by volume feedback in two sequential stages: Stage 1 - reversible, graded inhibition of inspiratory motor output; and Stage 2 - irreversible termination of inspiratory
activity. During lung inflation, Stage 1 inhibition correlates with lung volume
above FRC, independent of the rate of airflow. The apparent lack of influence of

flow rate probably derives from integrative delays within the CNS.

Solitary tract neurons can be identified whose discharge correlates with the magnitude of Stage 1 inhibition under a variety of conditions, suggesting that these specialized neurons mediate the inhibition. The neurons also fire during the apneustic plateau.

ACKNOWLEDGEMENTS

The authors express their appreciation to Ms. Angela Barksdale for technical assistance.

This research was supported in part by National Heart and Lung Institute Grant HL-18007. J. P. Baker, Jr. was supported by National Heart and Lung Institute Training Grant 1T32 HL-07217. J. E. Remmers is the recipient of a National Institute of Health Pulmonary Academic Award 5K07 HL-00131.

REFERENCES

(1) F. J. Clark and C. von Euler, On the regulation of depth and rate of breathing, J. Physiol. London 222, 267-295 (1972).

(2) C. von Euler, I. Marttila, J. E. Remmers and T. Trippenbach, Effects of lesions in the parabrachial nucleus on the mechanisms for central and reflex termination of inspiration in the cat, Acta Physiol. Scand. 96, 324-337 (1976).

(3) M. I. Cohen, Switching of the respiratory phases and evoked phrenic responses produced by rostral pontine electrical stimulation, J. Physiol. London 217, 133-158 (1971).

(4) C. von Euler and T. Trippenbach, Excitability changes of the inspiratory "off-switch" mechanism tested by electrical stimulation in Nucleus Parabrachialis in the cat, Acta Physiol. Scand. 97, 175-188 (1976).

(5) M. K. Younes, J. E. Remmers and J. Baker, Characteristics of inspiratory inhibition by phasic volume feedback in cats, J. Appl. Physiol. 45, 80-86 (1978).

(6) M. Younes, J. P. Baker, J. Polacheck and J. E. Remmers, Termination of inspiration through graded inhibition of inspiratory activity, In: The Regulation of Respiration During Sleep and Anesthesia, Plenum Press, New York, 383-395 (1978).

(7) H. L. Davis, W. S. Fowler and E. H. Lambert, Effect of volume and rate of inflation and deflation on transpulmonary pressure and response of pulmonary stretch receptors, Am. J. Physiol. 187, 558-566 (1956).

(8) G. Miserocchi, J. Mortola and G. Sant'Ambrogio, Localization of pulmonary stretch receptors in the airways of the dog, J. Physiol. London 235, 775-782 (1973).

(9) D. Bartlett, Jr., P. Jefferey, G. Sant'Ambrogio and J. C. M. Wise, Location of stretch receptors in the trachea and bronchi of the dog, J. Physiol. London 258, 409-420 (1976).

(10) D. Bartlett, Jr., G. Sant'Ambrogio and J. C. M. Wise, Transduction properties of tracheal stretch receptors, J. Physiol. London 258, 421-432 (1976).

(11) J. P. Baker, J. E. Remmers and M. Younes, Effect of instantaneous flow rate on inspiratory termination, Physiologist 20, 5 (1977).

(12) J. P. Baker, Jr. and J. E. Remmers, Characteristics of sustained inspiratory inhibition by controlled volume trajectory, Physiologist 21, 4 (1978).

(13) J. L. Feldman, M. I. Cohen and P. Wolotsky, Phasic pulmonary afferent activity drastically alters the respiratory modulation of neurons in the rostral pontine pneumotaxic centre, In: Respiratory Centres and Afferent Systems, INSERM, Paris, 95-105 (1976).

DISCUSSION

Lipski asked whether the neurons which were found to correlate with the graded inhibition would correspond to any of the previously known groups such as R_β neurons or early expiratory neurons. Remmers replied that in agreement with Feldman and Cohen, he believed that these neurons were of a different population since they did not show the criteria of R_β neurons nor of early expiratory cells.

Euler asked whether the results would be consistent with his idea that in the type of apneusis which can occur at certain levels of anaesthesia the apneustic plateau of inspiratory activity might reflect a regulated level of activity 'riding', as it were, on the threshold for graded inhibition: An increase in inspiratory activity and CIA would cause an increase in graded inhibition leading to a fall of CIA (and the inspiratory activity) to just below the threshold for graded inhibition. This in turn would permit CIA (and the inspiratory activity) to increase and again attain this threshold and be inhibited. This would be a model of another mechanism for apneusis in addition to, or instead of, the model depicting the apneustic activity due to that   the thresholds for the inspiratory 'off-switch' mechanisms is raised above reach for CIA. Remmers reported that they had obtained preliminary results which seemed to support this hypothesis. Their results, Remmers said, were also consistent with the hypothesis that R_α neurons are feeding into R_β cells and from there into the inspiratory 'off-switch' mechanisms.

REFLEX AND CENTRAL MECHANISMS CONTROLLING EXPIRATORY DURATION

C. K. KNOX

Laboratory of Neurophysiology, University of Minnesota,
Minneapolis, Minnesota, U.S.A.

INTRODUCTION

Although considerable attention has been paid to the brainstem
mechanisms underlying the generation of central inspiratory activity
(CIA) and the control of its rate of rise and final amplitude, there
exists the equally important question of how the expiratory (E) phase
of the respiratory cycle is controlled. At the simplest level of the
automatic control of eupneic breathing, where expiration is accomplished mainly by passive recoil of the lungs and chest wall with
little or no activity in the expiratory musculature, it can be assumed
that at the very least there are central mechanisms which serve to
set the expiratory duration (T_E) so the lungs can adequately empty.
With increased demand for ventilation, activation of the expiratory
musculature adds yet another dimension to the control problem. And
at the most complicated levels of control, it is known that the automatic mechanisms may be temporarily overridden by volitional control
via the corticobulbar and corticospinal pathways to the brainstem and
spinal cord.

In our studies we have been concerned with the brainstem mechanisms
responsible for the control of T_E at the simplest level of the automatic control of breathing, and have attempted to characterize the
system by examining its reflex behavior. Among many reflexes affecting T_E, we have chosen to study the Breuer-Hering lung inflation and
deflation reflexes because of the ease with which lung volume changes
can be produced and quantitated, and because the two reflexes provide
both inhibitory and excitatory inputs to the system. Our method of
study has been to determine the dynamic characteristics of these
reflexes, in the anesthetized or decerebrate cat, by applying servo-
controlled changes in lung volume and noting the resultant changes in
T_E, as defined neurally by cessation and onset of phrenic nerve discharge. This technique has also been used in conjunction with electrical stimulation and discrete lesioning of rostral and caudal
pontine structures in an effort to determine the possible contributions of these portions of the brainstem respiratory complex to the
control of T_E.

In general, our results support the hypothesis set forward by Larrabee

and Hodes (1) thirty years ago that at the bulbo-pontine level of
control, T_E is determined by the time course of activity in a pool of
central inspiratory inhibitory (CII) neurons whose activity is largest
early in expiration and then gradually decays during expiration to a
level at which inspiratory (I) neurons are released. The well known
properties of the Breuer-Hering reflexes (2,3), that inflations produce graded increases in T_E and deflations decrease T_E, suggest that
the afferent inputs from slowly adapting stretch and irritant receptors
which are responsible for the reflexes (4,5,6), have relatively unim-
peded access to the CII pool during expiration. These reflex properties are much different from those during the I phase, where, as has
been well documented (7), there exists an "off-switch" threshold for
the inhibition of I neurons to which inputs from slowly adapting
stretch receptors contribute. As to the neural correlates for this
hypothetical CII pool, and whether or not it also serves as the I
off-switch mechanism, I shall speculate on later. Suffice it to say
for now that our results to date would indicate that it resides in
the medulla and is modulated by, but does not depend on, inputs from
the pons.

PROPERTIES OF THE CII POOL

The Inflation Reflex

Inflation of the lungs above functional residual capacity (FRC) during expiration in the pentobarbital anesthetized or the decerebrate
cat increases T_E, and the magnitude of the increase depends on both
size and duration of the inflation (8). Pulse inflations of rather
short duration will increase T_E. The increase is somewhat dependent
on the time into expiration (T_P) when the pulse is applied, becoming
greater with increasing T_P. Inflations are effective only during the
initial approximately 70% of a control expiratory duration (T_{EC})
(Fig. 1). The inhibitory ratio T_E/T_{EC} is greater than one and related

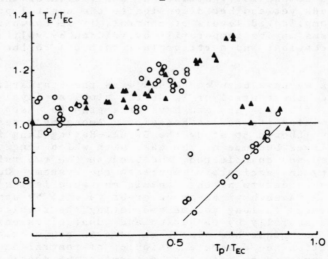

Fig. 1 Prolongation of T_E produced by pulse
inflations. Results from two deeply anesthetized cats (T_{EC}=2.0 and 2.1). Inflation pulses
were of tidal volume size and 200 msec in

duration. Filled triangles are responses
typically observed. Open circles show results
from one cat in which rapid inflations late
in expiration activated the deflation reflex
mediated by irritant receptors. Redrawn from
Knox (8).

to the product of pulse amplitude and pulse duration. These data
imply that the effect of inflations on CII activity is a modulatory
one with properties of integration over time, and they rule out other
types of mechanisms such as resetting of activity to some baseline
level. The integrative property of the reflex suggests a mechanism
with a rather long internal time constant and is consistent with a
slow decay of CII activity during expiration in the absence of vagal
feedback.

Step inflations of varying amplitude applied at variable times (T_S)
in the E phase again result in values of T_E/T_{EC} which are larger
with larger step sizes; however, dependency on T_S is also evident.
For small step inflations, T_E/T_{EC} decreases with T_S, but for step
inflations of control eupneic tidal volume amplitude (V_{TC}) and larger,
T_E/T_{EC} tends to increase with T_S. The response to small steps again
indicates that integration occurs within the CII pool. The progressive deviation from integrative behavior as step size increases suggests
an additional transient component in the activity of the CII pool in
response to stretch receptor input.

The Deflation Reflex

When the lungs are deflated below FRC T_E decreases. This reflex has
both graded and threshold properties and it is the threshold property
which is of some interest, since it provides more direct evidence for
a slowly decaying CII activity. Early in the E phase the deflation
pressure required to reach the threshold for E to I switching is
largest (typically -6 to -10 cm H_2O) and with time into expiration
progressively declines until it reaches zero some 100 to 200 ms before
the onset of the next inspiration.

Previous investigators have emphasized that irritant receptors are
called into play by inhaling irritant substances (9,10), or by forced
deflations or by atelectasis of the lungs (6). However, our studies
suggest that because the deflation reflex threshold is low late in
expiration they may normally facilitate E to I switching as lung
volume returns to FRC.

The Inflation Sensitive Phase

As mentioned above, when the lungs are inflated T_E is increased only
if the inflation falls during the initial approximately 70% of T_{EC}.
During the final 30% of the phase, inflations up to two or three
times V_{TC} are without effect on T_E (T_E/T_{EC}=1). This raises two questions: (1) are there mechanisms for actively inhibiting stretch
receptor input late in expiration, or (2) is the inhibitory effect of
stretch receptor input eventually offset by discharge of irritant
receptors responding to lung inflations? Several kinds of evidence
favor the first alternative: (1) changing the amount of CO_2 in the
inspired gas or the depth of anesthesia (8), or the body temperature
(11) changes T_E but not the proportion of the inflation sensitive

phase to T_{EC}. (2) The duration of the sensitive phase is independent of inflation size for inflations up to twice V_{TC}. A response of irritant receptors to inflations might be expected to progressively reduce the duration of the sensitive phase as inflation size increased (3) Electrical stimulation in the medial parabrachial nucleus (NPBM) which increases T_E (see below) is effective only during the initial inflation sensitive phase. (4) The proportion of the inflation sensitive phase to T_{EC} may be altered by discrete lesions in the caudal pons (see below). (5) Normally, with lung inflations, values of T_E/T_{EC} abruptly return to one during the final 30% of T_{EC}. When there is evidence of irritant receptor activation the data fall on the deflation reflex threshold curve late in T_E (Fig. 1).

Coupling of the Inspiratory and Expiratory Phases

In their studies of the mechanisms controlling rate and depth of breathing, Clark and Euler (12) concluded that T_E is partly determined centrally by the factors which determine T_I, independent of vagal feedback during expiration. Thus, if inspiration is terminated prematurely, by inflating the lungs or electrically stimulating the vagus nerves, the following T_E is shortened. The "timing-relationship" also holds true as T_I shortens during conditions of increased CO_2 with the vagus nerves intact. Zechman, et al. (13), studying the volume-time relationships in anesthetized cats using resistive loads, failed to find a correlation of T_E with the preceding T_I. When V_T was reduced and T_I increased with an added resistance during inspiration, T_E remained unaltered from control values.

Resistive loads differ from lung inflations, however, in that they result in decreased pulmonary stretch receptor activity and increased CIA at the time of I off-switch, whereas inflations produce just the opposite pattern of activity. Taken together, these results would suggest that the linkage between the T_I and T_E controlling mechanisms is perhaps more directly related to the amount of stretch receptor feedback existing at the time of I cutoff and its effect on subsequent CII activity. To test this hypothesis we have examined the step response characteristics of the inflation and deflation reflexes during the E phase following premature termination of the preceding inspiration with inflation pulses. The effect of such a maneuver on the unperturbed T_E is to shorten it. Even so, when the lungs are inflated with a step volume change during the conditioned expiration, the inhibitory ratio remains unchanged from the case of a normal expiration (8). This behavior is shown by the data of Fig. 2, taken from a pentobarbital anesthetized cat, in which the E phase inflation reflex characteristics were determined with ¼ V_{TC} steps for three different values of preceding V_T-T_I. The inhibitory ratio is referred to the T_{EC} of the unperturbed, unconditioned expiration. Although the inflation sensitive phase changes with the conditioned T_E, the inhibitory ratio early in E remains essentially constant at 1.3 to 1.4. These data suggest that in the face of such a decreased T_E there is an increase in the gain of the inflation reflex which results in a nearly constant prolongation of T_E. Evidence that inflating the lungs during inspiration does result in increased excitability of the CII pool during the E phase was obtained in similar types of experiments in which the deflation reflex threshold was determined in conditioned expirations, as shown in Fig. 3. Here the tracheal deflation pressure below ambient required to produce E to I switching is plotted against time into expiration (referred to the unconditioned T_{EC}) for three

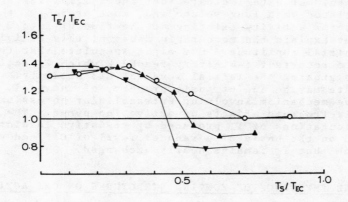

Fig. 2 E phase inflation reflex characteristics after prematurely terminating the
preceding inspiration with an inflation pulse.
Circles: Normal inspiration, V_{TC}=30 ml, T_{IC}=
1.3 sec, T_{EC}=1.2 sec; Filled triangles: V_T=
45 ml, T_I=0.85 sec; Filled inverted triangles:
V_T=65 ml, T_I=0.5 sec. Redrawn from Knox (8).

different values of preceding V_T-T_I. The threshold increases significantly with increased I phase vagal feedback and decays more rapidly
with time.

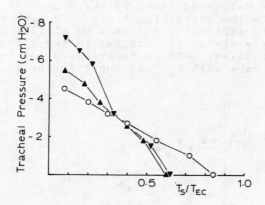

Fig. 3 E phase deflation reflex threshold.
Circles: Normal inspiration, V_{TC}=35 ml, T_{IC}=
1.25 sec, T_{EC}=1.25 sec; Filled Triangles:
V_T=40 ml, T_I=1.1 sec; Filled inverted triangles:
V_T=50 ml, T_I=0.95 sec (Knox, unpublished).

Thus far, then, our data indicate that the initial level of CII activity is correlated with lung volume and, most probably, the amount of stretch receptor activity existing at the time of I to E switching. We cannot yet explain the more rapid decay of this activity with increased initial amplitude. One might speculate that the CII pool is subject to recurrent inhibitory feedback which is activated more strongly the greater the initial level of CII activity. Alternatively the decay rate may be an intrinsic property of the pool, e.g., an accommodative mechanism involving extracellular potassium ion accumulation or electrogenic effects of active ion pumps. The constancy of T_E with prolongations of T_I produced by resistive loading (13) could be explained on the basis of a reduced level of CII and a slower rate of decay such that T_E remains nearly unchanged.

THE INFLUENCE OF PONTINE STRUCTURES ON CII ACTIVITY

The Rostral Pons

It is well established that neurons in the parabrachial/Kölliker-Fuse nuclear complex (NPB) play a role in modulating the activities of lower brainstem respiratory neurons. A number of studies employing electrical stimulation and discrete lesioning of NPB have revealed that it exerts both inhibitory as well as facilitatory influences on medullary I neurons (14,15,16,17,18,19,20,21). During the E phase, electrical stimulation of the more ventral portions of NPB results in prolongation of T_E. The effects of short stimulus trains are quite similar to those of pulse inflations (15, cf. Fig. 1), that is, T_E is increased even though the stimulus ends well before the end of expiration, and there is a tendency for the prolongation to increase as the stimulus is delivered later in the phase. As shown in Fig. 4, the effects of stimulus trains applied to the same site beginning at varying times T_S in expiration and left on until E to I switching occurs (crosses) are again very similar to the effects of step lung inflations (open circles). There is evidence for integration (the prolongation decreases with T_S) and the stimulus is effective only

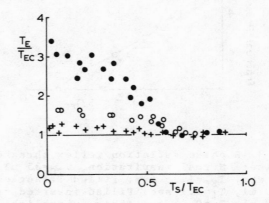

Fig. 4 Interaction of lung inflation reflex
and electrical stimulation applied to ventral
NPB. Redrawn from Knox and King (21).

during the inflation sensitive phase. The combined effects of stimulation and lung inflation (filled circles) are greater than the sum
of either input applied alone. These results are all consistent with
a summation of the excitatory effects of the two separate inputs at a
common functional pool of neurons whose output is directed to I inhibitory neurons. Electrical stimulation of more dorsal and lateral
regions of the NPB complex produces I-facilitatory effects, with a
threshold characteristic for E to I switching similar to that for the
lung deflation reflex (14,15).

The results obtained using electrical stimulation of the NPB complex
are suggestive of this structure playing a role in control of T_E;
however, they are not conclusive. There is no reason to suppose that
the responses to electrical stimulation are similar to normal patterns
of activity generated within NPB. Furthermore, the use of electrical
stimulation is complicated by the fact that, as King has shown (22),
the reciprocal pathways which interconnect the respiratory regions of
the medulla and NPB intermingle and course together, running through
the ventrolateral medulla, turning dorsally and rostrally between the
7th nerve and superior olive, and anterior to the trigeminal complex.
Thus, in stimulating near this pathway one cannot rule out the possibility that the effects seen are not due to antidromic activation of
neurons in the medulla which project to NPB.

By placing discrete lesions in the NPB complex it has been possible
to deduce something of its normal function, at least in the anesthetized or the decerebrate cat. Such lesions result in an elevation of
the vagal threshold characteristic for I off-switch (19,20,21) with
no change in the constant describing rate of decay of the curve (19,
21). This would imply that the NPB complex contributes a tonic threshold lowering input to the I off-switch, but does not affect the
time-dependency of this mechanism. During the E phase the gain of
the inflation reflex, as measured by the inhibitory ratio T_E/T_{EC} with
step inflations, is increased by a factor of approximately two.
Otherwise, the qualitative shape of the step response curves remains
the same, including the ratio of the inflation sensitive phase to T_{EC}
(21). This result suggests again that the NPB complex is not the
primary T_E controller, but rather contributes a modulating influence
which in this case may normally inhibit the CII pool. This finding
is somewhat paradoxical in view of the fact that the gain of the
inflation reflex is, in effect, decreased by lesion during the I phase.
The E phase deflation reflex threshold curve shows, however, that
lesions result in a much reduced rate of decay of CII activity late
in expiration, with no change from prelesion values early in the
phase (21). Thus, the same increment in CII activity in response to
any given inflation step could result in an increased prolongation of
T_E as compared to prelesion. One might speculate, then, that the NPB
complex is also involved in E to I switching, either through late
expiratory inhibition of CII activity or by late expiratory facilitation of I neurons.

The Caudal Pons

In the classical view of the neural control of respiration it has
been held that certain caudal pontine structures provide I facilitatory
influences to medullary neurons which produce apneusis after removal
of rostral pontine and vagal I inhibitory inputs (see Mitchell and
Berger (23) for a review of the earlier literature in this area).
After destruction of the rostral pons, a transection through the

caudal pons partially restores normal breathing patterns. Recently
it has been shown that bilateral lesion of a portion of the medial
reticular formation at the ponto-medullary junction in the cat has
the same effect (24). The site would appear to lie on either side of
the midline in the gigantocellular (FTG) and magnocellular (FTM)
tegmental fields at the level of the facial nucleus (P7 to P9) (nomen
clature after Berman, 25). This site is somewhat rostral to the
regions near the midline in the medulla which were described by Pitts
et al. (26) as the inspiratory and expiratory 'centers,' on the basis
of the effects of electrical stimulation. Anderson and Sears (27)
reexamined the question as to whether or not the I apneusis produced
by stimulation of more medial and ventral portions of the medullary
reticular formation could be considered a true respiratory response.
They concluded that it was not, but rather that it represented an
activation of the medullary contingent of the reticulospinal tracts
which interact at the segmental level with inputs carrying normal
respiratory rhythm. Electrophysiological studies (28,29) have shown
that there are two reticulospinal projection systems with cell bodies
located near the midline in FTG and FTM of the caudal pons and rostra
medulla. The FTG component lies more dorsal and rostral at the ponto
medullary junction and projects its axons mainly in the ventromedial
reticulospinal tract. The FTM component is situated more ventrally
and posteriorly projecting mainly in the ipsilateral lateral reticulo
spinal tract. It is apparently the rostral portion of FTM which,
when lesioned, partially restores normal breathing after apneusis
promoting lesions of NPBM (24). Electrical stimulation of FTG in the
decerebrate cat increases extensor rigidity while producing I to E
switching and prolongation of T_E, whereas, stimulation of FTM reduces
extensor rigidity and causes E to I switching and I apneusis (30,31,
32, and unpublished observations). These observations support
Stellas' (33) conclusions that decerebrate rigidity and I apneusis
result from different mechanisms.

Although there are undoubtedly interactions of the reticulospinal and
rhythmic respiratory inputs at the segmental level, the phase switching produced by electrical stimulation within FTG and FTM suggests
that interactions also occur within the medulla and/or caudal pons.
To test this hypothesis we have been examining the effects of discret
lesions of the medial tegmental field at the pontomedullary junction
on the vagal reflexes of decerebrate cats. The most consistent resul
of a bilateral lesion of FTG in the caudal pons, made at sites where
the electrical threshold is lowest for I to E switching, is a decreas
in T_E together with increased gain of the E phase deflation reflex an
decreased gain of the inflation reflex (Fig. 5). The proportion of
the inflation sensitive phase to T_{EC} also decreases. There are no
significant changes in V_T or T_I. Lesions placed more ventrally and
caudally in FTM, at sites where stimulation causes E to I switching
and I apneusis, result in similar E phase reflex changes and, also,
decreases in V_T and T_I and T_E. Minute volume actually increases,
because the decrease in V_T is not as great, proportionately, as are
the decreases in T_I and T_E.

These results provide evidence that the medial regions of the
reticular formation of caudal pons and rostral medulla are involved
in modifying activity within the respiratory phase switching mechanisms. Furthermore, these reticular influences act more specifically
than, say, generally exciting or inhibiting interneurons within the
vagal sensory pathways, because the lesions affect the two phases of

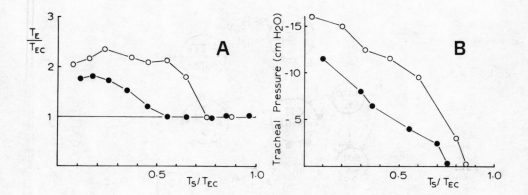

Fig. 5   Effects of FTG lesions on the inflation
and deflation reflexes. Open circles: prelesion,
filled circles, postlesion. A: Increase in T_E
produced by tidal volume size step inflations.
B: Deflation pressure required to produce short
latency E to I switching. Prelesion V_{TC}, T_{TC} and
T_{EC}: 40 ml, 1.2 sec, 1.2 sec; postlesion, 40 ml,
1.1 sec, 0.95 sec (Knox, unpublished).

the respiratory cycle differently. In the case of FTG lesions only
the E phase reflexes are altered. This suggests that neurons of FTG,
or perhaps pathways through FTG, normally provide facilitatory inputs
to the CII pool, which when removed result in less CII activity and,
hence, a decrease in T_E and a shift in the gains of the inflation and
deflation reflexes to favor the deflation reflex. These results also
provide evidence that the I off-switch neurons and the CII neurons
controlling T_E are different functional pools. The effects of FTM
lesions are rather more complicated. However, one could speculate
that FTM primarily inhibits the I off-switch mechanism and that the
changes in E phase reflexes which occur are due to interruption of
pathways from FTG to the lower medulla. In general, the lesion
results are consistent with the results of electrical stimulation of
FTG and FTM. Together they indicate that there are two reticular
pathways which can separately control the two respiratory interneuron
pools responsible for I termination and continued I inhibition during
the E phase.

CONCLUSION

Figure 6 presents in block diagram form some of the central and lung
reflex mechanisms involved in the automatic control of T_E as we have
come to understand them. Central to the scheme is the CII pool. It
is likely to be located in the medulla, and it is shown to receive
excitatory inputs from lung stretch receptors (SR), inhibitory inputs
from irritant receptors (IR) and to in turn inhibit central inspiratory
neurons. Inhibitory feedback from I neurons to the CII pool is included to account for the observations that subthreshold inflations

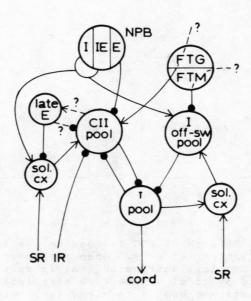

Fig. 6 Functional diagram of the basic control
of expiratory duration. Arrows denote excitation,
filled circles inhibition.

during inspiration have little effect on I activity (cf. 7). The CII
pool is shown as being different from the I off-switch pool for the
reasons discussed above. Late expiratory neurons are postulated to
inhibit stretch receptor inputs and possibly the CII pool, to account
for the inflation reflex sensitive portion of T_E and the more rapid
rate of decay of CII activity as this activity becomes larger. The
rate of decay could also be determined by intrinsic properties of the
pool as discussed above. The NPB complex provides inhibitory influences to the CII pool which accelerate the decline of CII activity
late in the E phase. In addition, there may also be excitatory pathways from NPB which sum with stretch receptor inputs. These are
apparently not normally active in the decerebrate cat but do respond
to electrical stimulation. FTG and FTM, or pathways through these
areas, excite and inhibit the CII and I off-switch pools, respectively

The scheme does not include many other inputs which can be assumed to
act on the system, e.g., central and peripheral chemoreceptors and
hypothalamic thermoregulatory inputs. Central chemoreceptive inputs
may facilitate CII activity, since with increased CO_2 the gain of the
E phase inflation reflex increases (8). Similarly, with increased
body temperature there is an increase in gain of the reflex as well
as increased rate of decay of CII activity, suggesting that thermoregulatory inputs act to excite the CII neurons (11). Reflexes from
the extrathoracic airways controlling expiratory air flow might also
modify CII activity (34).

There are a number of neural correlates and pathways that could be
suggested to account for our results. According to the model of

Fig. 6, CII neurons would normally be silent during inspiration,
discharge maximally just after I off-switch and gradually slow in
firing rate with time into expiration. Neurons having such firing
patterns, excited by lung inflation and located in the nucleus of the
solitary tract (NTS) in the rostral medulla have been described by
Feldman and Cohen (35), who reached similar conclusions regarding
their function. There is some evidence that stretch receptor inputs
to the CII and I off-switch pools are mediated by different NTS interneurons. The "P" cells of Berger (36) may transmit this input to the
CII pool, since these cells have quite low inflation thresholds during
the E phase and do not receive central inspiratory drive inputs. The
Iβ cells of NTS have been implicated in transmitting stretch receptor
inputs to the I off-switch pool (7,37). It is difficult to say, at
this point, if the reticulospinal projection neurons of FTG and FTM
are also the cells which influence the CII and I off-switch pools.
Midline tegmental lesions placed more rostrally than P7 in the
decerebrate cat do not significantly affect the lung reflexes (unpublished observations). It is possible, however, that more caudal
FTG/FTM lesions destroy propriobulbar neurons or interrupt crossing
fibers coming from the lateral tegmental field to respiratory interneurons. We have not placed lesions more laterally to test this
possibility because the pathways between the NPB complex and medullary
respiratory areas (22) would be interrupted and thereby complicate
the results. Recent neuroanatomical studies, using horseradish
peroxidase and radioactive amino acid tracing techniques, have so far
revealed no connections from FTG/FTM to the ventral respiratory group
of the medulla, from NPB to FTG/FTM or from FTG/FTM to NPB (22,38,39).
Nevertheless, Vibert, et al. (40,41) have found high density foci of
respiratory modulated units within the medial tegmental field of the
ponto-medullary junction. Whether or not these neurons subserve the
functions discussed here remains an open question.

Our own speculations on neural correlates for the results aside, the
model we have proposed based on functional properties of the lung
reflex mechanisms should provide, it is hoped, a useful framework for
further studies into the neural mechanisms involved in the control of
breathing.

This work was supported by Grant HL16430 from the U.S. Public Health
Service, National Institutes of Health.

REFERENCES

(1) M.G. Larrabee and R. Hodes, Cyclic changes in the respiratory
     centers, revealed by the effects of afferent impulses, Am. J.
     Physiol. 155, 147-164 (1948).

(2) J. Breuer, Die Selbststeurung der Athmung durch den Nervus
     vagus, Sitzungsber. Akad. Wiss. Wien 58 (II), 909-937 (1868).

(3) E. Hering, Die Selbststeurung der Athmung durch den Nervus
     vagus, Sitzungsber. Akad. Wiss. Wien 57 (II), 672-677 (1868).

(4) E.D. Adrian, Afferent impulses in the vagus and their effect on
     respiration, J. Physiol., London 79, 332-358 (1933).

(5)   H. Sellick and J.G. Widdicombe, Vagal deflation and inflation
      reflexes mediated by lung irritant receptors, Quart. J.
      Exptl. Physiol. 55, 153-163 (1970).

(6)   E.A. Koller and P. Ferrer, Studies on the role of the lung
      deflation reflex, Respir. Physiol. 10, 172-183 (1970).

(7)   C. von Euler, The functional organization of the respiratory
      phase-switching mechanisms, Fed. Proc. Am. Physiol. Soc. 36,
      2375-2380 (1977).

(8)   C.K. Knox, Characteristics of inflation and deflation reflexes
      during expiration in the cat, J. Neurophysiol. 36, 284-295
      (1973).

(9)   H. Sellick and J.G. Widdicombe, Stimulation of lung irritant
      receptors by cigarette smoke, carbon dust and histamine
      aerosol, J. Appl. Physiol. 31, 15-19 (1971).

(10) R. Buff and E.A. Koller, Studies on mechanisms underlying the
      reflex hyperpnoea induced by inhalation of chemical irritants,
      Respir. Physiol. 21, 371-383 (1974).

(11) C. von Euler and T. Trippenbach, Temperature effects on the
      inflation reflex during expiratory time in the cat, Acta
      Physiol. Scand. 96, 338-350 (1976).

(12) F.J. Clark and C. von Euler, On the regulation of depth and rate
      of breathing, J. Physiol., London 222, 267-295 (1972).

(13) F.W. Zechman, D.T. Frazier and D.A. Lally, Respiratory volume-
      time relationships during resistive loading in the cat, J.
      Appl. Physiol. 40, 177-183 (1976).

(14) F. Bertrand and A. Hugelin, Respiratory synchronizing function
      of nucleus parabrachialis medialis: pneumotaxic mechanisms,
      J. Neurophysiol. 34, 189-207 (1971).

(15) M.I. Cohen, Switching of the respiratory phases and evoked
      phrenic responses produced by rostral pontine electrical stim-
      ulation, J. Physiol., London 217, 133-158 (1971).

(16) C. von Euler and T. Trippenbach, Excitability changes of the
      inspiratory 'off-switch' mechanism tested by electrical
      stimulation in nucleus parabrachialis in the cat, Acta
      Physiol. Scand. 97, 175-188 (1976).

(17) S.H. Ngai and S.C. Wang, Organization of central respiratory
      mechanisms in the brain stem of the cat: localization by
      stimulation and destruction, Am. J. Physiol. 190, 343-349
      (1957).

(18) W.M. St. John, R.L. Glasser and R.A. King, Apneustic breathing
      after vagotomy in cats with chronic pneumotaxic center lesions,
      Respir. Physiol. 12, 239-250 (1971).

(19) C. von Euler, I. Marttila, J.E. Remmers and T. Trippenbach,
      Effects of lesions in the parabrachial nucleus on the mechan-

isms for central and reflex termination of inspiration in the
cat, Acta Physiol. Scand. 96, 324-337 (1976).

(20) J.L. Feldman and H. Gautier, Interaction of pulmonary afferents
and pneumotaxic center in control of respiratory pattern in
cats, J. Neurophysiol. 39, 31-44 (1976).

(21) C.K. Knox and G.W. King, Changes in the Breuer-Hering reflexes
following rostral pontine lesion, Respir. Physiol. 28, 189-
206 (1976).

(22) G.W. King, A neuroanatomical and neurophysiological investigation of the bulbo-pontine circuits contributing to the
rhythmicity of respiration in the cat, Ph.D. Thesis,
University of Minnesota (1978).

(23) R.A. Mitchell and A.J. Berger, Neural regulation of respiration,
Am. Review of Respir. Disease 3, 206-224 (1975).

(24) W.M. St. John and S.C. Wang, Integration of chemoreceptor stimuli by caudal pontile and rostral medullary sites, J. Appl.
Physiol. 41, 612-622 (1976).

(25) Berman, A.L. (1968) The Brain Stem of the Cat, Univ. of Wisconsin
Press, Madison.

(26) R.F. Pitts, H.W. Magoun and S.W. Ranson, Localization of the
medullary respiratory centers in the cat, Am. J. Physiol. 126,
673-688 (1939).

(27) P. Anderson and T.A. Sears, Medullary activation of intercostal
fusimotor and alpha motoneurones, J. Physiol., London 209,
739-755 (1970).

(28) M. Ito, M. Udo and N. Mano, Long inhibitory and excitatory
pathways converging onto cat reticular and Deiters' neurons
and their relevance to reticulofugal axons, J. Neurophysiol.
33, 210-226 (1970).

(29) B.W. Peterson, R.A. Maunz, N.G. Pitts and R.G. Mackel, Patterns
of projection and branching of reticulospinal neurons, Exp.
Brain Res. 23, 333-351 (1975).

(30) R. Rhines and H.W. Magoun, Brain stem facilitation of cortical
motor response, J. Neurophysiol. 9, 219-229 (1946).

(31) H.W. Magoun and R. Rhines, An inhibitory mechanism in the bulbar
reticular formation, J. Neurophysiol. 9, 165-171 (1946).

(32) R. Llinás and C.A. Terzuolo, Mechanisms of supraspinal actions
upon cord activities. Reticular inhibitory mechanisms on
alpha-extensor motoneurons, J. Neurophysiol. 27, 579-591 (1964).

(33) G. Stella, On the mechanism of production and the physiological
significance of 'apneusis,' J. Physiol., London 93, 10-23
(1938).

(34) J.E. Remmers and D. Bartlett, Jr., Reflex control of expiratory
airflow and duration, J. Appl. Physiol. 42(1), 80-87 (1977).

(35) J.L. Feldman and M.I. Cohen, Relation between expiratory dura-
     tion and rostral medullary expiratory neuronal discharge,
     Brain Res. 141, 172-178 (1978).

(36) A.J. Berger, Dorsal respiratory group neurons in the medulla of
     cat: Spinal projections, responses to lung inflation and
     superior laryngeal nerve stimulation, Brain Res. 135, 231-254
     (1977).

(37) M.I. Cohen and J.L. Feldman, Models of respiratory phase-switch-
     ing, Fed. Proc. Am. Physiol. Soc. 36, 2367-2374 (1977).

(38) M. Denavit-Saubié and D. Riche, Descending input from the pneumo-
     taxic system to the lateral respiratory nucleus of the medulla.
     An anatomical study with the horseradish peroxidase technique,
     Neurosci. Letters 6, 121-126 (1977).

(39) M. Kalia, Neuroanatomical organization of the respiratory centers
     Fed. Proc. Am. Physiol. Soc. 36, 2405-2411 (1977).

(40) J.F. Vibert, F. Bertrand, M. Denavit-Saubié and A. Hugelin,
     Discharge patterns of bulbo-pontine respiratory unit population
     in cat, Brain Res. 114, 211-225 (1976).

(41) J.F. Vibert, F. Bertrand, M. Denavit-Saubié and A. Hugelin,
     Three dimensional representation of bulbo-pontine respiratory
     networks architecture from unit density maps, Brain Res. 114,
     227-244 (1976).

DISCUSSION

Commenting on the role of 'irritant' receptors in the control of the
pattern of breathing, Widdicombe reported that they had arrived at
similar conclusions as now presented by Knox despite three main technical differences: Firstly, the London group used rabbits and not
cats; secondly they used short, 100 ms, pulses of inflation and deflation which are a more specific stimulus to 'irritant' receptors;
and thirdly they used the sulphur dioxide method to block pulmonary
stretch receptors. Widdicombe further emphasized that with respect
to the role of the 'irritant' receptors in quiet breathing, there
were two qualifications. In his laboratory the afferent activity had
always been recorded in vagotomized animals, whose tidal volume
would be greater than in eupnoea. Therefore, the pattern of inspiratory discharge is not known for the latter condition. Secondly,
Widdicombe expressed some doubt as to whether we would regard the
conditions of anaesthetized cats and rabbits as physiological, at
least with regard to their lungs which always will show some degree
of collapse.

Merrill emphasized the very striking difference between the transitions from inspiration to expiration and from expiration to inspiration which is so apparent when recording from many bulbar respiratory neurons. Whereas the inspiratory-to-expiratory phase transition
there is characterized by a substantial overlap in the firing of
inspiratory and expiratory neurons the expiration-to-inspiration
transition is very abrupt: Within about 50 msec there is an almost
complete cessation of all expiratory activity in the nucleus retroambigualis (NRA) and an abrupt onset of the early burst inspiratory
neurons.

CHARACTERISTICS AND FUNCTIONAL SIGNIFICANCE OF THE EXPIRATORY BULBAR NEURONE POOLS*

H. P. KOEPCHEN, D. SOMMER, CH. FRANK,
D. KLÜSSENDORF, A. KRÄMER, P. ROSIN
and K. FORSTREUTER

Institute of Physiology, Free University of Berlin, D-1000 Berlin 33, F.R.G.

Ventilation consists of inspiration and expiration. Thus, control of ventilation may be understood as control of inspiration and control of expiration. Both may be studied separately, but finally the question is inevitable, how and to what extent they are linked together. If we study respiratory control by recording from inspiratory (I) and expiratory (E) neurone populations, the same question arises at the central nervous level where three main aggregations of respiratory neurones are found: the dorsal inspiratory (2,3,4), the ventral inspiratory and the ventral expiratory neurone pools (1, 3, 4, 29, 34, 37). In view of the fact that the total amount of activity of I and E neurones is not very different, earlier concepts proposed a more or less symmetrical I-E oscillator (6, 10). But in the more recent development of central nervous respiratory control theories, rhythmogenesis and control of ventilation were reduced successfully to the question of generation of inspiratory excitation and the mechanism and timing of inspiratory switch-off (7,11). Consequently, the question has to be asked, if the electrophysiologically impressive expiratory neurone pools have any function at all in respiratory rhythmogenesis and, if not, which other purposes they may serve.

Under this aspect, we have recorded from the densely packed main expiratory retroambigual neurone pools caudal to the obex (1,29,34,37) in dogs and cats in comparison with the behaviour of ventrolateral (= retroambigual) I neurones. Computer analyses were performed to get quantitative information. These studies will try to answer three questions:

A. Which main drives and inhibitions act on the E neurones and what is their relative weight?
B. Which efferent actions take their origin from the E neurone pools?
C. Which conclusions may be drawn concerning the physiological function of medullary E neurones?

---

*Supported by Deutsche Forschungsgemeinschaft

A. <u>DRIVES AND INHIBITIONS</u>

1. <u>Basic and Chemical Drives</u>

E neurones are excited by peripheral and central chemoreceptors (8, 19, 23, 24, 35). This action is strongly confined to the expiratory time. In the case of CO_2 the activity - measured as impulses/burst or impulses/time is nearly linearly related to P_{ACO_2} in spontaneously breathing as well as in artificially ventilated cats (13,26). CO_2 response curves for the single neurone give quantitative information about the individual neuronal CO_2 sensitivity which is correlated to the basic activity at standard CO_2 level (12, 13). Ventral medullary alkalosis and hyperventilation reduce E neuronal activity (8,24), application of procaine at the ventral surface immediately reduce or abolish the E neuronal activity depending on the concentration of procaine (41). This dependency on ventral medullary drive is qualitatively similar as in other systems (I neurones, tonic reticular activity, arterial blood pressure), but with different quantitative and temporal characteristics (25).

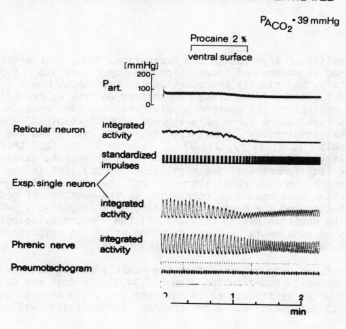

DOG HB17 PARALYSED, ARTIFICIALLY VENTILATED

Fig. 1. Response of reticular neurone, expiratory neurone and phrenic nerve to temporary addition of 2 % procaine to ventral medullary surface superfusion in an anaesthetized paralyzed artificially ventilated dog. Note the differences in the time courses of decrease of the different neuronal activities and blood pressure respectively with primary E inactivation followed by acceleration of central respiratory rhythm.
(From Koepchen, Schwanghart and Schröter, unpublished)

At low level of drive or general activity (deep anaesthesia (24), acapnia (8, 24), central hypoxia (5), reduced ventral medullary drive (41)), ventral E and I populations behave differently: E activity is gradually reduced like I activity but in all mentioned cases becomes continuous at lower levels if ventral I activity has ceased. If the level of activity rises again, rhythmic burst-like E activity never begins before rhythmic activity reappears in at least part of I neurones. Therefore, E neurones seem to play a secondary role in rhythmogenesis.

2. Lung Volume Perception

a) Volume above FRC

E neurones react very sensitively, even to small lung volume increase, with activation (9, 22). With higher volumes or steeper increase of volume, this reaction is converted to inhibition (22). We have not yet found primarily "paradoxical" E neurones in the caudal retroambigual E population.

b) Volume below FRC

The high sensitivity of E neurones to lung volume changes continues in the range of reduced volumes. E activity is linearly related to pneumothorax volume if graded pneumothorax is applied experimentally. The absolute decrease of E activity with increasing pneumothorax volume is bigger in neurones with higher control discharge rate, but the relative decrease is fairly similar in all E neurones studied. The percentage decrease may be expressed by the equation

$$\Delta act_E = -3{,}63 \cdot V_{ipl} \quad (r = 0{,}93, \ p < 0{,}001)$$

where Δact is the percentage diminution of mean impulse rate and V_{ipl} the volume in ml per kg body weight introduced into the interpleural space. The corresponding equation for the activation of I neurones by pneumothorax is

$$\Delta act_I = +1{,}65 \cdot V_{ipl} \quad (r = 0{,}74, \ p < 0{,}001).$$

That means that the reaction of I neurones to decrease of lung volume is about half as great as that of E neurones with no such strong correlation. Taking into account the expansion of entire thoracic volume under pneumothorax, diminution of lung volume in the order of magnitude of 0.5 ml in the cat may be detected by individual E neurones. The increase of phrenic discharge during pneumothorax does never follow in a similar precise manner to lung volume changes (42, 43, 44).

Thus, E neurones are highly sensitive volume receptors with continuous sensitivity around FRC and volume thresholds quite different from those known for phrenic nerve and I neurone activity (11,44). Their reaction is confined to their discharge time, i.e., T_E (Fig. 2). That means that the receptors responsible for this sensitive answer to lung volume changes under physiological conditions must be active during T_E at FRC. According to a recent re-investigation in our laboratory, the number of such low-threshold pulmonary stretch receptors may be estimated as about 15-20 % of the total number of pulmonary stretch receptors. At very high and very low lung volumes, other receptors, as irritant receptors or special lung deflation receptors, may contribute to the reaction of E neurones. The described reaction of E neurones to lung deflation disappears after vagotomy.

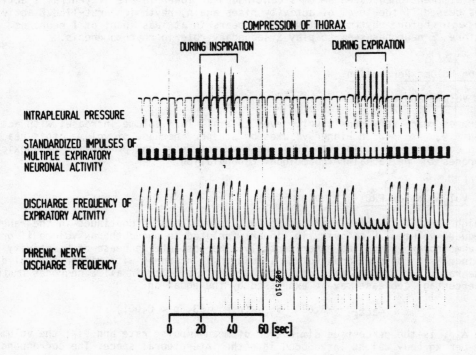

Fig. 2.   Effect of repeated identical short manual compressions of thorax during
          inspiratory (left) and expiratory (right) phase on multiple neurone acti-
          vity in caudal bulbar expiratory neurone population in a spontaneously
          breathing anaesthetized cat. Note strong inhibition of E activity by tho-
          racic compression during E phase but not during I phase and distinctly
          greater acceleration of respiration with compression during E phase.

3. Interaction Between Chemical Drive and Vagal Drive

One consequence of the above findings and considerations is that part of the drive
of E neurones comes from pulmonary vagal afferents. The relative contribution of
this vagal drive, in comparison with the chemical CO_2 drive, can be estimated on
the basis of the shift of single E neurone response curves under vagal cooling (12,
13). The cooling causes a parallel downward shift of the response curves in the majority of the studied E neurones. The relation between the slope of the response
curves and the amount of the shift gives a measure of the mean relation between the
CO_2 drive and the vagal drive (Fig. 3). It results that at normal P_{CO_2} more than
half of the E neurone drive comes from vagal afferences - presumably pulmonary
stretch receptors. This value varies considerably in individual neurones and may be
influenced by the condition of artificial ventilation. In this context, the question how far the CO_2 drive is identical with the ventral medullary surface drive remains to be settled.

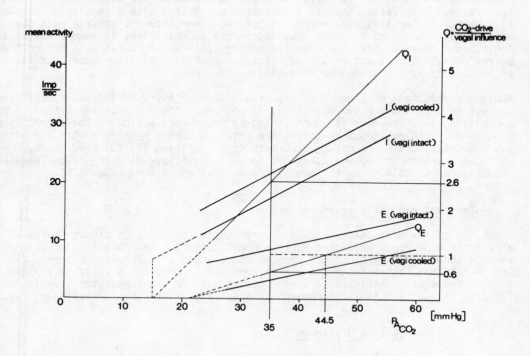

Fig. 3. Average course of single retroambigual I and E neurone CO_2 response curves
and their shifts by vagal cooling to 4 °C in anaesthetized artificially
ventilated cats. Vagal cooling causes upward shift of I and downward
shift of E response curves. Note the higher activity and greater slope of
I as compared with E response curves and the bigger shift of E response
curves under vagal cooling. The Q-lines indicate the relation between the
CO_2 drive and the vagal drive or inhibition calculated from the response
curves. The calculation is based on the observation of a sudden stop of
most of the I activity at about 15 mm Hg P_{ACO_2} and a continuous decrease
of E activity until zero under hyperventilation. This quantitative estimation shows that at the normal P_{ACO_2} of 35 mm Hg in the cat the vagal
drive is greater than the CO_2 drive in E neurones whereas in I neurones
the CO_2 drive is more than twice as strong as the vagal inhibition.
(Calculated from values measured by Frank (12)).

4. Inhibitory Influences on E Neurones

a) Inhibition by I neurones

The powerful inhibition of E neurones during inspiratory phase (2,32,38,40) presumably comes from I neurones. Consequently, one kind of activation of E neurones is
disinhibition if I neurones become less active. This can be observed frequently if

the I drive is weakened by inhibition or inactivation (5). With quantitative measurements of activity two types of E disinhibition may be discerned: if simply the previous inspiratory gaps in E discharge are filled with E impulses, the average number of impulses/time increases but the momentaneous discharge rate does not exceed that during E bursts measured before I inhibition. In some cases of I inhibition, however, also the mean E discharge rate during burst gets higher than before cessation of I activity. The latter kind of disinhibition speaks in favour of inhibition by I neurones which outlasts the I phase.

Ambiguous reactions of E neurones may result if excitatory or inhibitory afferences act on both I *and* E neurones (23). In that case the indirect inhibition or disinhibition via I neurones is counteracted by the direct action of the afferents on E neurones. Such ambiguous reactions are observed during hypoxia - with and without chemoreceptors - and during baroreceptor stimulation (5, 20) (see below). Strong activation of the whole brain stem through seizure-inducing drugs leads to reduction of E activity by the prevailing activation of I neurones (28).

b) Inhibition by baroreceptors

According to the mentioned ambiguity, baroreceptor stimulation causes equivocal effects on E neurones which are further complicated if the inhibition of respiration is accompanied by blood gas changes and changes of pulmonary afferents (14, 16). But if the latter factors are kept constant by constant artificial ventilation, unequivocal inhibition of E neurones results from baroreceptor stimulation (20,24). This effect is still present if inspiratory activity is abolished (24).

c) Inhibition by type J afferents

Strong pharmacological excitation of pulmonary type J afferents (36) immediately suppresses medullary I *and* E activity. Recovery of I activity is much faster than that of E activity, so that phases with prevalent inactivation of E neurones are observed (15,21). During such transitional states, the behaviour of inspiratory parameters hints at an inspiratory disinhibition with shortening of T_E and increase in respiratory frequency.

Summarizing the afferent actions on E neurones, we may state that in many respects they are similar to the reactions of surrounding reticular neurones with the exception of the response to pulmonary afferents.

B. EFFERENT ACTIONS OF E NEURONES

1. Descending Action on Spinal E Motoneurones

There is general agreement that caudal E neurones project to spinal E motoneurones and hence govern movement and tone of E muscles (e.g. 30,31). This function is mirrored by the parallelism between medullary E neurone activity and endexpiratory position, i.e. FRC (19). Moreover, electrical microstimulation in the centre of medullary E neurone pool leads to active expiratory movements below FRC (18,24).

2. Intracentral Effects of E Neurones (?)

With weaker stimuli at the same electrode position sudden arrest of ongoing inspiration occurs and the next inspiration begins earlier. If stimuli are applied in expiratory phase, T_E is prolonged. This prolongation or shortening of respiratory

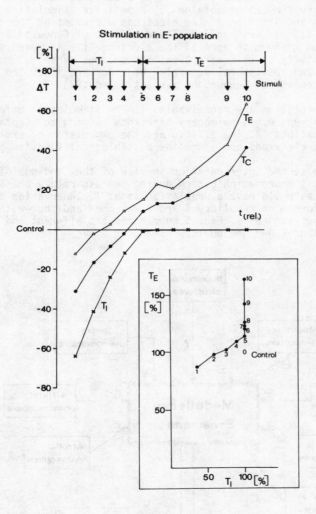

Fig. 4. Relative changes of inspiratory duration (T_I), expiratory duration (T_E)
and whole respiratory cycle duration (T_C) produced by short stimulus
trains applied through the previous recording electrode in the center of
caudal bulbar E neurone population at different times (1-10) in the respiratory cycle in spontaneously breathing anaesthetized cats. Note shortening of T_I, T_E and therewith T_C by stimulation in early inspiration and
prolongation of T_E and T_C by stimulation from the end of inspiration until
a maximum value at the end of expiration. The "neutral point" for changes
of respiratory frequency indicated by intersection of the T_C curve with
the control value lies near the end of inspiration. Inset: Relation between T_I and T_E under stimulation at the times indicated by the same ci-
phers as in the figures above.

cycle by stimulation in the E region is a reproducible function of the stimulation time within the respiratory cycle (Fig. 4). As a consequence, acceleration or slowing of respiratory rhythm can be obtained by repetitive stimulation with the same stimulus parameters and location of the electrode dependent on the respiratory phase in which the stimuli are applied. These effects of E neuronal region stimulation diminish from maximum to zero if the electrode tip is moved stepwise out of the centre of E activity in both directions. Recordings during stimulation show that contralateral and ipsilateral ventral I neurones are inhibited by the stimulation whereas contralateral E neurones are activated (27).

Two kinds of interpretation are conceivable: 1. The stimulation effects are caused by excitation of fibres, e.g., pulmonary afferents running accidentally through the E neurone populations. 2. The effects are the expression of excitation of bulbar E neurones or their axons and mimic the physiological function of E neurones.

We would prefer the second interpretation in view of the findings of other authors indicating synaptic I neurone inhibition during the expiratory phase (38,39). In this case, E neurones would have a double function: 1. Innervation of spinal E motoneurones, 2. influence on medullary I and E neurones and therewith interference with respiratory rhythmogenesis. Fig. 5 summarizes the afferent and efferent connections of the bulbar E neurone pools.

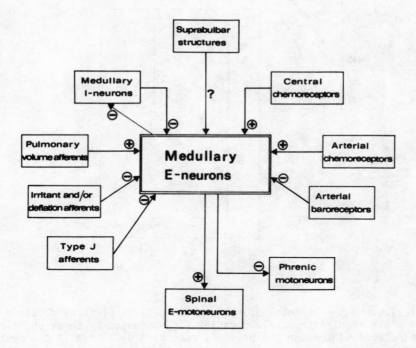

Fig. 5. Schematical survey on the afferent and efferent connections of E neurones. Excitatory connections are labelled by + , inhibitory connections by - .

C. MODELS AND CONCLUSIONS CONCERNING E NEURONE FUNCTIONAL SIGNIFICANCE

The following three models of respiratory neuronal control may be discussed on the basis of the described afferent and efferent connections of E neurones (the problem of generation and termination of central inspiratory activity will be excluded from the present considerations):

I. A symmetrical I-E oscillator where rhythmogenesis and timing are dependent on the reciprocal interaction between I and E neurones.

II. A model where rhythmogenesis and timing depend exclusively on I neuronal mechanisms and E neurones act on spinal E motoneurones only.

III. An intermediate asymmetrical model where rhythmogenesis and timing are due mainly to I mechanisms but E neurones contribute to respiratory timing in addition to their spinal actions.

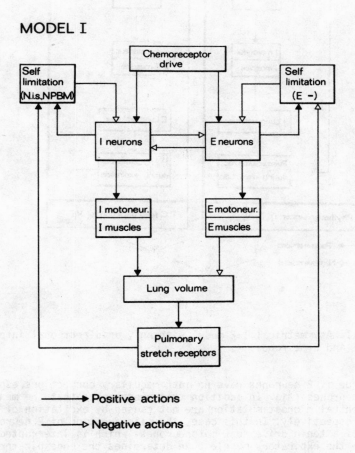

Fig. 6. Model I: Symmetrical I-E model.

Model 1 is extremely unlikely in view of the asymmetrical behaviour of I and E neurones, especially in the transitional states of beginning apnoea and reappearance of respiratory rhythm.

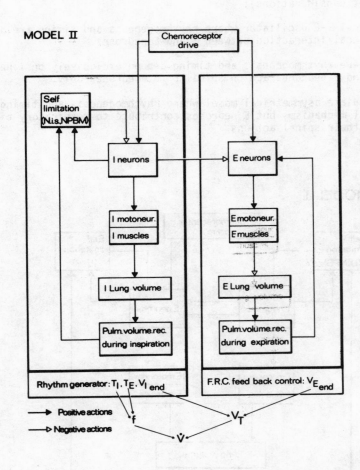

Fig. 7.   Model II: Asymmetrical I-E model with only unidirectional interaction between I and E neurones.

Model 2 comes true if E neurones have no intramedullary connections, especially none to medullary I neurones (31). In addition this presupposes that the mentioned effects of intracentral microstimulation are not caused by excitation of E neurones or their axons respectively. In this case, the main function of E neurones would be the generation of a tonic drive to E motoneurones, which is interrupted during inspiration. Since the expiratory muscle tone determines the endexpiratory position, this tonic drive governs FRC. Since caudal E neurones are extremely sensitive in a graded manner to lung volume changes around FRC, this population is optimally suitable to act as the central relay station of a feedback system controlling expira-

tory lung volume. For this function, it is dependent on low threshold pulmonary afferents. Since a regulator for constancy of lung volume cannot be permitted to work
during inspiration, its interruption during inspiration is a functional necessity.
The drive from chemoreceptor afferences determines the bias or set point of the regulator leading to lower FRC, i.e. deeper expiration at higher chemical drive. The
sensitive graded response to the weak expiratory low threshold stretch receptor
discharge within the E phase feedback circuit differs fundamentally in kind of action and functional meaning from the I phase feedback control governed by the
strong phasically active inspiratory pulmonary stretch receptor discharge.

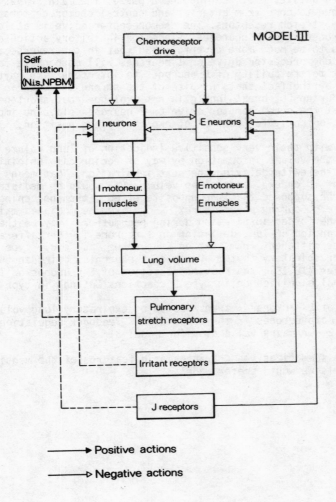

Fig. 8.   Model III: Asymmetrical I-E model with bidirectional, but asymmetrical interaction between I and E neurones.

Model 3 represents a modification of model 2 with the assumption that E neurones inhibit medullary I neurones in addition to their spinal action on E motoneurones. This model inevitably means that E neurones take part in timing of respiration and therewith the afferences acting upon them likewise gain influence on timing via the E neurones. The changes in respiratory rhythm seen during selective depression of E neurones in the second phase of J receptor excitation, during pneumothorax or during some kinds of ventral medullary anaesthesia, and the intracentral stimulation effects speak in favour of this interpretation.

The functional significance of a reciprocal inhibition of I neurones by E neurones may be judged according to the following considerations: It can be proposed that the action of E neurones on I neurones is effective primarily during that phase where E neurones are active, i.e., during the E phase. The main drives to E neurones have been shown to come from arterial and central chemoreceptors and low threshold pulmonary stretch receptors. The chemoreceptor drive is at least as much effective on I neurones as on E neurones. Since the inhibitory action of I neurones on E neurones seems to be much more powerful than that in the reverse direction (2,32,38,40), the chemoreceptor drive on I neurones will compensate for that on E neurones in respect to the ability of E neurones to interfere with rhythmogenesis. This is manifested by the fact that in spite of the strong increase in E discharge rate during burst during CO_2 breathing T_E is not prolonged but shortened (8,19,23, 26). That means that the chemoreceptor drive on E neurones plays no important role for rhythmogenesis, but only for control of expiratory end position, i.e. FRC.

But the E neurones with their very sensitive indication of lung volume during E phase may transmit the volume information by way of reciprocal inhibition to the silent I neurones, therewith delaying the next inspiration. That means that the graded dependency of T_E on expiratory lung volume (17) would be mediated mainly by E neurones. It can be supposed that the opposite effect, the shortening of T_E by reduction of FRC - e.g. during pneumothorax -, is likewise mediated mainly by E neurones, whereas the forced inspiration during pneumothorax may be the consequence of a direct action of lung deflation on I neurones. Other afferents with an action on I neurones different from that on E neurones, as, e.g., type J afferents, may also influence respiratory rhythm by way of E neurones. Using another terminology proposed earlier (18,19), the reciprocal action of E neurones on I neurones would gain functional significance in type B reactions but not in type A reactions.

The other function of E neurones - transmission of expiratory lung volume information on expiratory motoneurones in the sense of FRC feedback regulation as described under model 2 - remains valid also for model 3.

The following table summarizes the characteristic features of the mentioned models. From the three models we would prefer model 3.

	Main function of		Characteristic features of the model
	I neurones	E neurones	
Model I	Rhythmogenesis Control of: T_I T_E V_T	Rhythmogenesis Control of: T_I T_E V_T	Symmetrical model Symmetrical mutual reciprocal inhibition I and E rhythmogenesis I and E timing
Model II	Rhythmogenesis Control of: T_I T_E V_T	FRC feedback control center Control of: V_T through V_E end position	Asymmetrical model No E → I inhibition! I rhythmogenesis Interrupted FRC feedback control I timing, no E timing
Model III	Rhythmogenesis Control of: T_I, T_E (partly), V_T.	FRC feedback control center Reflex transmission to I neurones and E motoneurones Control of: T_E V_T	Asymmetrical model Asymmetrical mutual reciprocal inhibition I rhythmogenesis E → I pulmonary reflex influences I *and* E timing

REFERENCES

(1) H. L. Batsel, Localization of bulbar respiratory center by microelectrode sounding, *Exper. Neurol.* 9, 410 (1963).

(2) R. v. Baumgarten, K. Balthasar, H. P. Koepchen, Über ein Substrat atmungsrhythmischer Erregungsbildung im Rautenhirn der Katze, *Pflügers Arch. ges. Physiol.* 270, 504 (1960).

(3) R. v. Baumgarten, A. v. Baumgarten, K. P. Schaefer, Beitrag zur Lokalisationsfrage bulboreticulärer respiratorischer Neurone der Katze, *Pflügers Arch. ges. Physiol.* 264, 217 (1957).

(4) A. L. Bianchi, Localisation et étude des neurones respiratoires bulbaires. Mise en jeu antidromique par stimulation spinale ou vagale, *J. Physiol. (Paris)* 63, 5 (1971).

(5) J. Borchert, A. Dinter, H. P. Koepchen, A. Scharnke, The direct action of hypoxia on medullary respiratory neurones, *Pflügers Arch. ges. Physiol.* 355 (Suppl.), R 31 (1975).

(6) B. D. Burns, G. C. Salmoiraghi, Repetitive firing of respiratory neurons during their burst activity, *J. Neurophysiol.* 23, 27 (1960).

(7) F. J. Clark, C. v. Euler, On the regulation of depth and rate of breathing, *J. Physiol. (Lond.)* 222, 267 (1972).

(8) M. I. Cohen, Discharge patterns of brain-stem respiratory neurons in relation to carbon dioxide tension, *J. Neurophysiol.* 31, 142 (1968).

(9) M. I. Cohen, Discharge patterns of brain-stem respiratory neurons during He-ring-Breuer reflex evoked by lung inflation, *J. Neurophysiol.* 32, 356 (1969).

(10) M. I. Cohen, How respiratory rhythm originates: evidence from discharge patterns of brainstem respiratory neurons. In: R. Porter (ed.), *Breathing, Hering-Breuer Centenary Symposium*, Churchill, London 1970, p. 125.

(11) C. v. Euler, The functional organization of the respiratory phase-switching mechanisms, *Fed. Proc.* 36, 2375 (1977).

(12) Ch. Frank, Die Wechselwirkung zwischen CO_2-Antrieb und vagalen Afferenzen am bulbären respiratorischen Einzelneuron: Eine quantitative Analyse an der künstlich beatmeten Katze, *Thesis*, Berlin 1978.

(13) Ch. Frank, J. Borchert, D. Klüßendorf, H. P. Koepchen, Modes of interaction between vagal and CO_2 chemoreflex input at bulbar respiratory neurons, *Bull. Europ. Physiopathol. Resp.* 12, 223 P (1976).

(14) M. Gabriel, H. Seller, Excitation of expiratory neurons adjacent to the nucleus ambiguus by carotid sinus baroreceptor and trigeminal afferents, *Pflügers Arch. ges. Physiol.* 313, 1 (1969).

(15) M. Kalia, H. P. Koepchen, A. S. Paintal, Somatomotor and autonomic effects of type J-receptor stimulation in awake-freely moving and restrained cats, *Pflügers Arch. ges. Physiol.* 339 (Suppl.), R 80 (1973).

(16) D. Klüßendorf, U. Philipp, H. P. Koepchen, Studies on the central mechanism of reflex inhibition of respiration by baroreceptor afferents, *Pflügers Arch. ges. Physiol.* 319 (Suppl.), R 50 (1970).

(17) C. K. Knox, Characteristics of inflation and deflation reflexes during expiration in the cat, *J. Neurophysiol.* 36, 284 (1973).

(18) H. P. Koepchen, Concept of two general types of reflexogenic central respiratory drive and inhibition. In: W. Umbach, H. P. Koepchen (eds.), *Central Rhythmic and Regulation*, Hippokrates, Stuttgart 1974, p. 122.

(19) H. P. Koepchen, Quantitative approach to neural control of ventilation. In: H. H. Loeschcke (ed.), *Acid Base Homeostasis of the Brain Extracellular Fluid and the Respiratory Control System*, Thieme, Stuttgart 1976, p. 164.

(20) H. P. Koepchen, The respiratory-cardiovascular brainstem oscillator in the context of afferent and central excitatory and inhibitory systems. In: H. P. Koepchen, S. M. Hilton, A. Trzebski (eds.), *Central Interaction between Respiratory and Cardiovascular Control Systems*, Springer, Heidelberg (in press).

(21) H. P. Koepchen, M. Kalia, D. Sommer, D. Klüßendorf, Action of type J afferents on the discharge pattern of medullary respiratory neurons. In: A. S. Paintal (ed.), *Respiratory Adaptations, Capillary Exchange and Reflex Mechanisms*, New Delhi 1976, Vallabhbhai Patel Chest Institute.

(22) H. P. Koepchen, D. Klüßendorf, M. Bilan, N. Sapunarow, D. Sommer, Central transmission of pulmonary inflation and deflation reflexes, *Proc. IUPS*, XXV. Intern. Congr. Physiol. Sci. 1971, p. 312.

(23) H. P. Koepchen, D. Klüßendorf, J. Borchert, D.-W. Lessmann, A. Dinter, Ch. Frank, D. Sommer, Types of respiratory neuronal activity pattern in reflex control of ventilation. In: A. S. Paintal (ed.), *Respiratory Adaptations, Capillary Exchange and Reflex Mechanisms*, New Delhi 1976.

(24) H. P. Koepchen, D. Klüßendorf, U. Philipp, Mechanisms of central transmission of respiratory reflexes, *Acta Neurobiol. Exper.* 33, 287 (1973).

(25) H. P. Koepchen, K. Kolbe, D. Klüßendorf, R. Schröter, F. Schwanghart, CO_2 and the brain stem respiratory complex, *Bull. Europ. Physiopathol. Resp.* 12, 216 P (1976).

(26) K. Kolbe, M. Bilan, D. Klüßendorf, H. P. Koepchen, The different action of CO_2 on inspiratory and expiratory bulbar respiratory neurones, *Pflügers Arch. ges. Physiol.* 359 (Suppl.), R 44 (1975).

(27) A. Krämer, D. Sommer, P. Rosin, D. Klüßendorf, H. P. Koepchen, Ventilatory and neuronal responses to microstimulation in bulbar expiratory neuronal population, *Proc. IUPS*, Vol. XIII, No. 1207, p. 409, Paris 1977.

(28) V. Lieske, R. Schröter, F. Schwanghart, H. P. Koepchen, Central neuronal respiratory activity during seizures induced by pentylenetetrazol (Cardiazol), *Pflügers Arch. ges. Physiol.* 343 (Suppl.), R 9 (1973).

(29) E. G. Merrill, The lateral respiratory neurones of the medulla: their association with nucleus ambiguus, N. retroambigualis, the spinal accessory nucleus and the spinal cord, *Brain Res.* 24, 11 (1970).

(30) E. G. Merrill, Thoracic motor drives from medullary expiratory neurones in cats, *J. Physiol. (Lond.)* 222, 154 P (1972).

(31) E. G. Merrill, Finding a respiratory function for the medullary respiratory neurons. In: R. Bellairs, E. G. Gray (eds.), *Essays on the Nervous System. A Festschrift for Professor J. Z. Young*, Clarendon Press, Oxford 1974, p. 451.

(32) R. A. Mitchell, D. A. Herbert, Synchronized high frequency synaptic potentials in medullary respiratory neurons, *Brain Res.* 75, 350 (1974).

(33) S. Nakayama, R. v. Baumgarten, Lokalisierung absteigender Atmungsbahnen im Rückenmark der Katze mittels antidromer Reizung, *Pflügers Arch. ges. Physiol.* 281, 231 (1964).

(34) J. R. Nelson, Single unit activity in medullary respiratory centers of the cat, *J. Neurophysiol.* 22, 590 (1959).

(35) R. S. Nesland, F. Plum, J. R. Nelson, H. D. Siedler, The graded response to stimulation of medullary respiratory neurons, *Exper. Neurol.* 14, 57 (1966).

(36) A. S. Paintal, Mechanism of stimulation of type J pulmonary receptors, *J. Physiol. (Lond.)* 203, 511 (1969).

(37) U. Philipp, Die exspiratorische Neuronenpopulation im unteren Hirnstamm des Hundes: Lokalisation, Abgrenzung und funktionelle Beziehungen, *Thesis*, Berlin 1972.

(38) D. W. Richter, F. Heyde, M. Gabriel, Intracellular recordings from different types of medullary respiratory neurons of the cat, *J. Neurophysiol.* 38, 1162 (1975).

(39) D. W. Richter, H. Camerer, M. Meesmann, N. Röhrig, Reciprocal inhibition of bulbar inspiratory neurones in the cat, *This symposium*, Pergamon Press (in press).

(40) G. C. Salmoiraghi, R. v. Baumgarten, Intracellular potentials from respiratory neurons in brain stem of cat and mechanism of rhythmic respiration, *J. Neurophysiol.* 24, 203 (1961).

(41) F. Schwanghart, R. Schröter, D. Klüßendorf, H. P. Koepchen, The influence of novocaine block of superficial brain stem structures on respiratory and reticular neurones. In: W. Umbach, H. P. Koepchen (eds.), *Central Rhythmic and Regulation*, Hippokrates, Stuttgart 1974, p. 104.

(42) D. Sommer, Quantitative Analyse der Reaktion medullärer respiratorischer Neurone bei Veränderungen des Lungenvolumens unterhalb der FRC. Ein Beitrag

zur Funktion der exspiratorischen Neurone, *Thesis*, Berlin 1978.

(43) D. Sommer, M. Kalia, D. Klüßendorf, H. P. Koepchen, Effects of lung deflation and J-receptor excitation on central respiratory innervation in cats, *Pflü-gers Arch. ges. Physiol.* 339 (Suppl.), R 35 (1973).

(44) D. Sommer, D. Klüßendorf, H. P. Koepchen, Quantitative analysis of reactions of bulbar respiratory neurons to lung deflation, *Proc. IUPS*, Vol. XIII, No. 2103, p. 707, Paris 1977.

RECIPROCAL INHIBITION OF BULBAR RESPIRATORY NEURONES IN THE CAT

D. W. RICHTER, H. CAMERER, M. MEESMANN
and N. RÖHRIG

I. Department of Physiology, University of Heidelberg, D-6900 Heidelberg, F.R.G.

For the interpretation of experimental results and the understanding of the rhythmogenésis of respiration it is of fundamental importance to know whether the theory of reciprocal inhibition of inspiratory and expiratory bulbar neurones (Ref. 6,9) is correct. This theory was accepted for many years but has recently been questioned. It is still accepted that inspiratory neurones inhibit expiratory neurones, but evidence against expiratory inhibition of inspiratory neurones has been provided by Merrill (3) and Mitchell and Herbert (5). These negative results, however, were not supported by certain findings from this laboratory (Ref. 2,7).

Our purpose in the present experiments was to demonstrate expiratory IPSPs in bulbar inspiratory neurones, and so to prove that reciprocal inhibition does exist. This was done by the methods of Cl^- -and current injection into respiratory neurones in pentobarbital (40 mg $\cdot$ kg^{-1}) anaesthetized cats. As different types of neurone may react differently, the neurones of both the dorsal and ventral populations (Ref. 1) were classified by antidromic excitation following spinal cord and vagal nerve stimulation. By this method neurones were categorised as bulbospinal (BS), vagal (V) or not antidromically activated (NAA) neurones. R_β-neurones which belong to the group of inspiratory NAA-neurones were identified by their monosynaptic input from lung stretch receptor afferents (Ref. 8).

All types of inspiratory neurone showed postsynaptic noise activity (PSPs) almost throughout the respiratory cycle. Under control conditions, PSPs were largest during inspiration and so indicate an excitatory nature (EPSPs). During the period of cyclic membrane hyperpolarization, PSPs were small, but increased tremendously when the mean level of the membrane potential differed significantly from the IPSP equilibrium potential. This was done by membrane depolarization (Fig. 1) or Cl^- -injection (see below). The finding that expiratory membrane hyperpolarization is accompanied by strong PSP-activity indicates inhibitory postsynaptic potentials (IPSPs). Minima of PSPs occurred during the transition periods of the respiratory cycle.

IPSP were also revealed by their reversal when the IPSP

D. W. Richter *et al.*

equilibrium potential was changed in a depolarizing direction after
intracellular Cl⁻ -injection.

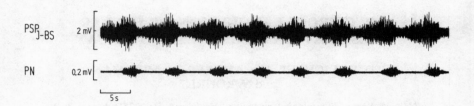

Fig. 1. Postsynaptic activity in an inspiratory bulbo-
spinal neurone of the ventral pool. The neurone was
depolarized to- 40 mV by damage after electrode penetration and the spike discharge was inactivated. PSP_{I-BS}:
membrane potential,as recorded after a 10 cps high pass
filter. PN: phrenic nerve activity.

The majority of the bulbar inspiratory neurones of all types revealed reversed IPSPs during expiration. The summed reversed IPSPs produced a wave of membrane depolarization and the neurones then depolarized not only during their period of synaptic activation but also
during their 'silent' period (Fig. 2,3,4).

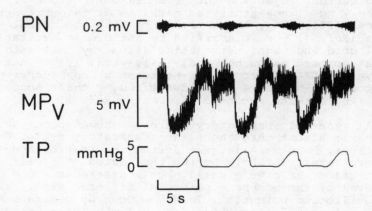

Fig. 2. Membrane potential of an inspiratory vagal neurone in which the IPSPs have already been reversed by Cl⁻ -
injection. PN: phrenic nerve activity. MP_V: membrane potential. TP: tracheal pressure.

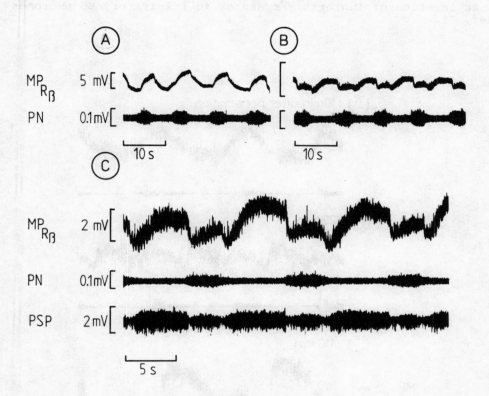

Fig. 3. Membrane potential of an R_β-neurone during control (A) and 10 min after Cl^--injection (B). The periodic changes in membrane potential ($MP_{R\beta}$) and the postsynaptic activity (PSP, recorded after a 10 cps high
pass filter) after Cl^--injection are shown in(C) at
higher amplification in a faster sweep recording. PN:
phrenic nerve activity.

The latency to a definite IPSP reversal varied in the different types of neurone. IPSP-reversal occurred promptly in inspiratory vagal
neurones (Fig. 2), some NAA-neurones and R_β-neurones (Fig. 3). In
these cases, the now depolarizing IPSPs could again be reversed to a
hyperpolarizing direction during injection of positive current which
depolarized the neurones below the new IPSP equilibrium potential.
The short latency of Cl-induced IPSP reversal and the finding that
the IPSPs could easily be influenced by current injection indicate synapses near to, or on the soma.

    The latency to IPSP-reversal was longest in inspiratory BS-
neurones of both dorsal and ventral pools, ranging between 20-60 min

(Fig. 4). During the process of reversal, IPSPs easily escaped notice. The wave of reversed IPSP during expiration, however, was fully
developed after 1-2 hrs. The long time of Cl^- -diffusion needed to
reverse IPSPs supports recent measurements indicating a remote dendritic location of inhibitory synapses in inspiratory BS-neurones
(Ref. 7).

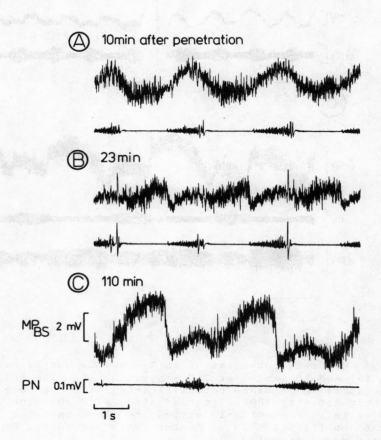

Fig. 4. Membrane potential of an inspiratory bulbospinal
neurone of the ventral pool of neurones. The hyperpolarizing IPSPs under control conditions (A) gradually reversed to depolarizing IPSPs (B+C). PN: phrenic nerve activity. MP_{BS}: membrane potential.

The only neurones in which IPSP reversal was not demonstrated were
those that could be recorded for only short periods. In these cases
the amount of Cl^- -injected and/or the time for Cl^- -diffusion was
probably insufficient.

One of the main arguments against 'expiratory' inhibition

of medullary inspiratory neurones was that expiratory BS-neurones
'never' possess 'long' axon collaterals which could reach the regions where inspiratory neurones are localized (Ref. 3). However,
axon collaterals shorter than 0.5 mm (Ref. 4), may possibly activate
medullary expiratory NAA-neurones, some of which may represent propriobulbar interneurones which transmit inhibition. This assumption
is supported by the finding that axons of several expiratory NAA-
neurones could be recorded within the ventrolateral nucleus of the
solitary tract, which discharge spikes in a pattern quite similar to
expiratory BS-neurones (Fig. 5).

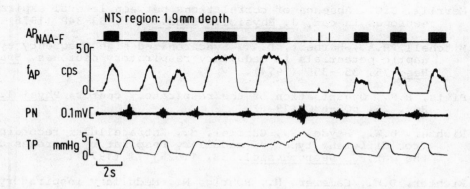

Fig. 5. Discharge of an expiratory axon which could not be
antidromically excited by spinal cord and vagal nerve stimulation. The axon was localized in close proximity of
inspiratory neurones of the dorsal pool. The expiratory
discharge showed a typical Hering-Breuer response to lung
inflation. Lung inflation prolonged the expiratory discharge and the spike frequency was increased. After inflation ended, firing was depressed. AP_{NAA-F}: normalized spikes
of the fibre discharge. f_{AP}: discharge frequency.
PN: phrenic nerve activity. TP: tracheal pressure.

A crucial finding in these experiments was of an axon of an expiratory BS-neurone which was recorded within the region of the nucleus
of the solitary tract. This finding contradicts Merrill's (3) general argument.

        The present results, therefore, show that axons or axon
collaterals of expiratory neurones certainly can reach the pool of
inspiratory neurones and provide a possible anatomical basis for expiratory inhibition of inspiratory neurones at the bulbar level.
However, further experiments are needed to define the exact pathways
of reciprocal inhibition, now it has been shown to exist.

This work was supported by the Deutsche Forschungsgemeinschaft.

REFERENCES

(1) Bianchi, A.L., Localisation et étude des neurones respiratoires
     bulbaires. Mise en jeu antidromique par stimulation spinale
     ou vagale, J. Physiol. (Paris) 63, 5-40 (1971).

(2) Kreuter, F., Richter, D.W., Camerer, H., Senekowitsch, R., Mor-
     phological and electrical description of medullary respira-
     tory neurons of the cat, Pflügers Arch. 372, 7-16 (1977).

(3) Merrill, E.G., Finding a respiratory function for the medullary
     respiratory neurones, In: Essays on the nervous system,
     Bellairs, R. and Gray, E.G. eds., pp 451-486,Clarendon Press,
     Oxford (1974).

(4) Merrill, E.G., Absence of correlations between lateral expiratory
     neurones in cat, J. Physiol. (Lond.) 276, 33-34P (1978).

(5) Mitchell, R.A., Herbert, D.A., Synchronized high frequency sy-
     naptic potentials in medullary respiratory neurones, Brain
     Res. 75, 350-355 (1974).

(6) Pitts, R.F., Organization of the respiratory center, Physiol.
     Rev. 26, 609-630 (1946).

(7) Richter, D.W., Heyde, F., Gabriel, M., Intracellular recordings
     from different types of medullary respiratory neurones of
     the cat, J. Neurophysiol. 38, 1162-1171 (1975).

(8) Richter, D.W., Camerer, H., Röhrig, N., Medullary inspiratory
     interneurons receiving a monosynaptic input from lung
     stretch receptors, Pflügers Arch. 373, R75 (1978).

(9) Salmoiraghi, G.C., Burns, B.D., Notes on mechanism of rhythmic
     respiration, J. Neurophysiol. 23, 14-26 (1960).

Discussion after the next paper

IS THERE RECIPROCAL INHIBITION BETWEEN MEDULLARY INSPIRATORY AND EXPIRATORY NEURONES?

E. G. MERRILL

Department of Anatomy, University College London, U.K.

ABSTRACT

The presence of reciprocal inhibition between medullary inspiratory and expiratory neurones in the cat was assessed with four types of experiments: (a) axonal projections between respiratory neurone populations were determined electrophysiologically; (b) selective lesions were employed to disrupt possible collateral interconnections, and changes in activity determined; (c) the expiratory neurone population was selectively activated and effects on inspiratory activity measured; and (d) correlations were performed on simultaneously recorded inspiratory and expiratory neurones. None of these experiments produced evidence for a true reciprocal inhibition between inspiratory and expiratory neurones.

INTRODUCTION

Respiratory Unit Locations and Activity Patterns

It is generally agreed that the medullary respiratory neurones are concentrated in two nuclei: the lateral part of Nucleus Tractus Solitarius (NST), and more laterally and ventrally in Nucleus Retro-ambiqualis (NRA). (There are in addition populations of cells with respiratory activity in the pons, but these cells do not appear to be active under the conditions of the experiments described here.)

The cells of NRA have one of three basic firing patterns: (a) early burst inspiratory, (b) late peak inspiratory, and (c) expiratory. Examples of these patterns are shown in Fig. 1. The inspiratory units are found in the rostral part of NRA, while the caudal part is exclusively expiratory (ref. 6). In the transition region, just caudal to the obex, inspiratory and expiratory cells are intermingled. In careful searches of the rostral part of NRA, in cats deeply anaesthetized with pentobarbital, no expiratory neurones are recorded, while a few are present in some less deeply anaesthetized cats, or in cats anaesthetized with chloralose or dial-urethane. Many of these rostral ex-

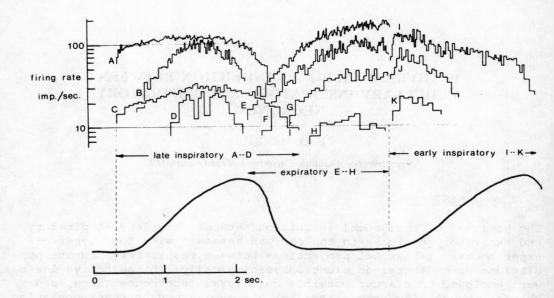

Fig. 1. Instantaneous firing rate patterns for
typical NRA respiratory neurones, plotted for a
single respiratory cycle. A-D are late peak units,
E-H are expiratory neurones, and I-K are early
burst inspiratory cells. The bottom trace is chest
circumference, with the inspiratory deflection upwards. (reprinted from ref. 10).

piratory neurones are laryngeal or pharyngeal motoneurones; in addition, facial and trigeminal motoneurones with respiratory activity can
be recorded from the rostral medulla and pons under light anaesthesia
or with elevated respiratory drives (ref. 6).

Virtually all of the cells of the NST have an inspiratory firing patt
ern, though a very small percentage of expiratory cells has been reported (ref. 3,4). (I have not recorded any NST expiratory neurones
in the deeply anaesthetized cat.) Von Baumgarten and Kanzow (2) subdivided the NST inspiratory population into R_β cells, which are activated by moderate lung inflation in expiration, and R_α's, which are
not activated.

The Salmoiraghi-Burns Model

Salmoiraghi and Burns (ref. 1, 18 and 19) recorded from medullary ins
atory and expiratory neurones (ie. mainly the cells of NRA), which
they regarded as two functionally homogeneous populations. They

attempted to explain the generation of the breathing pattern by post-
ulating certain interactions between these two groups of cells.   The
features of their model are: (a)   units within each population have
accomodative or fatigue properties which eventually result in the termination of activity in each respiratory phase; (b)   cells in each
population are connected to each other via excitatory collaterals so
that activity, once begun in the lower threshold units, spreads to
higher threshold cells throughout the population in a regenerative
manner; and (c)   the two populations reciprocally inhibit each other
so that activity alternates between the two populations.   This model
is extremely attractive because it is simple, because it is based on
accepted classical concepts, and because respiratory physiology is
desperate for something to replace the largely discredited "centres"
model.

Approximately seventeen years of further investigations in the medulla
have shown the Salmoiraghi-Burns model to be inadequate.   Firstly,
several workers have shown that respiratory neurones are among the
least accomodative of central nervous system cells (refs. 10, 17).
Secondly, mutual synaptic excitation within the expiratory population
in NRA does not appear to be an important mechanism (if it exists at
all)(Refs. 11, 13).   Re-excitation within inspiratory populations
appears to be a selective rather than a general mechanism, since NRA
inspiratory units do not have projections to NST (ref. 12), and, insp-
iratory--inspiratory firing pattern correlations only occasionally
exhibit excitatory interactions in the deep pentobarbital cat (Merrill,
unpublished observations).

The experiments in this paper investigate the third (and probably
most important) feature of the Salmoiraghi-Burns model: reciprocal
inhibition between medullary inspiratory and expiratory cells.   Because this is an almost universal tenet in theories of respiration,
the evidence against reciprocal inhibition must, it seems, be not
merely persuasive, but incontrovertible.   Therefore several sorts of
of experiments will be described in addition to the antidromic mapping
ones already described elsewhere (Refs. 6,7 and 10), and summarized
here.

METHODS

Experiments were conducted on cats (1.7 to 3.0 kg) anaesthetized with
pentobarbital (45-55 mg/kg) i.p., supplimented i.v. during the experiment.   Deep pentobarbital anaesthesia was used exclusively in the
present experiments in order to 'simplify' the experimental situation
by eliminating respiratory activity in the pons, and expiratory activity in the NST and rostral NRA.   The preparation is otherwise intact,
has excellent pulmonary reflexes, a regular, slightly slowed breathing
pattern, but with no accessory respiratory activity and much reduced
sensitivity to CO_2.   The three groups of NRA cells shown in Fig. 1,
as well as the two NST inspiratory populations, are active in substan-

tial numbers. The foramen magnum was enlarged and laminectomies at
various spinal levels performed. In some experiments, medullary lesions were produced using a sliver of razor blade mounted in a micro-
manipulator. Respiratory neurones were recorded with platinum plated
tungsten-in-glass microelectrodes (Ref. 14); unplated monopolar tungsten microelectrodes were used for microstimulation and antidromic
mapping. Pretriggered Post-Stimulus Time (PPST) histograms were computed with a NeuroLog NL 750 Averager-NL 730 Pulse Delay combination.

RESULTS

The Axonal Projections of NRA and NST Cells

The axonal anatomy of medullary respiratory neurones has been determined in an extensive series of experiments using the technique of
antidromic (AD) mapping (Refs. 5,6,7 and 12). A summary of these
results follows (see Fig. 2):

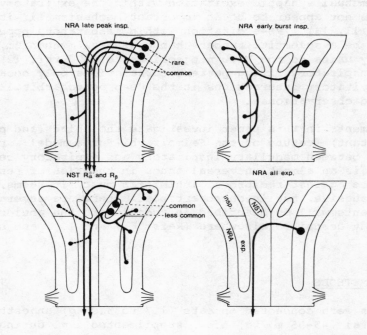

Fig. 2. Schematic diagrams of the projections of the four
major groups of medullary respiratory neurones, as determined by AD mapping. Except for the early burst inspiratory
group, all have axons whose main branch terminates in the
spinal cord. Large filled circles represent cell bodies-
small filled circles axon terminations.

(a) All late peak inspiratory neurones in NRA have axons which descend into the spinal cord, terminating in thoracic segments. Approximately 25% have collaterals which arborize in the Phrenic Nuclei.
Most of the axons (about 90%) cross in the medulla at, or rostral to,
the obex; the rest are uncrossed spinal projections. A few of these
cells have medullary collaterals which arborize among contralateral
NRA expiratory cells--more often the collaterals arborize among NRA
inspiratory cells of both sides. None have collaterals in the ipsilateral expiratory region of NRA, or in the NST of either side.

(b) In contrast to the late peak units, NRA early burst inspiratory
cells commonly have rich arborizations in the contralateral expira-
tory NRA region, as well as collaterals in the inspiratory region.
There is a very sparse projection to ipsilateral expiratory cells.
None of these cells appear to have spinal axons (or projections to
NST, but this has not yet be carefully examined).

(c) All NRA expiratory cells have crossed descending spinal axons
without any medullary collaterals. The absence of medullary collaterals projecting to NRA inspiratory or expiratory regions, or to the
NST, has been established with the most exhaustive experiments in the
series (whilst collaterals for other cells were demonstrated with relative ease).

(d) NST cells of both types have crossed spinal axons which terminate in thoracic cord; some of these axons also have collaterals which
arborize in the Phrenic Nuclei, but not enough cells have been tested
to establish the extent of this projection. Many NST cells of both
types have collaterals which project into the NRA inspiratory region;
only a few arborize among expiratory neurones. In contrast to the
NRA to NRA projections (which are mainly crossed), the NST to NRA
projections are almost totally ipsilateral.

It seems clear from these observations that the one interaction between respiratory neurone groups which is ruled out is the inhibition
of NRA or NST inspiratory neurones by NRA expiratory units.

Lesion Experiments

Even a good lesion experiment is a bad sort of an experiment, especially in a part of the brain with as many diverse intermingled systems as are found in the medulla. The results of these lesion experiments are however moderately compelling with regard to the issue of
expiratory--inspiratory interactions. Figure 3. shows the two lesions
employed. In the first, single or bilateral transverse lesions com-
separated the lateral quarter(s) of the medulla. These lesions passed just beyond the medial boundary of the caudal part of the inspiratory region of NRA. (Prior to making the lesions. NRA was carefully
mapped rostro-caudally, determining the boundaries between the inspiratory, mixed and expiratory populations.) Further, a series of pene-

trations were made with medio-lateral separations of 0.2 mm at three
levels on one side, as shown in Fig. 3. These maps established the
depths and borders of NRA. The three series of penetrations were
repeated immediately after each lesion.

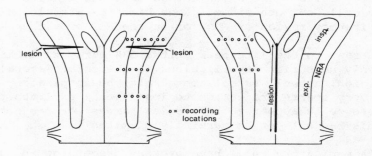

Fig. 3. These diagrams show the locations of the
lesions used to interrupt the inputs to the caudal
NRA expiratory units (left) and their crossed axons
(shown at the right).

With a unilateral transverse lesion, the hemi-diaphragm on the side of
the lesion was immediately silenced (as shown by recordings from in-
dwelling EMG electrodes). The respiratory pattern and contralateral
diaphragmatic contractions were virtually unchanged. What is important, however, is that the NRA cells caudal to the lesion were silenced
--both inspiratory and expiratory cells, even in the most caudal part
of NRA. With the bilateral lesion, all respiratory movements immediately stopped, and all NRA units caudal to the lesions were silenced.
Inspiratory neurones rostral to the lesions continued to fire with the
usual periodic patterns, hardly altered if artificial ventilation was
begun promptly (and if the arteries on the ventral surface of the medulla were spared, as was usually the case). Such results have been
obtained in 6 experiments.

In the second lesion experiment, a sagittal cut was made from the obex
to C_1, separating the dorsal halves of the medulla, but sparing most of
the pyramidal decussation. This lesion interrupts all the crossing
axons of NRA expiratory cells, and removes the descending excitatory
inputs to expiratory motoneurones (Refs. 8, 20). This lesion also
transects collaterals to contralateral inspiratory populations, if
such collaterals exist. It is the case, however, that the breathing
pattern is virtually unaffected by the lesion, and the firing patterns
of the NRA inspiratory and expiratory cells unchanged by this procedure

Massive Selective Activation of NRA Expiratory Neurones

The converse of the lesion experiments described above is to elevate
the activity in the NRA expiratory population, rather than eliminate
it. Stimulation within the expiratory region as a means of doing this
is (a) _ineffective_ (since only a few cell bodies will be within the
effective radius of the stimulus, and further, since their axons run
immediately medial and dorsal, rather than along the NRA column, so
that very few axons or cell bodies will be activated) and (b) _non-
selective_ (since the many large, low threshold fibres which pass along
and through the nucleus, especially those which are _inputs_ to these
cells, will be preferentially activated, Ref. 16). Fortunately, however, the axons of NRA expiratory cells form a reasonably discrete
tract at C_3 (Refs. 7 and 10); this can be selectively stimulated in
inspiration with low intensity stimuli which, for all practical purposes, leave other systems unaffected.

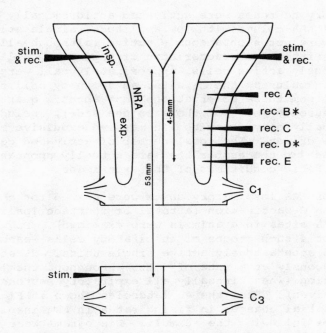

Fig. 4. This diagram shows the placement of recording and
stimulating microelectrodes (all were in fact vertical penetrations). Six independently positioned electrodes were
used; simultaneous recordings were obtained from two opposite sites in the inspiratory region of NRA, and three in
the expiratory region. Electrode C was subsequently moved
to locations B* and D*. The stimulating electrode at C_3
was used to antidromically activate the crossed tract of
descending expiratory axons.

Figure 4 shows this experiment diagramatically. Three independently
positioned recording microelectrodes were placed in the expiratory
part of NRA, at 1 mm spacings. Two further microelectrodes were placed in ipsilateral and contralateral inspiratory regions of NRA--these
were arranged so that they could be used both for stimulation and recording. The contralateral spinal cord at C_3 was explored with a stimulating microelectrode until the expiratory tract was located. This
electrode was then used to activate the contralateral expiratory population.

Figure 5 shows just how effective the C_3 stimulus was: a single 25μA
100μs duration stimulus activated at least twenty expiratory neurones
at the three NRA sites (A,C and E). Electrode C was moved 0.5 mm
rostrally and caudally from its original position, to the same depth,
(traces B* and D*), and at least eleven additional antidromically
activated expiratory neurones could be recorded (with the volleys at
A and E unchanged).

Thus expiratory neurones were activated antidromically all along the
contralateral NRA column with low amplitude, single stimuli. Many of
these cells were not spontaneously active (although all showed periodic latency variations characteristic of expiratory cells, Ref. 8). Of
the spontaneously active cells, approximately half were activated by
this single stimulus at the C_3 site, as shown by collision tests. It
is estimated from these observations that about a quarter of all NRA
expiratory neurones (or ½ of those on one side), including many units
which are usually only recruited in massive expulsive movements such
as cough, are driven. The total number of activated cells is thus
probably close to the number that are actually spontaneously active
in the anaesthetic conditions of the experiment.

Many groups of NRA inspiratory units were tested for changes in firing
rate using the C_3 activation (a total of fourteen ipsilateral and contralateral NRA sites in 4 animals were examined). Figure 6 shows PPST
histograms for 4 such groups of inspiratory cells--each group had between 2 and 5 spontaneously active single units. C_3 stimuli were presented continuously at a rate of 5 Hz. throughout the last 2/3's of
each inspiration (when virtually all expiratory neurones can be antidromically driven). From the AD latencies shown in Fig. 4., one would
expect substantial changes in firing rates in NRA inspiratory cells
from 1 to 8 ms following the stimuli. Histograms were also computed
for periods following the C_3 stimuli of up to 100 ms. No alterations
in inspiratory activity were ever demonstrated with this experiment,
even though some histograms contained as many as 20,000 inspiratory
spikes.

The absence of NRA expiratory axon collaterals in the rostral NRA
inspiratory regions was tested at each inspiratory site (as well,
of course, as on countless occasions in AD mapping experiments).
Trace C', Fig. 5., shows the absence of activation of any of the units
in trace C, with a large stimulus (100μA, 100μs duration) at the ipsi-

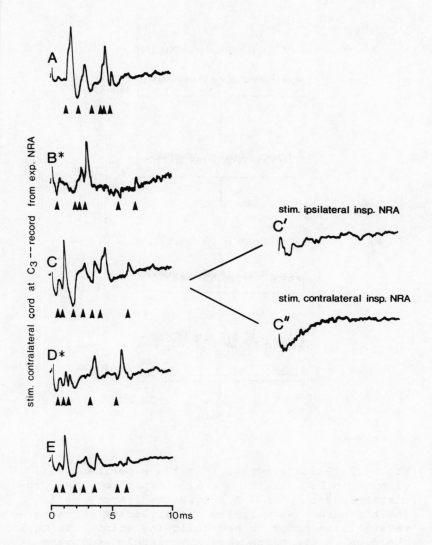

Fig. 5. Single traces recorded from the microelectrode placements
shown in Fig. 4. A, C and E were simultaneously recorded following
a single C_3 stimulus (which occured at the beginning of each trace).
Trace C' was obtained at location C with a single stimulus at the
ipsilateral inspiratory NRA site; C" was produced with a stimulus at
the contralateral inspiratory NRA site. Traces B* and D* were obtained by moving electrode C halfway between, first, A and C, and then
between C and E. The arrows indicate the presence of single antidromically activated expiratory neurones, as determined by slowly
decreasing the stimulus strength and noting the abrupt disappearance
of each unit.

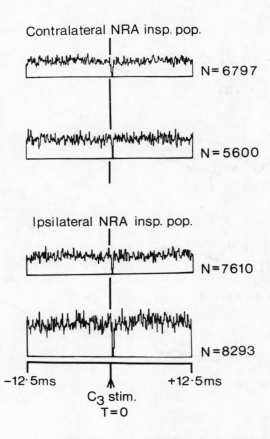

Fig. 6. PPST histograms from the experiment diagrammed in Fig. 4. for 4 small inspiratory NRA populations, each with 2-5 active inspiratory cells.
The histograms show firing probabilities for intervals 12.5 ms prior to and following stimuli at C_3.
The dips in the histograms immediately following
the C_3 stimuli are due to the overshoot of the stimulus artifact, when inspiratory spikes could not be
discriminated. (Examination of photographs of the
spike trains show that the inspiratory populations
are in fact active during this interval.)

lateral NRA site where dense inspiratory activity was recorded (corresponding to the bottom ipsilateral histogram in Fig. 6). Volleys in
passing axon tracts are evident in trace C', Fig. 5.; these are not
expiratory units. Some orthodromic activation of expiratory units
can usually be produced by stimuli at all levels of NRA, both ipsi-
laterally and contralaterally, but this is easily distinguished from

AD activation (see histogram D, Fig. 7). Trace C" shows the lack of
effect at site C of a contralateral inspiratory NRA stimulus.

If synchronous activation of a quarter of the expiratory population
does not alter NRA inspiratory activity, then (consistent with the
AD mapping results), these expiratory cells cannot be the cause of
the silent periods in NST .or NRA inspiratory units.

Correlations between NST and NRA Inspiratory Units and Expiratory Units

The anatomy leads one to expect that some inspiratory neurones must
make synaptic contact with caudal NRA expiratory cells. Three classes
of potential interactions have been examined, based on the AD maps
(Fig. 2): (a) ipsilateral inputs to NRA expiratory cells from NST units
of both sorts, (b) contralateral inputs from NRA late peak units, and
(c) contralateral inputs from NRA early burst inspiratory units. In
these experiments, a microelectrode was positioned in the expiratory
region of NRA so that 2-4 easily discriminated single units were recorded. A search was then made with a second microelectrode until a
single inspiratory unit of the desired type was found, and then
the PPST histogram was computed, using the inspiratory unit to trigger the histogram time base (ie. as the "stimulus"). Spikes from the
expiratory units were delayed so that the mean firing rate prior to
the occurence of the inspiratory spike is included at the beginning
of the histogram as control data. Figure 1 shows that there is a
substantial overlap in inspiratory and expiratory activities at the
transition from inspiration to expiration, when interesting inhibitions might be expected. The histograms are constructed from data obtained during this overlap. Additionally, since NST R_β cells can be
activated during expiration with gentle lung inflations, histograms
can be computed for these cells throughout expiration, using continuous lung inflations of about a third of a tidal volume (these produce steady, somewhat irregular, low firing rates in the R_β cells).

PPST histograms were computed both for inspiratory cells which could
be shown to send collaterals to the expiratory sites (9 cases) as
well as for a rather larger number (34) which did not. (The latter
histograms are relevant evidence if the input from inspiratory cells
is transmitted through an interposed neurone--possibly an unrecord-
able one). Figure 7 shows histograms for inspiratory cells (A and B)
which did have collaterals among the recorded expiratory units. Histogram C is for a small population of inspiratory cells, several of
which had collaterals in the expiratory region from which the spikes
in the histogram were recorded. None of the 43 histograms obtained
showed any statistically significant interactions between inspiratory
and expiratory cells in NRA.

Another commonly used way to test for inputs from one group of cells
to those in another region is to stimulate one group electrically.

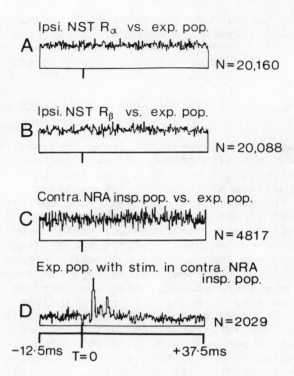

Fig. 7. PPST correlations in which the spikes of
single inspiratory neurones (A and B) or of a small
inspiratory population (C) were used to trigger the
histogram time base (T=0). Firing probabilities
are shown for small expiratory populations to which
axon collaterals from the inspiratory units project-
ed. A 12.5 ms interval prior to the occurrence of
the inspiratory spikes is included to indicate control activity levels. In D, the microelectrode at
the inspiratory location in C was used to stimulate
rather than record, and the firing of the expiratory
units in C used to construct the histogram in D.
Note the absence of any significant correlations in
C, but the obvious excitation of expiratory units
shown in D.

Objections to the use of electrical stimulation were briefly discussed above with respect to the choice of the stimulation site for expiratory cell activation. An example of the data obtained by directly
stimulating NRA is shown in Fig. 7., histogram D. The small stimulus
used (15μA, 100μs duration) clearly activated (rather than inhibited)

the expiratory units at short latency (about 3 ms). This excitatory
effect is certainly due to stimulation of fibres other than those
of the inspiratory cells, since the effect can be produced at many
neighboring locations where none of the inspiratory cells project
to the vicinity of the recorded expiratory units. Note also the absence of a correlation in C consistent with excitatory inputs. Similar powerful activations of both inspiratory and expiratory neurones
can be produced by microstimulation at sites in the pyramidal decussation. These observations underline the difficulties in interpreting
the effects of stimulation, even when the stimuli are small and well
localized among cells of interest.

DISCUSSION

Experiments are described in this paper which attempt to determine
whether reciprocal inhibition exists between the inspiratory neurones
of NST and NRA and the expiratory neurones of NRA. The NRA expiratory
cells, the cells studied by Salmoiraghi and Burns, are the most numerous group of expiratory neurones in the brainstem, even under very
light anaesthesia or with elevated respiratory drives. It is therefore essential in any consideration of reciprocal inhibition to establish, first, whether it is these expiratory cells that cause the
silent periods in the inspiratory firing patterns. These determin-
ations are, as well, specific tests of the Salmoiraghi-Burns model,
and others like it, which are based on evidence obtained from NRA
expiratory cells.

Since, in my experience, the NRA expiratory neurones are the only
active, recordable expiratory cells in the deep pentobarbital cat,
these results are of more general importance than merely tests of the
Salmoiraghi-Burns model (which is unacceptable on the grounds listed
in the Introduction, in any case). If the breathing pattern is generated only by interactions between the groups so far identified with
extracellular techniques, then that pattern cannot be the result of
reciprocal inhibitions between these cells, since my experiments conclusively show that NRA expiratory neurones do not interact in any way
with the NRA or NST inspiratory neurones. One is free, of course, to
speculate about the existence of other, as yet unrecorded, groups of
medullary expiratory units, and their possible roles in the generation
of the breathing pattern, but in the absence of any data, such speculations are completely open-ended.

The evidence that medullary inspiratory cells inhibit NRA expiratory
cells is somewhat more complicated than for the reverse interaction,
but still at variance with the general, massive population interactions
postulated in the Salmoiraghi-Burns model. The AD mapping experiments
show that several inspiratory populations can be distinguished (ie.
that they are not functionally homogeneous), with only a few NST and
late peak NRA units arborizing in the NRA expiratory region. Even
those cells which can be demonstrated to arborize there do not appear

to profoundly influence the nearby respiratory neurones (Fig. 7).

The failure to demonstrate an effect of inputs from NST and NRA inspiratory units on expiratory neurones, even in the most favorable circumstances, may however be a reflection of the insensitivity of the
analysis using the PPST histogram technique (even with 20,000 events!)
(This reservation about the PPST histogram analysis cannot however
explain the lack of effect seen with C_3 stimulation on inspiratory
populations, since, instead of attempting to detect the changes in
activity due to one cell, as in Fig. 7., changes due to the synchronous activation of very large numbers of cells were sought).

The early burst NRA inspiratory population (Figs. 1 and 2) is the
most likely group to provide a potent inhibition to the NRA expiratory
population. These cells arborize extensively among expiratory cells,
but are not involved in transmitting the motor pattern to spinal motoneurones. Their firing patterns match the patterns of hyperpolarization in expiratory neurones (Refs. 9,10 and 15). Correlations between expiratory units and early burst inspiratory neurones are extremely difficult to obtain, primarily because very few early burst
units (relatively rare in the first place) have overlapping firing
patterns with even the earliest onset expiratory neurones (Fig. 1).
The goal of a series of experiments now in progress is to assess
directly the importance of the early burst inspiratory input in the
production of the NRA expiratory firing pattern.

REFERENCES

1. B. D. Burns and G. C. Salmoiraghi, Repetitive firing of respiratory neurons during their burst activity, J. Neurophysiol. 23, 27-46
(1960).

2. R. von Baumgarten and E. Kanzow, The interaction of two types of
inspiratory neurons in the region of the tractus solitarius of the cat
Arch. Ital. Biol. 96, 361-373 (1958).

3. C. von Euler, J. N. Hayward, Irja Marttila and R. J. Wyman, Respiratory neurones of the ventrolateral nucleus of the solitary tract
of cat: vagal input, spinal connections and morphological identification, Brain Res. 61, 1-22 (1973).

4. Jack L. Feldman and Morton I. Cohen, Relation between expiratory
duration and rostral medullary expiratory neuronal discharge, Brain
Res. 141, 172-178 (1978).

5. E. Jankowska and W. Roberts, An electrophysiological demonstration of the axonal projections of single spinal interneurones in the
cat, J. Physiol. 222, 597-622 (1972).

6. E. G. Merrill, The lateral respiratory neurons of the medulla:

their associations with nucleus ambiguus, nucleus retroambigualis, the spinal accessory nucleus and the spinal cord, Brain Res. 24, 11-28 (1970).

7. E. G. Merrill, The descending pathways from the lateral respiratory neurones in cats, J. Physiol. 218, 82-83P (1971).

8. E. G. Merrill, Thoracic motor drives from medullary expiratory neurones in cats, J. Physiol. 222, 154-155P (1972).

9. E. G. Merrill, Temporal patterns of antidromic invasion latencies for the respiratory neurones of nucleus retroambigualis in cats, J. Physiol. 223, 18-20P (1972).

10. E. G. Merrill (1974), Finding a respiratory function for the medullary respiratory neurons, Essays on the Nervous System, Clarendon Press, Oxford.

11. E. G. Merrill, Antidromic activation of lateral respiratory neurones during their silent periods, J. Physiol. 241, 118-119P (1974).

12. E. G. Merrill, Preliminary studies on nucleus retroambigualis--nucleus of the solitary tract interactions in cats, J. Physiol. 244, 54-55P (1974).

13. E. G. Merrill, Absence of correlations between lateral expiratory neurones in cat, J. Physiol. 276, 33-34P (1978).

14. E. G. Merrill and A. Ainsworth, Glass-coated platinum-plated tungsten microelectrodes, Med. Biol. Eng. 10, 662-672 (1972).

15. R. A. Mitchell and D. A. Herbert, Synchronized high frequency synaptic potentials in medullary respiratory neurons, Brain Res. 75, 350-355 (1974).

16. J. B. Ranck, Which elements are excited in electrical stimulation of mammalian central nervous system: a review, Brain Res. 98, 417-440 (1975).

17. D. W. Richter and F. Heyde, Accommodative reactions of medullary respiratory neurons of the cat, J. Neurophysiol., 38, 1172-1180 (1975).

18. G. C. Salmoiraghi and B. D. Burns, Localization and patterns of discharge of respiratory neurones in brain-stem of cat. J. Neurophysiol., 23, 2-13 (1960).

19. G. C. Salmoiraghi and B. D. Burns, Notes on mechanism of rhythmic respiration, J. Neurophysiol., 23, 14-26 (1960).

20. T. A. Sears, C. R. Bainton and P. A. Kirkwood, On the transmission of the stimulating effects of carbon dioxide to the muscles of respiration, J. Physiol., 280, 249-272 (1978).

DISCUSSION

of the papers by Richter et al. and Merrill

In the discussion both Merrill and Richter further emphasized that
there was little real disagreement between the two speakers.Richter
had presented strong evidence that reciprocal inhibition of bulbar
inspiratory neurons is a prominent feature of their operation but he
had no information on which group of neurons are responsible for
this inhibition or by which pathways this inhibition is transmitted.
Merrill, on the other hand, had presented strong evidence against
the presence of reciprocal coupling between the large population of
expiratory bulbo-spinal neurons in the caudal part of nucleus retroambigualis, NRA, and the inspiratory bulbo-spinal neurons in the
more rostral part of NRA or in nucleus tractus solitarius, NTS. It
was emphasized both by Euler and Sears that it is almost impossible
to conceive of a rhythm generation without inhibitory and excitatory
couplings between different parts of the network. Also the asymmetrical models of respiratory rhythmogenesis (e.g. Bradley et al., Biol.
Cybernetics 19, 105, 1975) include as an absolutely essential part
inhibition of the central inspiratory activity by the inspiratory
'off-switch' mechanisms which are responsible for the graded and the
final inhibition of the inspiratory activity (see e.g. Remmers et al.
p. 195, this volume) and for the silence of inspiratory activity
during the phase of expiration.

Both Merrill and Richter agreed that it was necessary, now, to pay
attention to other populations of expiratory neurons than that of the
caudal part of NRA. Attention was drawn to the findings of a sizeable
population of expiratory neurons in the NTS complex reported by
Feldman and Cohen (Respiratory Centers and Afferent Systems, INSERM,
Paris, 1976) and to the type of neurons analysed by Remmers et al.
(p. 195, this volume) the activity of which was related to the graded
inhibition of central inspiratory activity.

Merrill and others emphasized that the extracellular technique by no
means provide an exhaustive sample of all the spontaneously active
cells in the medulla. It only gives a more or less selective sample,
the selectivity being different in character in different nervous
structures depending on several different factors, not only on the
properties of the electrodes employed.

Mention was also made of the possibility that non-spiking neurons
(see Bruce et al., p. 177, this volume) might play an important role
in the reciprocal couplings which are an inevitable prerequisite for
rhythm generating networks whether 'symmetrical' or 'asymmetrical'.

THE CENTRAL TRANSMISSION OF RESPIRATORY SIGNALS: A PHARMACOLOGICAL STUDY

M. DENAVIT-SAUBIÉ, J. CHAMPAGNAT and J. C. VELLUTI

*Laboratoire de Physiologie Nerveuse, Département de Neurophysiologie Appliquée,
C.N.R.S., 91190 Gif-sur-Yvette, France*

ABSTRACT

In order to characterize the synaptic inputs which are involved in the modulation
of bulbar respiratory neurones, juxtacellular iontophoretical applications of
drugs were performed. Two types of agents were used. Some of them mimic the effect
of tonic excitations (e.g. L-glutamate) or inhibitions (e.g. GABA), and others can
act through modifications of synaptic transmission (e.g. picrotoxin, bicuculline,
opiates).

Strong periodic inhibitions related to the respiratory cycle were demonstrated.
They were able to rhythmically cut off tonic excitations and could be reduced by
drugs considered as antagonists of depressant amino-acids (picrotoxin or strychnine). Data suggest the involvement of strong inhibitory transmitters such as
depressant amino-acids. These results are in agreement with the hypothesis of a reciprocal inhibition of inspiratory and expiratory neurones at the bulbar level.

Periodic excitations related to the respiratory cycle were also demonstrated.
Opiates which depress excitatory afferents suppressed these periodic excitations
without affecting the tonic background. This effect is important since it
can explain the respiratory depression observed after morphine administration.
However excitations do not appear in the model of reciprocal innervation.

Keywords : <u>Bulbar respiratory neurones</u> – <u>Reciprocal inhibition</u> – <u>Gating mechanisms</u>
Excitatory afferences – Pharmacology – Microiontophoresis.

INTRODUCTION

The present work is a part of a series of studies intended to elucidate the central
respiratory mechanisms. This rhythmic activity, as recorded from respiratory
neurones (RN) located in the medulla at the level of the obex, is determined by
afferents acting on these neurones during a constant and restricted part of the
respiratory cycle (Mitchell and Herbert, 1974 ; Richter et al., 1975). The use of
juxtaneuronal applications of pharmacological tools is of interest to demonstrate
whether these afferents are inhibitory or excitatory and to determine during which
part of the respiratory cycle these afferents are the most active.

Occurence and functional significance of respiratory inhibitions are tested in RN

using L-glutamate. This agent, which is known to postsynaptically depolarize neurones in the CNS (Curtis and Johnston, 1974 ; Zieglgänsberger and Puil, 1973), was
applied iontophoretically in the vicinity of a single recorded RN. It induced a reproducible and stable increase in firing that can be used as a model of increased
tonic excitatory inputs. If a natural, strong, rhythmic, inhibitory mechanism gates
the firing of RN, it is also expected to be able to gate the effectiveness of L-
glutamate during the same restricted part of the respiratory cycle.

Pharmacological tools that block transmission from the presynaptic afferents to
the postsynaptic neurone were also used. Inhibitory transmission was studied using
iontophoretical applications of picrotoxin and strychnine. These are known to block
the inhibitory effect of some amino-acids which are possible transmitters of inhibitions in the mammalian CNS (Curtis and Johnston, 1974 ; Krnjevic et al., 1977 ;
Sonnhof et al., 1975). The natural occurence of respiratory rhythmic inhibitions is
demonstrated when picrotoxin or strychnine are able to disinhibit the firing of RN
during a restricted part of the respiratory cycle. Excitatory transmission was
studied in a similar way using iontophoretical application of opiates or opioid
peptides (morphine, levorphanol, enkephalin). The observations reported here
support the theory of a reciprocal inhibition of bulbar inspiratory (IN) and expiratory neurones (EN) (Pitts et al., 1939 ; Salmoiraghi and Burns, 1960). Furthermore, periodic respiratory excitations are also present in RN and are depressed by
opiate applications.

METHODS

Experiments were performed on cats either under pentobarbitone sodium (30 mg/kg)
anaesthesia or prepared with a spinal section at the C_7T_1 level. The animals were
bivagotomized, paralyzed with gallamine triethiodide and artificially ventilated.
Phrenic nerve activity was recorded with bipolar electrodes. Extracellular recordings of respiratory neurones were obtained after stereotaxic placement of a multibarrelled electrode at the level of the obex. The explored area extends laterally
from 1 to 4 mm to the midline and at a depth from 2 to 4 mm from the dorsal surface
of the medulla (see Denavit-Saubié et al., 1978 b). The tip diameter of the micro-
pipette could vary with the number of adjacent barrels (usually 7), each one having
a diameter of about one micron. The barrels of the micropipettes were filled with
NaCl (3M, recording barrel), methyl blue (0.1 %, pH 5.8, for histological localization) and the following solutions of agents to be applied iontophoretically :
L-glutamate (0.5 M, pH 8.0), GABA (1M, pH 4.2), glycine (0.5 M, pH 3.7), and, dissolved in 165 mM NaCl solution (pH 5.0) : picrotoxin (4.5mM), strychnine (10 mM),
morphine-HCl (50 mM), levorphanol-SO4 (50 mM), dextrorphan-SO4 (50 mM), naloxone-
HCl (50 mM), methionine-enkephalin (12.5 mM).

Microiontophoresis was used to apply substances in the vicinity of a single
neurone which was simultaneously recorded. Spike shape was continuously monitored
on oscilloscopes and recorded on a moving film in order to insure that only single
units were studied. Steady current of very low intensity was applied through the
solution in order to eject small amounts of the drug. The relative value of
dosages was proportional to the intensity of iontophoretic current and expressed
in nano-ampères (nA, range of currents used 5-100 nA). Possible artefactual
effects were systematically tested using a barrel containing no active agents (for
details, see Kelly, 1975).

RESULTS

1. Evidence for periodic gating mechanisms

All bulbar RN in this study were excited by 5-50 nA of L-glutamate and thus considered to be recorded from the somato-dendritic part of the neurones (see

Denavit-Saubié et al., 1978 b). The pattern of discharge of RN is characterized by high ("maximal") frequency periods which alternate during each respiratory cycle with low ("minimal") frequency periods. In most cases the effectiveness of L-glutamate on RN was apparently not the same throughout the cycle. Under L-glutamate application the maximal frequency was increased while the minimal frequency remained at a very low level. This must be due to the fact that excitations produced by a constant dose of L-glutamate cannot balance the effect of strong inhibitions occurring in a special part of the cycle. These strong inhibitions can be the basis for a gating mechanism. Their temporal position in the respiratory cycle is very well localized for a given cell and, even under L-glutamate, cannot be shifted.

Figure 1 illustrates the effect of L-glutamate on an early EN, discharging during the first half of expiration. L-glutamate increased the maximal frequency at the beginning and caused spike firing during the second half of expiration. However, even with a high dosage of L-glutamate, no spike was elicited during a constant part of inspiration. Such a gating of L-glutamate effect was found during inspiration in late and the majority of early EN (Fig. 1) and during expiration in about half of IN. Conversely, in the remaining IN and in some early EN, relatively low dosages of L-glutamate (5-50 nA) increased both basal and maximal frequencies, and no gating of the glutamate effect was evident during any part of the cycle.

REF

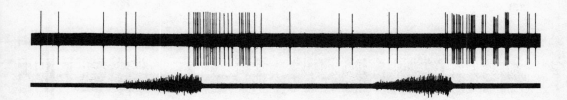

GLUT 50

500 ms

Fig. 1 : Effect of L-glutamate on the discharge of an early expiratory bulbar neurone. In the reference (REF, upper part), the discharge (upper) begins at the end of each inspiration indicated by the discharge of phrenic nerve activity (lower). During application of L-glutamate with an ejection current of 50 nano-amperes (GLUT 50), the discharge was increased at the beginning of expiration and spike occurred during the remaining part of expiration. Note that a "silent" period remained during inspiration and that the rapid increase in spike frequency remained located at the very end of inspiration.

2. Evidence for periodic inhibitory transmission

Pharmacologically induced inhibitions of bulbar RN were performed using applications of GABA or glycine (5-50 nA). Picrotoxin or strychnine (20-100 nA) were generally found sufficient to reversibly reduce or abolish respectively the GABA or
glycine induced inhibitions. Considering the pattern of discharge during the respiratory cycle, evidences were obtained suggesting that strychnine or picrotoxin were
selectively active on naturally occurring respiratory periodic inhibitions without
affecting the discharge in the remaining part of the respiratory cycle. Different
effects demonstrated a weakening of respiratory inhibitory processes of IN and EN
under strychnine or picrotoxin :

    a) The minimal frequency occurring during the respiratory cycle was increased ;
    b) The onset of this minimal frequency or "silent" period was delayed ;
    c) The effectiveness of L-glutamate on the minimal frequency was increased.

These effects, occurring without change in maximal frequency, tend to decrease the
gating inputs to RN.

3. Evidence for excitatory transmission

Pharmacologically induced excitations of bulbar RN were performed using applications of L-glutamate (5-50 nA). Opiate agonists, morphine and levorphanol, and the
endogenous ligant to the opiate receptors, methionine-enkephalin, applied with

REF

MO 50

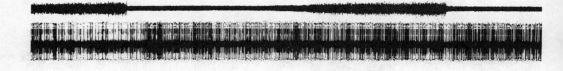

500 ms

Fig. 2 : Effect of morphine on the discharge of a tonic early expiratory bulbar
neurone. In the reference (REF, upper part) at the end of each inspiration indicated by the discharge of phrenic nerve (upper tracing), an increase of neuronal discharge (lower tracing) was recorded and was suppressed by iontophoretic application of morphine with a current of 50 nanoamperes (MO 50, lower part). Note that
this neurone discharged continuously throughout the respiratory cycle and that
morphine did not decrease firing occurring during the end of expiration and during
inspiration.

current ranging from 20 to 75 nA were found able to reduce or abolish the L-glutamate induced excitation on the majority of bulbar RN. Considering the pattern of
discharge during the respiratory cycle, evidences were obtained suggesting that
opiates were selectively active on naturally occurring respiratory periodic excitations :
    a) Opiates depressed the mean discharge of RN by reducing maximal frequency ;
    b) In tonic early EN (Fig. 2) and tonic IN, maximal frequency was clearly
lowered by dosages of opiates that did not change the minimal frequency. These
effects were shown to involve stereospecific opiate receptors because they were
antagonized by a selective opiate antagonist (naloxone), and they were not mimicked by applications of the physiologically inactive D^+-enantiomer of levorphanol
(dextrorphan).

DISCUSSION

Present studies suggest that strong inhibitions with a respiratory periodicity
modulate the discharge of the majority of bulbar RN. One can postulate that they
arise from the activity of either presynaptic IN, when occurring during inspiration, or presynaptic EN when occurring during expiration. These results are in
accordance with what is postulated in the theory of reciprocal innervation. Functionally these inhibitions are able to maintain the modulation of RN discharges
when they are submitted to strong tonic excitations similar to those induced
pharmacologically by L-glutamate applications. These data are in agreement with
other results demonstrating changes in antidromic (Bianchi, 1971 ; Lipski et al.,
1978 ; Merril, 1974) and orthodromic vagal (Von Euler, 1973) responses during this
type of inhibitions. Pharmacologically the finding that these inhibitions are
sensible to strychnine or picrotoxin suggest that they are at least partly due to
strong inhibitory transmitters which have properties in common with depressant
amino-acids. Such inhibitory amino-acids (GABA, glycine, taurine) were previously
shown to be active on bulbar RN (Denavit-Saubié and Champagnat, 1975). It is of
interest to note that intracellular studies performed at different levels of the
mammalian CNS (Curtis and Johnston, 1974 ; Krnjevic et al., 1977 ; Sonnhof et al.,
1975) demonstrated that the depressant amino-acids induced membrane hyperpolarisat-
ion associated with an increase in conductance probably to chloride ions.
Intracellular analysis demonstrated that similar mechanisms are underlying the
periodic inhibition of bulbar RN (Richter et al., 1975).

Opiates were shown to be active on excitatory transmission to bulbar RN. In tonic
RN, opiates do not change the minimal frequency and act selectively during the
period of maximal frequency. Opiates probably reduce the effectiveness of excitatory transmission occurring during a restricted part of the respiratory cycle, and
lacking during the remaining part of the cycle. These data suggest that excitatory
afferences, with a respiration related periodic activity, may also be implicated
in the modulation of bulbar RN. The functional importance of excitatory transmission in the central respiratory mechanisms are further suggested by the occurence
of severe respiratory depressions after opiate administration in cats with vagi
intacts or bilaterally cut (Denavit-Saubié et al., 1978 a).

REFERENCES

Bianchi, A. L. (1971). Localisation et étude des neurones respiratoires bulbaires.
    Mise en jeu antidromique par stimulation spinale ou vagale. J. Physiol. (Paris),
    63, 5-40.
Curtis, D. R. and G.A.R. Johnston (1974). Aminoacid transmitters in the mammalian
    central nervous system. Ergebn. Physiol. Biol. Chem., 69, 97-188.
Denavit-Saubié, M. and J. Champagnat (1975). The effect of some depressing amino-
    acids on bulbar respiratory and non-respiratory neurones. Brain Res., 97,
    356-361.

Denavit-Saubié, M., J. Champagnat and W. Zieglgänsberger (1978 a). Effects of
    opiates and methionine-enkephalin on pontine and bulbar respiratory neurones
    of the cat. Brain Res., 155, 55-67.
Denavit-Saubié, M., D. Riche and J. Champagnat (1978 b). Anatomo-functional study
    of pontine afferents to the bulbar respiratory area of the Cat. This volume.
Euler, C. Von, J. N. Hayward, I. Martilla and R. J. Wyman (1973). Respiratory
    neurones of the ventrolateral nucleus of the solitary tract of cat : vagal
    input, spinal connections and morphological identification. Brain Res., 61,
    1-22.
Kelly, J. S. (1975). Microiontophoretic application of drugs onto single neurons.
    'In' L. L. Iversen, S. D. Iversen and S. H. Snyder (Eds.), Handbook of Psycho-
    pharmacology, 2, Plenum Press, New York and London, pp. 29-67.
Krnjevic, K., E. Puil and R. Werman (1977). GABA and glycine actions on spinal
    motoneurons. Can. J. Physiol. Pharmacol., 55, 658-669.
Lipski, J., J. Kedra and L. Kubin (1978). A method for averaging response latency
    patterns of antidromically excited neurons. Acta Neurobiol. Exp., 38, 79-84.
Merrill, E. G. (1974). Finding a respiratory function for the medullary respiratory
    neurons. 'In' R. Bellairs and E. G. Gray (Eds.), Essays on the nervous system,
    Clarendon Press, Oxford, pp. 451-486.
Mitchell, R. A. and D. A. Herbert (1974). Synchronized high frequency synaptic
    potentials in medullary respiratory neurons. Brain Res., 75, 350-355.
Pitts, R. F., H. W. Magoun, S. W. Ranson (1939). Localization of the medullary
    respiratory centers in the Cat. Am. J. Physiol., 126, 673.
Richter, D. W., F. Heyde and M. Gabriel (1975). Intracellular recordings from
    different types of medullary respiratory neurons of the Cat. J. Neurophysiol.,
    38, 1162-1171.
Salmoïraghi, G. C. and B. D. Burns (1960). Notes on mechanism of rhythmic
    respiration. J. Neurophysiol., 23, 14-26.
Sonnhof, U., P. Grafe, J. Krumnikl, M. Linder and L. Schindler (1975). Inhibitory
    post-synaptic actions of taurine, GABA and other aminoacids on motoneurons of
    the isolated frog spinal cord. Brain Res., 100, 327-341.
Zieglgänsberger, W. and E. A. Puil (1973). Actions of glutamic acid on spinal
    neurones. Exp. Brain Res., 17, 35-49.

Acknowledgements : The authors wish to thank G. Ghilini and G. Levesque for their
technical assistance.

This study was supported by an ATP from the DGRST n° 78.7.2776 and an ATP from
the CNRS n° 3176.

LUNG STRETCH RECEPTOR INPUTS TO Rβ-NEURONES: A MODEL FOR "RESPIRATORY GATING"

H. CAMERER, D. W. RICHTER, N. RÖHRIG
and M. MEESMANN

I. Department of Physiology, University of Heidelberg, D-6900 Heidelberg, F.R.G.

"Respiratory gating", i.e. failure of neurones to respond to excitatory afferent inputs during certain periods of the respiratory cycle, as seen when investigated extracellularly, or variations in the postsynaptic effect in parallel with the respiratory cycle, as seen in intracellular recordings, has been described for several inputs to different types of respiratory neurone. The afferent inputs tested were from lung stretch receptors (Ref. 4), chemoreceptors (Ref. 7,8) and baroreceptors (Ref. 9).

The afferent input from lung stretch receptors to R_β-neurones acts monosynaptically (Ref. 11,12). This input has been used as a model to investigate the mechanisms underlying "respiratory gating", since variations of postsynaptic effects cannot then be due to changes in interneuronal spike transmission. In this model "respiratory gating" may be explained by three mechanisms: (a) Presynaptic depolarization of the afferent terminals of lung stretch receptors during central expiration, as suggested by Hildebrandt (5), (2) weak convergence of lung stretch receptor afferents or a high threshold for excitation of R_β-neurones, which would mean that this input would need to be superimposed on an inspiratory postsynaptic depolarization to reach firing levels (Ref. 3) or (c) postsynaptic inhibition of R_β-neurones during central expiration.

Electrical excitation of lung stretch receptor fibres generates rather steeply rising EPSPs in R_β-neurones which often give rise to one or more action potentials, whose thresholds are not abnormally high. The amplitude of the EPSPs varied with the respiratory cycle: during inspiration they were largest and revealed only small fluctuations in steepness, but during expiration they decreased continuously (Fig. 1).

Since subthreshold events are also "gated", weak convergence or an abnormal high threshold for excitation cannot be the basic mechanism of "respiratory gating" (c.f. mechanism b).

In order to explain the variations of the amplitude of EPSPs, we started to investigate the mechanisms acting at the post-

synaptic site of R$_\beta$-neurones in synchrony with the respiratory cycle .

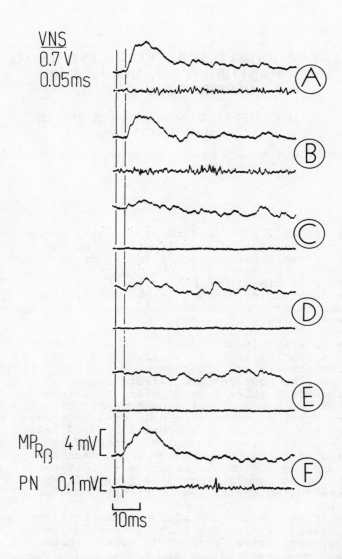

Fig. 1. Excitatory postsynaptic potential (EPSP) in an
R$_\beta$-neurone evoked by single pulse stimulation of the
vagal nerve. The recordings A-F were made at different
phases of the respiratory cycle. In A the recordings were
made during early inspiration, in B during the second half
of inspiration, in C at early expiration, in D at mid-ex-
piration, in E at late expiration and in F at early inspiration of the following respiratory cycle. MP$_{R\beta}$: membrane potential of the R$_\beta$-neurone. PN: phrenic nerve activity. The vertical lines indicate the time of vagal nerve
stimulation and the onset of the EPSP.

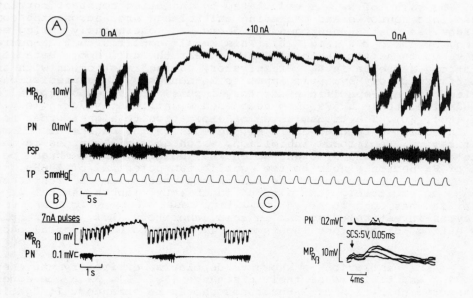

Fig. 2. R$_\beta$-neurone. A: Demonstration of expiratory IPSPs:
The IPSPs had been reversed to a depolarizing direction
by Cl$^-$ -injection before the start of the trace and were
again reversed to a hyperpolarizing direction by positive
current injection (shown above the trace). B: Negative
current pulses were repetitively injected into the soma.
The input resistance was calculated by the voltage drop
across the membrane (IPSPs were reversed, i.e. depolarizing). The bridge circuit for current injection was over-
compensated by 1 MΩ in A and B. C: The spinal cord was
stimulated at the C$_2$ - level by single shocks. A short-
latency EPSP varied in amplitude and steepness in synchrony with the respiratory cycle. MP$_{R\beta}$: membrane potential. PN: phrenic nerve activity. PSP: postsynaptic activity as recorded using a 10 Hz high pass filter. TP: tracheal pressure. SCS: spinal cord stimulation.

R$_\beta$-neurones show an augmenting pattern of IPSPs during expiration
and the inhibitory synapses responsible appear to be close to the
soma (Ref. 13, see Fig. 2A). IPSPs are known to be generated by a
significant increase in the chloride and potassium conductivity of
the subsynaptic membrane. The amplitudes of the EPSPs, i.e. the voltage drop across the soma membrane due to the synaptic current produced by excitation of lung stretch receptor afferents, must therefore vary in synchrony with the changes in neurone input resistance

(R_N). The value of R_N was calculated by injecting constant current pulses into neurones and measuring the voltage drop across the soma membrane. In most R_β-neurones, R_N decreased continuously during expiration, by up to 80% (Fig. 2B). This result confirms that R_β-neurones receive postsynaptic inhibition at or near the cell body. Because of the strong decrease in R_N, "respiratory gating" must occur with any type of excitatory synaptic input to R_β-neurones. This prediction was verified for non-specific excitatory inputs activated by spinal cord stimulation: these EPSPs also decreased significantly during expiration (Fig. 2C). The transmission of excitation to higher order neurones, in addition to changes in R_N, depends on the degree of membrane polarization. Reciprocal inhibition, which acts via changes in membrane resistance and membrane potential, "holding" the membrane potential of R_β-neurones near to the equilibrium potential of IPSPs, therefore, seems to represent the fundamental mechanism of "respiratory gating" of excitatory (and also of inhibitory) inputs. As reciprocal inhibition has been found in medullary respiratory neurones of all types investigated so far in this laboratory (Ref. 1), "respiratory gating" of afferent inputs clearly seems to be a general phenomenon.

Lung inflation is known to depolarize expiratory neurones (Ref. 10) and to increase their discharge (Ref. 2). As a consequence, expiratory inhibition of R_β-neurones should be enhanced. If "gating" depends on the strength of reciprocal inhibition, not only should the EPSPs now be more effectively short-circuited during expiration but IPSPs may even dominate. During lung inflation lasting for several respiratory cycles, the central inspiratory drive is also reduced, so R_β-neurones (like R_α-neurones) may then show decreased excitation during inspiration and increased inhibition during expiration (Fig. 3) in spite of the excitatory input of lung stretch receptors.

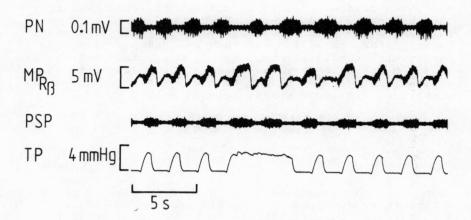

Fig. 3. Effect of lung inflation upon an R_β-neurone. The IPSPs have been reversed by Cl^--injection. Synaptic inhibition, therefore, produced depolarization. (The IPSPs reached large amplitudes as seen in the PSP trace). Lung inflation started during late inspiration. The following

inspiration was delayed and weaker. The net effect on this R_β-neurone was a reduction in inspiratory membrane depolarization in spite of the excitatory input of lung stretch receptors. The amplitude of the summed (depolarizing) IPSPs during expiration, however, increased. PN: phrenic nerve activity. $MP_{R\beta}$: membrane potential. PSP: postsynaptic activity, as recorded using a 10 Hz high pass filter. TP: tracheal pressure.

A similar reversal of effects is described for the chemoreceptor input to inspiratory R_α and R_β -neurones (Ref. 7) when depolarized by excitant amino acids. Since chemoreceptor afferents are also known to activate both inspiratory and expiratory neurones (Ref. 6), this effect can be explained in a similar way.

Because non-specific inputs to R_β-neurones are also "gated" and there appears to be no significant variation in the excitability of lung stretch receptor afferent terminals in parallel with the central respiratory cycle (preliminary results), we assume that presynaptic inhibition, if present here at all, plays only a minor functional role.

This work was supported by the Deutsche Forschungsgemeinschaft.

REFERENCES

(1) Camerer, H., Meesmann, M., Richter, D.W., Röhrig, N., Reciprocal inhibition of bulbar respiratory neurones in the cat, J. Physiol. (Lond.), in press.

(2) Cohen, M.I., Discharge patterns of brain-stem respiratory neurones during Hering-Breuer reflex evoked by lung inflation, J. Neurophysiol. 32, 356-374 (1969).

(3) Cohen, M.I., Feldman, J.L., Models of respiratory phase switching Fed. Proc. 36, 2367-2374 (1977).

(4) von Euler, C., Hayward, J.N., Marttila, I., Wyman, R.J., Respiratory neurones of the ventrolateral nucleus of the solitary tract of cat: vagal input, spinal connections and morphological identification, Brain Res. 61, 1-22 (1973).

(5) Hildebrandt, J.R., Gating: a mechanism for selective receptivity in the respiratory center, Fed. Proc. 36, 2381-2385 (1977).

(6) Koepchen, H.P., Klüssendorf, D., Philipp, U., Mechanisms of central transmission of respiratory reflexes, Acta Neurobiol. Exp. 33, 287-299 (1973).

(7) Lipski, J., McAllen, R.M., Spyer, K.M., The carotid chemoreceptor input to the respiratory neurones of the nucleus of tractus solitarius, J. Physiol. (Lond.) 269, 797-810 (1977).

(8) Mitchell, R.A., Herbert, D.A., The effect of carbon dioxide on the membrane potential of medullary respiratory neurons,

Brain Res. 75, 345-349 (1974).

(9) Richter, D.W., Seller, H., Baroreceptor effects on medullary
      respiratory neurones of the cat. Brain Res. 86, 168-171
      (1975).

(10)Richter, D.W., Seller, H., Response of medullary respiratory neu-
      rones to lung inflation and vagal nerve stimulation, Pflü-
      gers Arch. Suppl. 362, R40 (1976).

(11)Richter, D.W., Camerer, H., Röhrig, N., Medullary inspiratory in-
      terneurons receiving a monosynaptic input from lung stretch
      receptors, Pflügers Arch. Suppl. 373, R75 (1978).

(12)Richter, D.W., Camerer, H., Röhrig, N., Monosynaptic transmission
      from lung stretch receptor afferents to R_β-neurones, Wenner
      -Gren Center Symposium (1978).

(13)Richter, D.W., Camerer, H., Meesmann, M., Röhrig, N., Studies on
      the synaptic interconnection between bulbar respiratory neu-
      rones of cats, in preparation.

Discussion after the next paper.

MONOSYNAPTIC TRANSMISSION FROM LUNG STRETCH RECEPTOR AFFERENTS TO Rβ-NEURONES

D. W. RICHTER, H. CAMERER and N. RÖHRIG

I. Department of Physiology, University of Heidelberg, D-6900 Heidelberg, F.R.G.

v. Baumgarten and Kanzow (1) first described the R_β-neurones which lie in the ventrolateral nucleus of the solitary tract (VL-NTS). These neurones receive excitatory synaptic inputs during both inspiration and lung inflation. The synaptic connection between lung stretch receptor afferents (LA) and R_β-neurones was investigated by v. Euler et al. (2) using extracellular recording techniques. They suggested that R_β-neurones might represent second order pulmonary afferent neurones.

In the present investigation we tried to verify monosynaptic transmission from LA to R_β-neurones using intracellular recordings (Ref. 4). Both LA fibres and R_β-neurones were recorded from within a region 1-2 mm cranial to the obex, 1-2 mm lateral to midline and a depth of 1.3-2.1 mm. LA fibres were identified functionally by their discharge following changes in artificial ventilation and electrophysiologically by the established criteria.

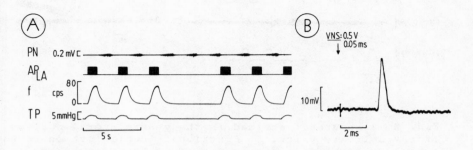

Fig. 1. Lung stretch receptor afferent fibre recorded in the ventrolateral nucleus of the solitary tract. A: Functional identification of the fibre. B: Electrophysiological

identification of the fibre and duration of orthodromic
conduction when stimulating the ipsilateral vagal nerve
with single pulses of 0.5V and 0.05ms. PN: phrenic nerve
activity. AP_{LA}: normalized spike discharge. f: discharge
frequency. TP: tracheal pressure.

Stimulating the ipsilateral vagal nerves, the threshold for excitation of LA fibres was found to range between 0.1 and 0.8 V (0.05ms).
Repetitive electrical stimulation (20-100 cps) of the vagal nerves
elicited a typical Hering-Breuer response. The latency to excitation
of LA fibres which were recorded within the VL-NTS region was 2.9 ±
0.8 ms (mean ± S.D., n= 44, Fig. 1B). The extracephalic distance was
65-70 mm. Assuming an intracephalic conduction distance of 8-10 mm,
a velocity of 17-37 m · s^{-1} was calculated for conduction along the
whole pathway. The extracephalic conduction velocity was measured by
two methods: 1.) By the latency to the LA-volley recorded at the
rootlets of vagal nerves. 2.) By the differences in latencies to LA-
fibre excitation within the VL-NTS region when stimulating the vagal
nerves at different positions. All these values were within the same
range and in agreement with those measured by Paintal (3). The results indicate that there is no significant slowing of conduction
along the intracephalic course of LA-fibres.

In intracellular recordings, R_β-neurones were identified by
their excitatory synaptic input (also subthreshold EPSPs) during both
inspiration and lung inflation (Fig. 2A).

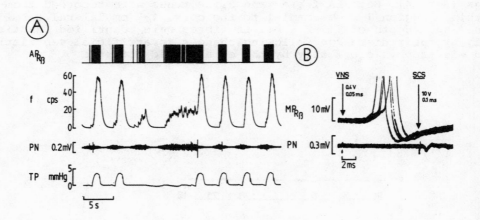

Fig. 2. R_β-neurone recorded in the ventrolateral nucleus
of the solitary tract. A: Functional identification revea-
ling a synaptic inspiratory drive and lung stretch receptor input, which disappears during deflation. B: Excitatory postsynaptic potential (EPSP) elicited by ipsilateral vagal nerve stimulation with single shocks at 0.4 V and
0.05 ms. Four traces are superimposed in the AC-recording.

Note that the latency of the EPSP remains constant,
whereas the steepness of the EPSP and the latency of the
spike discharge vary significantly. Spinal cord stimulation (SCS) does not antidromically excite the neurone
(this was also true without preceding vagal nerve stimulation). $AP_{R\beta}$: normalized spike discharge. f: discharge frequency. PN: phrenic nerve activity. TP: tracheal
pressure. $MP_{R\beta}$: membrane potential.

These neurones could not be antidromically activated by spinal cord
stimulation at the C_2 - C_3 -level (Fig. 2B). Stimulating the ipsilateral vagal nerve with single shocks of 0.2-0.5 V produced a steeply
rising EPSP (Fig. 2B). The time necessary to reach the threshold for excitation varied by as much as 2.6 ms within a single neurone (Fig. 2B+3). The shortest latencies of the spike discharge were
measured during the period of inspiration. The latency of the EPSP
itself, however, remained constant. In different R_β-neurones it was
3.1 ± 0.8 ms (mean $\pm$ S.D., n=40; Fig. 2B). The differences in EPSP
latencies when stimulating at different positions of the vagal nerve
revealed that the EPSPs were evoked by afferent fibres conducting at
$23-32$ m $\cdot$ s^{-1}, i.e. a range of conduction velocities as found for
LA-fibres. Using the data from several experiments, the average difference in the latencies to the excitation of LA-fibres within the
VL-NTS and the start of EPSPs in R_β-neurones was 0.2 ms. This time
delay is far too short to permit an interneurone being involved in
synaptic transmission. This interpretation was verified by the results of one experiment in which 11 LA-fibres and 10 R_β-neurones
were recorded within the VL-NTS region some of which are shown in
Fig. 3.

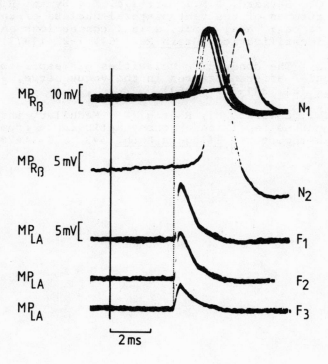

Fig. 3. R_β-neurones and lung stretch receptor afferent fibres recorded in the ventrolateral nucleus of the solitary tract in a single experiment. The ipsilateral vagal nerve was stimulated with single shocks (0.2-0.7 V and 0.05 ms) at the time marked by the vertical line. Recordings of two R_β-neurones (N_1 and N_2) are shown and the latency of their EPSPs is compared with the latency of three of the fastest conducting lung stretch receptor fibres (F_1-F_3). Note that they are almost identical (dashed vertical line). $MP_{R\beta}$: membrane potential of R_β-neurones. MP_{LA}: membrane potential of lung stretch receptor fibres.

The minimum latencies to excitation of LA-fibres within the VL-NTS and the shortest latency to the start of EPSPs within R_β-neurones were nearly identical.

Therefore, there must be a monosynaptic coupling between LA-fibres and R_β-neurones.

This work was supported by the Deutsche Forschungsgemeinschaft.

REFERENCES

(1) von Baumgarten, R., Kanzow, E., The interaction of two types of inspiratory neurones in the region of the tractus solitarius of the cat, Arch. ital. Biol. 96, 361-373 (1958).

(2) von Euler, C., Hayward, J.N., Marttila, I., Wyman, R.J., Respiratory neurones of the ventrolateral nucleus of the solitary tract of cat: vagal input, spinal connections and morphological identification, Brain Res. 61, 1-22 (1973).

(3) Paintal, A.S., The conduction velocities of respiratory and cardiovascular afferent fibres in the vagus nerve, J. Physiol. (Lond.) 121, 341-359 (1953).

(4) Richter, D.W., Camerer, H., Röhrig, N., Medullary inspiratory interneurons receiving a monosynaptic input from lung stretch receptors, Pflügers Arch. 373, R75 (1978)

DISCUSSION

of the papers by Camerer et al. and Richter et al.

The problem on whether or not the R_β neurons project to the spinal cord was discussed at some length. Earlier Euler et al. (Brain Res. 61, 23, 1973) had arrived at the conclusion that the R_β:s do not have bulbo-spinal projections. Now Richter from intracellular recordings provided further evidence for this view whereas Lipski, Merrill and Bianchi referring to earlier work expressed the opinion that R_β:s do project to the spinal cord in agreement with the original work by Baumgarten and Kanzow. The different techniques used in these different studies were discussed. Richter pointed out the possibilities for mistaking orthodromic for antidromic activation but no clear understanding was reached as to the nature of the reported discrepancies.

There was general agreement, however, that there was virtually no direct excitatory or inhibitory effects exerted on the phrenic motoneurons by activating pulmonary stretch receptor afferents neither by lung volume changes nor by threshold stimulation of the large vagal afferents. It may thus be concluded either that R_β neurons do not project down to the spinal cord, or their descending axons project to other neurons than the inspiratory motoneurons. This would imply, as pointed out by Feldman, that the R_β and R_α neurons cannot be lumped together and be regarded as forming one population of neurons with a range of properties from almost exclusive CIA input at the other extreme of almost pure vagal input.

It was agreed on that besides the population of R_β neurons which are largely inhibited during expiration there must exist other groups of neurons which transmit pulmonary stretch receptor information during expiration, since in this phase pulmonary stretch receptors exert a potentially powerful action by causing prolongation of the expiratory phase and retarding the onset of next inspiration.

Sears drew attention to the fact that the employment of pneumothorax for the improvement of stability of the recording conditions might possibly have caused considerable differences between different laboratories in the outcome of the inflation tests used for the identification of R_β cells. Starting from relative low levels of lung volume would increase the likelihood to co-activate also 'irritant' and other receptors provoking inspiratory facilitatory reflexes. This would not apply to the work of Euler et al. (Brain Res. 61, 1, 1973) who for this very reason did not employ pneumothorax in their experiments.

There was general agreement with Lipski that available evidence is not in harmony with the original view of Baumgarten and Kanzow that R_β neurons inhibit directly the R_α neurons. If the R_β cells transmit the inspiration-inhibiting action of the pumonary stretch receptors they would have to exert this effect indirectly by the way of other groups of neurons constituting the inspiratory 'off-switch' mechanisms. The group of neurons in the solitary tract complex discussed earlier in this session in the paper by Remmers et al. were considered to be likely candidates for the connection between R_β and R_α neurons.

INTRAMEDULLARY COURSE OF AFFERENT AND EFFERENT FIBERS OF THE VAGUS NERVE: A STUDY USING THE TETRAMETHYL BENZIDINE REACTION FOR HORSERADISH PEROXIDASE

M. KALIA and M.-M. MESULAM

*Department of Physiology, Hahnemann Medical College, Philadelphia, PA, and
The Bullard and Denny-Brown Laboratories, Harvard Neurological Unit,
Beth Israel Hospital, Boston, MA, U.S.A.*

The vagus nerve contains some of the most significant connections concerning the central integration of respiratory, cardiovascular and gustatory function (9, 21, 32). The central termination of these sensory fibers have been the subject of intense attention and over the past seventy years a considerable amount of work has been done on tracing these fibers into the nervous system in different species including man (1, 2, 3, 6, 7, 10, 12, 13, 14, 15, 16, 21). All these studies have been done using either the anterograde degeneration techniques or Golgi methods, and have provided us with the current state of understanding concerning the sites of relay for vagal sensory fibers.

Afferent vagal fibers enter the medulla in association with emerging efferent fibers. Cutaneous fibers contained in the auricular branch of the vagus nerve enter the dorsal part of the spinal trigeminal tract along with similar general somatic afferent fibers of other branchiomeric cranial nerves. These fibers terminate in caudal portions of the spinal trigeminal nucleus. More numerous visceral afferent fibers pass dorsomedially to the nucleus of the tractus solitarius where some fibers terminate; other fibers bifurcate into small ascending and large descending components which enter the solitary fasciculus. Descending vagal fibers in the fasciculus solitarius give off terminals to the cells of the nucleus solitarius but some fibers descend caudal to the obex where the solitary nuclei of the two sides join to form the commissural nucleus of the vagus. A considerable number of descending vagal fibers decussate and enter the contralateral half of the commissural nucleus (2, 3, 5, 6, 10, 14).

The tractus solitarius is formed by visceral afferent fibers contributed by the vagus, glossopharyngeal and facial nerves. The upper portion of the fasciculus solitarius, rostral to the entry of the vagus nerve, contains fibers related primarily to taste, while caudal portions of the fasciculus contain mainly general visceral afferent fibers from structures innervated by the vagus nerve. Thus, the fasciculus solitarius constitutes a composite bundle of visceral afferent fibers comparable to the spinal trigeminal tract which contains general somatic afferent fibers (2, 3, 5, 6, 10, 14, 31, 32).

273

The nucleus tractus solitarius (nTS), in which fibers of the fasciculus solitarius terminate, can be divided into two parts: a medial portion, dorsolateral to the dorsal motor nucleus of the vagus, known as the "dorsal sensory nucleus of the vagus" and a lateral portion situated along the lateral border of the fasciculus solitarius referred to as the "ventral nucleus of the fasciculus solitarius". The medial portion of the nTS consists of a column of small, densely packed cells within a fine intrinsic fiber plexus. Rostrally, it extends to levels slightly above the oral pole of the dorsal motor nucleus of the vagus: caudally, it merges with the same cell group of the opposite side to form the commissural nucleus of the vagus. The lateral portion of the nucleus consists of slightly larger multipolar cells scattered in a rich fiber plexus; some cells lie ventrolateral to, or within, the fasciculus solitarius, while at rostral levels, portions of the nucleus completely surround the fasciculus. Rostrally, the lateral portions of the nucleus increases in size and extends almost to the inferior border of the pons. This portion of the nucleus parallels the fasciculus solitarius throughout most of its length but in caudal regions, cells diminish in number and are difficult to delimit from neurons of the reticular formation. The most significant projections of the caudal part of the medial nucleus solitarius are to portions of the dorsal and lateral reticular formation of the medulla which have been implicated in the central regulation of respiratory, cardiovascular and emetic function (5, 12, 31).

The location of cell bodies of motor fibers of the vagus nerve have been investigated by many workers using the classical degeneration and electrophysiological techniques (1, 2, 3, 5, 6, 13, 14, 15, 19, 21, 28). The central vagal complex is known to consist of two motor nuclei--a dorso-medial nucleus (dmnX) and a ventrolateral nucleus (nucleus ambiguus, nA) (48), and both nuclei are active in the integration of cardiopulmonary function. Recent electrophysiological studies on medullary neurons related to respiratory activity have shown that the nucleus retroambigualis (nRA),(27) is also involved in respiratory activity (23, 24). However, anatomical relationship of this nucleus to the vagus nerve has not been delineated.

Important questions still remain to be answered as far as the central connections of the vagus nerve are concerned. The present study was undertaken to see if the recently available sensitive neuroanatomical techniques using the axonal transport of horseradish peroxidase (HRP) can be used to determine the central neuronal connections of the vagus nerve. Various laboratories have recently been using the retrograde transport of HRP to determine the cell bodies of origin in peripheral nerve fibers and dorsal and ventral roots, (7, 8, 11, 17, 18) and more recently diffusion of HRP from dorsal roots into the spinal cord has been used to determine the central distribution of sensory fibers (22, 29). All these procedures have utilized the diamino benzidine (DAB) reaction for HRP (26) which is not very sensitive and produces variable results even under very similar conditions.

The development of the tetramethyl benzidine (TMB) reaction for HRP (25) which is extremely sensitive, now enables the visualization of very small amounts of the enzyme HRP. Recently Brushart and Mesulam (4) have demonstrated labeling in nerve terminals in the substantia gelatinosa of the spinal cord and in the nucleus gracilis of the medulla following exposure of the sciatic nerve to HRP. The tissue was reacted with TMB technique and demonstrated trans-perikaryal passage of HRP from peripheral nerve through the dorsal root ganglion into the spinal cord and brain stem. This work has opened up the possibility of using the TMB reaction for HRP to trace central connections of sensory fibers in other peripheral and cranial nerves. Consequently, this investigation was undertaken to determine if the cells of origin and central sensory terminations of the vagus nerve could be demonstrated simultaneously with the TMB method for HRP neurohistochemistry.

METHODS

Experiments were carried out on eighteen adult cats. The animals were anesthetized with chloralose-urethane (chloralose 40 mg/kg and urethane 250 mg/kg) administered intravenously following an initial intramuscular injection of Ketamine (Ketaset Bristol Laboratories). The vagus nerve of one side was exposed and sectioned low in the neck. The nerve was then separated from the underlying tissue up to 10-15 mm rostrally and reflected to one side. A length of polyethylene tubing (2 mm internal diameter) 10-15 mm long was heat-sealed at one end and filled with 33% horseradish peroxidase (HRP) type VI Sigma in triz buffer pH 8.3. This tubing was then sutured into position in the place originally occupied by the vagus nerve with the open end directed rostrally. The vagus nerve was carefully desheathed and eased into the HRP-filled polyethylene tubing. Such a procedure helped to prevent the nerve from being pulled out of the tubing when the animal regained consciousness. The superficial muscles were sutured in layers and the skin closed. The animals recovered from anesthesia and survived 48-52 hours post-operatively, following which they were re-anesthetized and perfused transcardially with the following solutions: 1) one liter of normal saline at 21°C , and 2) 4 liters of 2.5% glutaraldehyde in 0.1 M phosphate buffer at 21°C, and 3) 10% sucrose solution in 0.1 M phosphate buffer at 4°C. The rationale and advantages associated with this sucrose-buffer post-perfusion procedure have been discussed elsewhere (30). The vagus nerve was reexposed to check for the position of the cut end of the nerve in relation to the polyethylene tubing. The brain and upper cervical cord and the nodose ganglia of both sides were removed and stored in 10% sucrose solution in 0.1 M phosphate buffer for 4-48 hours at 4°C. The pia was carefully removed and the brain stem and spinal cord were sectioned into 50μ thick sections, using a freezing microtome. Sections were collected serially into 0.1 M phosphate buffer.

The tissue was then reacted histochemically within 2 hours of the sectioning.   All enzymatic reactions were carried out on free-floating tissue sections at 21°C. The entire reaction procedure was carried out on a rocker table with gentle agitation. The reaction was begun by three washes in distilled water for 1 minute each. This was followed by pre-incubation of the sections for 20 minutes in freshly made solutions A and B made in the following manner: Solution A - 92.5 ml distilled water, 100 mg sodium nitroferricyanide and 5 ml of acetate buffer at pH 3.3.   Solution B - 5 mg tetramethyl benzidine and 2.5 ml of absolute alcohol. Solutions A and B were mixed in the reaction vessel only seconds before the sections were introduced. After 20 minutes of pre-incubation, the enzymatic reaction was started by adding 3.0 ml of 0.3% H_2O_2 solution to each 100 ml of the reaction solution. Gentle agitation was continued for another 20 minutes. Without an intervening wash, the sections were transferred to a chilled stabilization solution at $0-4^\circ$C. Each 100 ml of the stabilization solution contained 9 grams of sodium nitroferricyanide, 5 ml of acetate buffer (pH 3.3), 45 ml of distilled water and 50 ml absolute alcohol.The method is discussed in detail elsewhere (25).

The sections were gently agitated for another 20 minutes in this stabilization solution and then transferred through several rinsing solutions of distilled water at room temperature (21°C). Sections were mounted in sets onto slides subbed with chrome-alum..   Once dry, the slides were coverslipped using Permount (Fisher Scientific) mounting medium. Each section was methodically scanned for the presence of HRP labeled neuronal structures using both dark and bright field illumination. A few alternate sets were counterstained with 1% aqueous neutral red solution. The distribution of HRP labeled neuronal structures was plotted using an electronic plantograph (X-Y Plotter, Hewlett Packard) connected by means of rectilinear potentiometers to the X and Y axes of the microscope stage.

RESULTS

The HRP reaction-product was detected in perikarya, axons and axonal terminals.
(Fig. 1).

1. Perikarya retrogradely labeled with HRP (cells of origin for vagal efferents):
The most dense population of perikarya labeled with HRP was found in the region
of the ipsilateral dorsal motor nucleus of the vagus (dmnX). These neurons are
shown in Figs. 2 and 3. It seems that practically every dmnX neuron is labeled
with HRP and these are tightly packed together. The presence of extraperikaryal
HRP granules around these neurons is noteworthy (Fig. 2). This extraperikaryal
reaction-product may reflect labeling in dendrites or recurrent collaterals of
dmnX motoneurons. Alternatively, this may represent HRP in the central processes
of sensory neurons in the nodose ganglion and may establish a reflex arc subserving
vital autonomic reflexes.

Labled perikarya were also present on the ipsilateral nucleus ambiguus (nA) and
Fig. 4 shows the morphology of these neurons. Labeled neurons in the nucleus
ambiguus were scattered rather than clustered with many unlabeled neurons intervening. In contrast to the dmnX which contains a dense concentration of extraperikaryal HRP reaction-product, the nA contained reaction product almost exclusively
within the perikarya (Figs. 3 and 4). A number of isolated HRP labeled neurons
were seen in parts of the reticular formation, along the path of HRP labeled nerve
fibers. Whether these are aberrant members of the dmnX or nA or neurons of the reticular formation could not be established in these experiments.

The rostro-caudal extent of the nucleus ambiguus is noteworthy. At the rostral
end of the medulla the HRP labeled neurons of the nucleus ambiguus became larger
and occupied a more ventral position. In some sections the neurons lay as close
as 250µ to the surface of the ventral medulla. This is directly under the chemosensitive area of the medulla (26) and the possibility of these neurons being
involved in the genesis of central chemosensitivity exists. Caudally, the labeled
neurons of the nucleus ambiguus extended into the nucleus retroambigualis (Fig. 1).
The morphology of these neurons was different as compared with the neurons in the
nucleus ambiguus: these neurons were smaller and not as multipolar. The HRP
labeled neurons in the nucleus retroambigualis extended well into the upper
part of the spinal cord. Isolated neurons with the HRP label were found as
caudally as the level of the C2 spinal cord.

2. HRP-labeled fibers (central course of vagal fibers): Several fascicles of
labeled fibers entered the lateral aspect of the medulla. Each of these fascicles
could be followed dorso-medially towards the dmnX and the tractus solitarius (TS).
In the vicinity of the dmnX, these fascicles trifurcated. One component (axons
of vagal motoneurons) joined the dmnX; a second component (central processes of
sensory neurons in the nodose ganglion) joined the TS; a third component (axons
of motoneurons in the nA) looped ventro-laterally to join the nA (Figs. 1, 3, 4).
In no case did we observe a nerve fiber travelling towards the lateral side of
the medulla directly from the nA. In all instances the nA axons had an obligatory
dorsal course until they looped laterally in the vicinity of the dmnX and joined
axons of vagal motoneurons and central processes of the nodose ganglion in order
to form intramedullary fascicles of the vagus nerve (Fig. 3). This is somewhat
surprising since earlier investigators (15) had described the efferent nA axons
as travelling laterally at more ventral levels than the efferent dmnX axons.

3. The HRP reaction-product at extraperikaryal sites within medullary nuclei
(central sensory connections of the vagus nerve): The superior sensitivity of the
TMB reaction enables the consistent visualization of anterogradely transported
HRP within axonal terminals (25). Furthermore, the same neurohistochemical method

has enabled the visualization of central sensory terminals following the application of HRP to peripheral nerves (4). In those experiments, the movement of HRP could be followed from the peripheral processes of sensory nerves into the neurons of the dorsal root ganglia and then into their central processes up to the terminal fields within central sensory nuclei. A similar phenomenon of transperikaryal HRP movement was visualized in these experiments.

First, the HRP reaction product was seen in the peripheral and central processes of the nodose ganglion as well as in the perikarya of this ganglion (Fig. 5). Then a component of the HRP-labeled intramedullary fiber fascicles which most probably consisted of central processes of the nodose ganglion entered the TS. Finally, extraperikaryal and granular reaction-product was seen in the medial, lateral and subnucleus gelatinosus subdivisions of the nucleus of the tractus solitarius (nTS). In all likelihood, this represents HRP reaction-product within terminations of central processes of the nodose ganglion. Thus, this extraperikaryal HRP reaction-product may indicated the central sensory terminations of the vagus nerve. (Figs. 1, 2, 3).

In sections rostral to the level of the obex this extraperikaryal labeling was limited to the ipsilateral side. However, caudal to the obex, a fairly dense collection of granular reaction-product was seen in the nucleus commissuralis of Cajal and in the contralateral medial nucleus of the TS. In fact, at some levels, a labeled nerve fiber was seen to cross the midline en route to the contralateral medial nTS.

As noted above, the dmnX contained extraperikaryal HRP reaction-product (Fig. 3). This could be due to the presence of HRP in dendrites, in recurrent collaterals or in sensory endings from central processes of neurons in the nodose ganglion. We intend to distinguish among these and other possibilities by means of tritiated amino acid injections within the nodose ganglion. The nA did not contain significant concentrations of extraperikaryal reaction-product (Fig. 4), thus indicating either that it has a different pattern of dendrites or of axonal collaterals or that it does not receive direct sensory input from the nodose ganglion.

In each case, the contralateral nX, dmnX, nA, TS and most of the nTS remained free of reaction-product, thus eliminating the possibility that these structures are prone to surreptitious labeling in the absence of exogenous HRP activity.

DISCUSSION

These findings suggest that the TMB method for HRP neurohistochemistry is useful in the simultaneous visualization of central efferents and afferents of mixed nerves. The present work has been done on the whole vagus nerve and shows that a demonstration of afferent terminations is possible even when the nerve is exposed to HRP several centimeters away from the medulla. This makes it feasible to design future studies on the central projections of specific groups of sensory afferent fibers of known functional significance. DeVito, Clausing and Smith (1974) applied HRP to the central cut end of the vagus nerve and described HRP labeled perikarya in the medulla but did not report having seen any sensory terminals. On the other hand, in studies that have demonstrated sensory terminals with HRP histochemistry, the enzyme has been applied proximal to the sensory ganglion (22, 29). In all these studies the Lavail modification of Graham and Karnovsky method has been used to demonstrate HRP activity (20). In the experiments described in the present study the more sensitive TMB method has been used and consequently it has been possible to demonstrate more extensive retrograde labeling as well as the presence of sensory terminations even though the HRP was applied distal to the sensory ganglion.

Many of the methodological limitations of HRP neurochemistry do not apply to investigations on peripheral nerves. In specific, uptake of HRP by damaged fibers of passage or the difficulty inherent in defining the exact injection site do not effect these experiments. On the other hand, in using the cut end of a peripheral nerve dipped in HRP solution, it can be argued that the HRP seen in distal regions could result not from transport but from the passive diffusion of the enzyme. Such a possibility does indeed exist but the recent studies of Light and Perl (1977) on lumbar and sacral rootlets in the cat and monkey have shown that as far as nerve terminals are concerned, diffused HRP was not recognizable for more than 15 mm from the application point (22). In our experiments we have observed excellent labeling in nerve terminals that were more than 10 cms from the point of application of HRP. Furthermore it has been suggested that the diffusion of HRP (as seen from the use of intracellular iontophoreses as a marker for neurons (22) is likely to appear as a uniform stain within the entire neuronal structure involved. In our experiments the HRP reaction-product was finely granular. It would seem, therefore, that the experiments reported above demonstrate the active transport and not the passive diffusion of HRP from the vagus nerve into its central sensory and motor components.

The HRP label in the contralateral medial nucleus of the tractus solitarius supports the existence of commissural fibers originally described by Cajal (1909). It has been demonstrated by many workers that the medial nucleus of the nTS is concerned primarily with afferent input from pulmonary vagal branches. As far as the rostro-caudal organization of the nTS is concerned, evidence based on degeneration studies indicated that both the intermediate and caudal portions receive projections from vagal afferent fibers (5, 6, 10, 14, 15). While pulmonary afferents seem to project predominantly to the caudal portion of the nTS, cardiovascular afferents terminate more rostrally in the intermediate region. The lateral nucleus of the nucleus of the tractus solitarius is the location from where respiratory neurons have been recorded by many workers (9, 23, 24, 26). It is interesting from a physiological point of view to find that both medial and lateral divisions of the nucleus of the tractus solitarius (nTS) receive primary afferent terminations as indicated by the presence of extraperikaryal reaction-product in these experiments. In this study we have not attempted to study specific afferent projections differentially and we cannot be certain that the projection to the lateral (nTS) is from pulmonary afferents; yet, the location of the extraperikaryal HRP in the rostro-lateral nTS corresponds very closely with the regions from where we have previously recorded inspiratory activity. Another interesting aspect of this study is the finding of extraperikaryal HRP in the dmnX. The presence of vagal sensory input to these motoneurons does not seem in the least unreasonable when one considers that these connections are most important in modulating various cardiovascular reflexes. However, the possibility that this extraperikaryal reaction product merely indicates the presence of HRP in dendrites or recurrent axonal collaterals of the motoneurons must also be considered. The contribution of efferents to the vagus nerve from the nucleus retroambigualis (nRA) has not been reported by any of the earlier workers in this field. Retrograde degeneration studies could have missed single nRA neurons that may have degenerated. This caudal region of the medulla has often been considered as being a region that has direct connections with spinal motoneurons -- Torvik (1956) and Merrill (1970) -- and may provide an important link between the medullary and spinal control of autonomic function.

ACKNOWLEDGEMENTS

It is a pleasure to thank Mr. Michael Biebel for technical assistance and Ms. Kathleen Barry for assistance in photography. This work was supported by USPHS grants HL 17800, and NS 09211 and RCDA HL 00103 (to MK); and the Scottish Rite Freemasonary of North America.

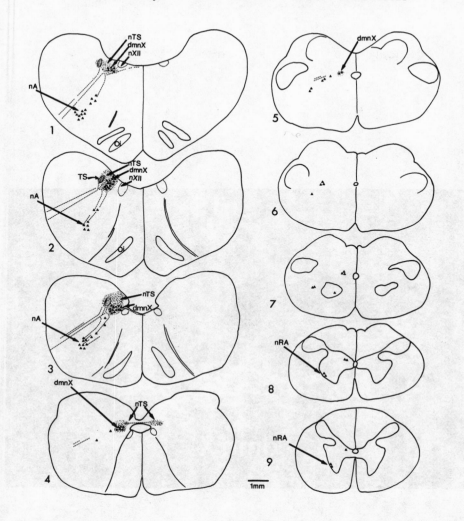

Fig. 1

Figure 1. Projection drawings of tranverse sections through the medulla and upper cervical spinal cord are shown in sections 1 through 9. Section 1 is most rostral and section 9 is most caudal. Interval between sections is 900μ nTS, nucleus tractus solitarii; dmnX, nucleus nervi dorsalis motorius; nA, nucleus ambiguus; nRA,nucleus retroambigualis; nXII, nucleus nervi hypoglossi; Oi, nucleus olivaris inferior. Interrupted lines indicate central sensory and motor fibers of the vagus nerve labeled with the enzyme HRP. Notice how all the fibers are directed dorso-medially towards the dorsal motor nucleus of the vagus nerve, and then some of the fibers loop ventro-laterally into the nucleus ambiguus. Notice an occasional fiber in section 4 crossing the midline dorsal to the central canal to end in nerve terminals in the contralateral medial nucleus of the tractus solitarius. Stippled areas shows sensory nerve terminals labeled with HRP in the various sub-nuclei of the nucleus of the tractus solitarius. Solid triangles indicate the positions of perikarya retrogradely labeled with the HRP enzyme.

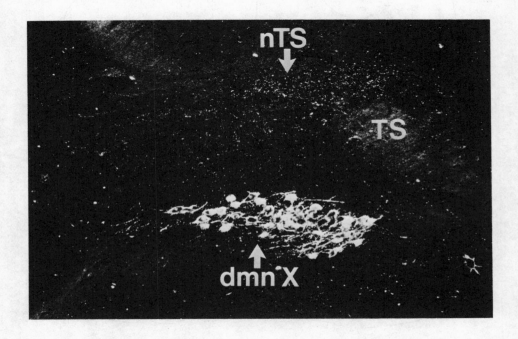

Fig. 2

Figure 2. This is a dark field photomicrograph at a level that corresponsds to
section 4 of Fig. 1. Virtually each perikaryon in the dorsal motor nucleus of
the vagus nerve (dmnX) is labeled. The HRP label is also clearly seen in sensory
fibers of the tractus solitarius (TS) and in sensory endings within the nucleus
of the tractus solitarius (nTS). Magnification at the film plane was X104.

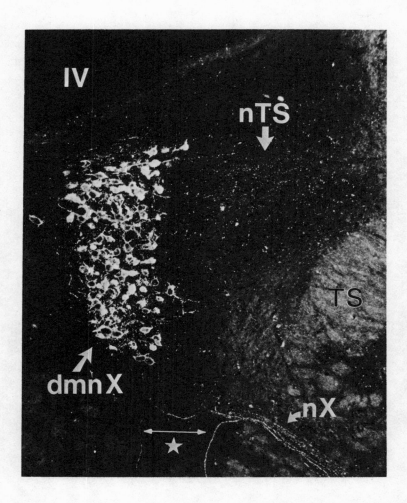

Fig. 3

Figure 3. This is a dark-field photomicrograph at a level that corresponds to
level 2 of Fig. 1. A fascicle of the vagus nerve (nX) has three destinations.
One component reaches the dorsal motor nucleus of the vagus (dmnX) and virtually
every neuron in the dmnX is labeled. Another component of the nX loops ventrally
(arrowheads with star) towards the nucleus ambiguus. A third component of the nX
enters the tractus solitarius (TS). From the TS, fibers reach the nucleus of the
tractus solitarius (nTS) and extraperikaryal sensory endings in the nTS are labeled
with the HRP reaction product. There are dense depositions of extraperikaryal
reaction-product within the dmnX. Magnification at the film plane was X104.

Fig. 4

Figure 4. This is a dark-field photomicrograph of the nucleus ambiguus (nA) from
the same tissue section as Fig. 3. In contrast to the pattern in the dmnX, the
labeled perikarya are less tightly packed and there is very little extraperikaryal
reaction-product. Note the labeled axon which does not travel directly laterally
but which must first course dorsally towards the dmnX (see Fig. 3). Magnification
at the film plane was X104.

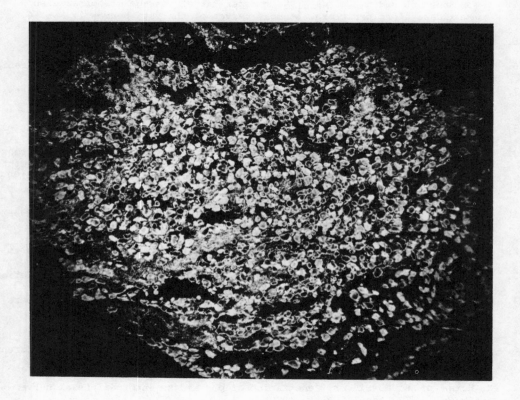

Fig. 5

Figure 5. This is a dark-field photomicrograph of the nodose ganglion. Virtually every neuron is labeled with HRP. Magnification was X52 at the film plane.

REFERENCES

1. E. Agostini, J.E. Chinnock, M. de B. Daly and J.G. Murray, Functional and
    histological studies of the vagus nerve and its branches to the heart, lungs
    and abdominal viscera in the cat, J. Physiol. 135, 182 (1957).
2. W. F. Allen, Origin and distribution of the tractus solitarius in the guinea
    pig, J. comp. Neurol. 35, 171 (1923).
3. K. E. Astrom, On the central course of afferent fibres in the trigeminal,
    facial, glossopharyngeal, and vagal nerves and their nuclei in the mouse,
    Acta Physiol. Scan. 29, (Suppl. 106) 209, (1953).
4. T. M. Brushart and M.-M. Mesulam Transperikaryal passage of horseradish
    peroxidase along peripheral sensory nerves of the rat, Neurosci. Abs. 4,
    (1978).
5. Cajal, S. R. (1909) Histologie due Systeme Nerveux de l'Homme et des
    Vertebres, A. Maloine Paris.
6. M. K. Cottle, Degeneration studies of primary afferents of IXth and Xth cranial
    nerves in the cat, J. comp. Neurol. 122, 329 (1964).
7. M. de B. Daly and D. H. L. Evans, Functional and histological changes in the
    vagus nerve of the cat after degenerative section at various levels,
    J. Physiol. 120, 579 (1953).
8. J. L. DeVito, K. W. Clausing and O. A. Smith, Uptake and transport of horse-
    radish peroxidase by cut end of the vagus nerve, Brain Res. 82, 269 (1974).
9. C. von Euler, J. N. Hayward, I. Marttila and R. J. Wyman, Respiratory neurons
    of the ventrolateral nucleus of the solitary tract of the cat: vagal input,
    spinal connections and morphological identification, Brain Res. 61, 1 (1973).
10. J. O. Foley and R. S. Dubois, An experimental study of the rootlets of the
    vagus nerve in the cat, J. comp. Neurol. 60, 137 (1934).
11. L. Furstman, S. Saporta and L. Kruger, Retrograde axonal transport of horse-
    radish peroxidase in sensory nerves and ganglion cells of the rat,
    Brain Res. 84, 320 (1975).
12. A. van Gehuchten, Recherches sur la Terminaison Centrale des Nerfs Sensibles
    Peripheriques: Le Faisceau Solitaire, Nevraxe 1, 173 (1900).
13. F. Harrison and S. R. Bruesch, Intramedullary potentials following stimulations
    of the cervical vagus, Anat. Rec. 91, 280 (1945).
14. W. R. Ingram and E. A. Dawkins, The intramedullary course of afferent fibers
    of the vagus nerve in the cat, J. comp. Neurol. 82, 157 (1945).
15. F. W. L. Kerr, Facial, vagal, and glossopharyngeal nerves in the cat,
    Arch. Neurol. 6, 264, 1962).
16. D. L. Kimmel, C. B. Kimmel and A. Zarkin, Central distribution of the afferent
    nerve fibers of the facial and vagal nerves in the guinea pig,
    Anat. Rec. 139, 245 (1961).
17. N. Krishnan and M. Singer, Penetration of peroxidase into peripheral nerve
    fibers, Am. J. Anat. 136, 1 (1973).
18. K. Kristensson, Y. Olsson and J. Sjostrand, Axonal uptake and retrograde
    transport of exogenous proteins in the hypoglassal nerve, Brain Res. 32,399(19
19. R. L. Lam and H. R. Tyler, Electrical responses evoked in the visceral afferent
    nucleus of the rabbit by vagal stimulation, J. comp. Neurol. 97, 21 (1952).
20. J. H. Lavail and M. M. Lavail, The retrograde intraaxonal transport of horse-
    radish peroxidase in the chick visual system: a light and electronmicroscopic
    study, J. comp. Neurol. 157, 303 (1974).
21. A. M. Lawn, The localization, in the nucleus ambiguus of the rabbit, of the
    cells of motor nerve fibers in the glossopharyngeal nerve and various branches
    of the vagus nerve by means of retrograde degeneration, J. comp. Neurol. 127,
    307 (1966).
22. A. R. Light and E. R. Perl, Differential termination of large-diameter and
    small-diameter primary afferent fibers in the spinal dorsal grey matter as
    indicated by labeling with horseradish peroxidase, Neurosi. Let. 6, 59 (1977).

23. E. G. Merrill, The lateral respiratory neurons of the medulla: their association with nucleus ambiguus, nucleus retroambigualis, the spinal accessory nucleus and the spinal cord, Brain Res. 24, 11 (1970).

24. E. G. Merrill, Finding a respiratory function for the medullary respiratory neurons, IN: Essays on the Nervous System, Clarendon Press, Oxford, 451 (1974)

25. M. M. Mesulam, Tetramethyl benzidine for horseradish peroxidase neurohisto-chemistry: a non-carcinogenic blue reaction-product with superior sensitivity for visualizing neural afferents and efferents, J. Histochem. Cytochem. 26, 106 (1978).

26. S. Nakayama and R. von Baumgarten, Lokalisierung absteigender Atmungsbahnen, im rückenmark der katze mittels antidromer Reizung, Pflugers Arch. 281, 231 (1964).

27. J. Olszewski and D. Baxter (1954) Cytoarchitecture of the Human Brain Stem, S. Karger A. G.

28. R. Porter , Unit responses evoked in the medulla oblongata by vagus nerve stimulation, J. Physiol. 168, 717 (1963).

29. E. Proshansky and M. D. Egger, Staining of the dorsal root projection to the cat's dorsal horn by anterograde movement of horseradish peroxidase, Neurosci. Let. 5, 103 (1977).

30. D. L. Rosene and M. M. Mesulam, Fixation variables in horseradish peroxidase neurohistochemistry. J. Histochem. Cytochem. 26, 28 (1978).

31. H. G. Schwartz, G. E. Roulhac, R. L. Lam and J. L. O'Leary, Organization of the fasciculus solitarius in man, J. comp. Neurol. 94, 221 (1951).

32. A. Torvik, Afferent connections to the sensory trigeminal nuclei, the nucleus of the solitary tract and adjacent structures, J. comp. Neurol. 106, 51 (1956).

ANATOMO-FUNCTIONAL STUDY OF PONTINE AFFERENTS TO THE BULBAR RESPIRATORY AREA OF THE CAT

M. DENAVIT-SAUBIÉ, D. RICHE and J. CHAMPAGNAT

*Laboratoire de Physiologie Nerveuse, Département de Neurophysiologie Appliquée,
C.N.R.S., 91190 Gif-sur-Yvette, France*

ABSTRACT

An anatomical study has demonstrated the presence of a direct projection from the
parabrachialis Kölliker–Fuse complex (PMKF) to the bulbar respiratory area. This
result has been obtained using both the techniques of retrogradely transported
horseradish peroxidase (HRP) and anterograde labelling with tritiated proline.
Perikarya located in the PMFK project to the medulla at the level of the obex.
Labelled fibers and terminals are located radially according to the fourth ventricle in an area extending from the nucleus hypoglossus to the nucleus ambiguus.
Functionally the importance of this projection has been confirmed using pharmacological tools. Iontophoresis of L-glutamate on respiratory activity enables us to
differentiate the somatodendritic spike from the fiber spike. With this technique
we obtained a precise localization of an inspiratory background activity related
to the activity of inspiratory fibers or terminals at the level of the obex. A
very good correlation exists between the localization of this inspiratory activity
and the labelled fibers and terminals. Furthermore, kainic acid, a compound which
is thought to selectively destroy the soma, has been injected into the PMKF and
produced apneusis in bivagotomized cats as well as an interruption of respiration
in intact anesthetized animals.

Keywords : Pontobulbar connections – Autoradiography – H.R.P. – kainic acid –
       Microiontophoresis.

INTRODUCTION

The central respiratory activity is essentially elaborated in the medulla where
respiratory neurones (RN) can be recorded. The rhythmic activity of the RN depends
upon the nature of inputs which reach them during the respiratory cycle. Two types
of afferents can be presumed : 1) the short ones coming from neurones located in
the medulla (propriobulbar); 2) the long ones coming either from the periphery or
from a more rostral part of the brain. While short connections can be the basis of
a bulbar circuitry, the direct afferents coming from distant structures may contribute to step changes in the discharge rate occuring at a specific point within
the respiratory cycle.
Among rostral afferents those coming from the upper part of the pons are of interest since a section located between the pontine and bulbar levels produces modifications of the rhythmic activity (Lumsden, T., 1922) which do not appear when

the section is done rostrally to the pons.
We undertook the following pluridisciplinary study in order to see if there is a
direct connection between pontine and medullary respiratory areas, and if so, to
evaluate the functional importance of this connection.

METHOD

Anatomical Approach

1) Horseradish peroxidase (HRP) technique. At the bulbar level unilateral slow
injections of a 25 % solution of HRP in distilled water were done with a Hamilton
syringe. Injected quantities varied from 0.2 to 0.5 µl. After 19-26 hours the cats
were perfused with a solution of 1 % glutaraldehyde and 1 % paraformaldehyde. Most
of the brains were prepared for light microscopy and one for electron microscopy.
Coronal sections 40 µm thick were made continuously from the injection site to the
level of PMKF. The sections were all processed according to the Graham and
Karnovsky method for demonstrating the presence of peroxidase. Frozen sections
were lightly stained with Cresyl violet before observation.

2) Tritiated proline technique. Unilateral injections of tritiated proline were
done in PMKF with a Hamilton syringe. Each animal received 60 µCi dissolved in
1 µl of normal saline of L-Proline 3H (specific activity : 27 Ci/mM). The brains
were fixed by perfusion, 70-74 hours post-operatively, with 2 % paraformaldehyde,
0.5 % glutaraldehyde in phosphate buffer. Brains were embedded in paraffin. Sections 10 µm thick were coated with diluted K5 emulsion (Ilford), stored in light-
tight containers at 4°C for 3-9 weeks, developed, and stained with Cresyl violet.

Functional Approach

1) Microiontophoretic application of L-glutamate at the bulbar level. Experiments
were similar to those described in the associated article (Denavit-Saubié, M. et
al., 1978). They were performed on bivagotomized, paralyzed and artificially ventilated cats. Bipolar recording of the left phrenic nerve was an index of central
respiratory rhythm. Multibarrelled glass micropipettes were used to extracellularly record respiratory neurones at the level of the obex and to simultaneously
apply L-glutamate (0.5 M, pH 8) in the vicinity of the recorded unit. Methyl blue
was applied to localize the recording site.

2) Microinjections of kainic acid at pontine level. Experiments were performed
on two groups of animals. Cats from group 1 were bivagotomized, curarised, and
artificially ventilated under halothane anesthesia. The respiratory periods were
recorded from the central cut end of the phrenic nerve using bipolar electrodes.
Cats from group 2 were anesthetized by intravenous injection of sodium pentobarbitone (30 mg/kg), and the spontaneous respiration was monitored by recording
the electrical activity of respiratory muscles.
One PMKF was injected with 0.5 µg of kainic acid dissolved in 0.5 µl of Ringer
(pH 7.4). The same amount of Ringer alone was injected as control. Cats from group
1 were studied during 7-20 hours. In group 2 a bilateral vagotomy was performed
6-11 days after the experiments. Animals from both groups were then perfused for
histological control and anatomical study.

RESULTS

Anatomical Approach

1) HRP labelling. HRP is an enzyme well known to be retrogradely transported from
the terminals at the injection site to neuronal somata. Neurons were considered

as labelled when the brown granules thought to be the reaction product of retrogradely transported HRP appeared in their cytoplasm and dendritic processes.
The enzyme was transported from the injection site (bulbar level) to the upper
part of the pons in PMKF. Marked cells were found throughout the entire PMKF from
its most posterolateral part to its anteromedial limit. Scattered marked cells
were observed on the contralateral complex. However no labelled cells were found
between the injection site and caudal limit of PMKF.

2) Tritiated proline labelling. This technique, very useful in neuroanatomy, has
been employed in order to localize terminals and axons. It has been demonstrated
by numerous authors (Grafstein, 1969; Cowan et al., 1972) that radio actively
labelled amino acids injected in the vicinity of neuronal somata are taken up by
the cells, incorporated into macromolecules and transported down the axons to
accumulate in the terminals.
From the injection site at the level of the pons (Fig.1.1.) ipsilateral descending
projections showed heavy labelling of terminals as well as fibers running through
the dorsolateral reticular formation. When the injection site was restricted to
superficial structures of the pons (Fig. 1.1b), labelling stopped in the plane
4 mm. anterior to the obex. When the injection site included the PMKF (Fig. 1.1a),
labels appeared in more caudal planes in a longitudinal bundle extending beneath
the spinal trigeminal nucleus. A section of this bundle appeared in frontal planes
at the level of the obex as an elongated area extending radially with respect to
the fourth ventricle, between the nucleus hypoglossus and the nucleus ambiguus
(Fig. 1.1a).
Rostrally an ascending pathway (mostly ipsilateral) ran through the ventromedial
midbrain tegmentum to the diencephalon. Labelled fibers and terminals could be
traced close to the nucleus ruber, the superficial part of the substantia nigra
pars compacta, the subthalamic nucleus, the entopeduncular nucleus and the lateral hypothalamic area. In the central nucleus of the amygdala only terminals were
found.

Functional Approach

1) Localization of a L-glutamate resistant inspiratory activity at the level of
the obex. L-glutamate was reported to be selectively active on neurones when applied in the vicinity of soma or dendrites but inactive on axonal fibers (Fries
and Zieglgansberger, 1974).
Single respiratory neurones studied at the level of the obex in the accompanying
article (Denavit et al., 1978) were excited by low dosages of L-glutamate and thus
presumed to be studied at the somatodendritic level. Conversely, other respiratory
neuronal activities were found to be unaffected by L-glutamate applied by means
of ejecting currents of up to 200 nanoamperes. This was the case of respiratory
activities that appeared in extracellular recordings as large rhythmic changes in
the background noise (respiratory background activity, RBA). RBA unaffected by
L-glutamate could not be a multiunitary somatodendritic recording and was thus
considered to be a multiaxonal discharge, a sum of synaptic potentials, or both.
During explorations of the medulla performed perpendicularly to the dorsal bulbar
surface, a L-glutamate resistant inspiratory RBA was constantly found under dorsal
column nuclei which were identified by ipsilateral tactile stimulation. This RBA
could be recorded along a depth of 0.5 - 1 millimeter. A histological study using
localized ejection of methyl blue demonstrated that this inspiratory RBA was located in an area extending continuously from the nucleus hypoglossus to the nucleus ambiguus (Fig. 1.2).

2) Microinjections of kainic acid into PMKF. Since it was found that PMKF neurons
project to the respiratory bulbar area, kainic acid was injected into this structure.

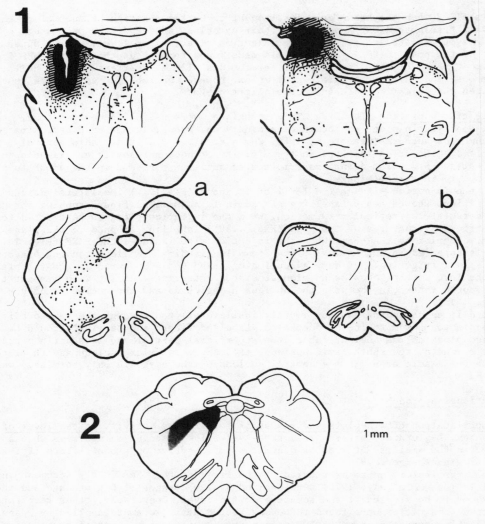

Fig.1.1 : The locations of injection sites are semi-schematically indicated in two different cases : in PMKF (a) and superficial structures (b). For the injection the head is titled ventrally at an angle of 45° relative to the Horsley-Clarke reference plane. Histological sections are done in this plane. Between a and b there is a slight variation of angle. In solid black : injection site with heavy concentration of silver grains. Cross-hatched area : zone with diffuse labelling. Dot-patterns : efferent pathways traced from the deposit.
- In a : almost all the PMKF region is involved. Labelling is found in caudal planes, at the level of the obex. Silver grains are found from the hypoglossus nucleus to the ambiguus nucleus.
- In b : only the superficial part of the PMKF is injected. Labelling is found only until plane 4 mm anterior to the obex.
     1.2 : Histological localization of inspiratory background activity recorded in the medulla at the obex level. Data obtained from 50 explorations of both sides are schematically summarized by the dotted area on one side.

Irreversible changes in the respiratory function were observed after each unilateral application of kainic acid a the level of the PMKF.
In bivagotomized cats (group 1) apneustic breathing occured a few minutes after
kainic acid application into the PMKF. (Fig.2). This type of breathing was stable
and could be observed during the remaining time of the experiment (7-20 hours).
When another injection of kainic acid was performed in the symetrical PMKF the
severity of apneusis could be further increased.

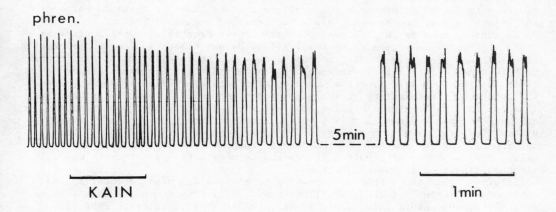

Fig.2: Effect of microinjection of kainic acid into the PMKF on the integrated phrenic nerve discharge (phren.). Kainic acid (KAIN) is injected (0.5 µg/0.5 µl)
during the time indicated by a bar under the recording.

In spontaneously breathing cats with intact vagi and barbiturate anesthesia
(group 2), kainic acid applications in the PMKF were followed after 15 to 60
seconds by an important reduction in the rhythm of breathing and then by a complete cessation of respiration. Animals were intubated and artificially ventilated
for 1-4 hours. As the effects of the anesthesia lessened spontaneous respiration
recovered and artificial ventilation could be discontinued. Animals could then be
let free for several days. Six to eleven days later a minimal analgesic dose of
barbiturate was given intravenously. A bilateral vagotomy was then performed which
in all cases induced apneusis, indicating that PMKF was also irreversibly severed
in these experiments. Such irreversible changes in respiration were not reproduced
in control experiments when kainic acid was applied 1-2 millimeters more caudally
or more medially to the PMKF, or when only Ringer was injected in PMKF. Under
those circumstances slight reversible apneusis was occasionally observed. This was
probably related to the compression of the nervous tissue inherent to the application procedure, as it was obtained after Ringer injection and even after inser-
tion of the needle. In these cases normal respiration recovered within 1-2 minutes.

DISCUSSION

The present results demonstrate that perikarya located in PMKF project directly
to the medulla at the level of the obex. They also suggest that both PMKF and its
area of bulbar projections are related to the central respiratory mechanisms.
Anatomical data were ascertained by means of two complementary methods : 1) the
uptake by terminals of injected HRP and its retrograde transport towards the corresponding perikarya; 2) the uptake by somata of injected tritiated proline and

its orthograde transport towards the corresponding axons and terminals. In both cases the substances to be transported were microinjected in a volume adjusted to involve, after diffusion, a sufficient sample of the neuronal structure under study to enable clear anatomical localization. Comparisons could be made with control experiments where the injection did not involve the area of interest, but only adjacent structures. (See fig.1.1 and, Denavit-Saubié and Riche, 1977). Anatomical connections were demonstrated between PMKF and bulbar structures located at a distance of more than 5 mm in the caudal direction. Transport at such distances is not due to simple diffusion but rather to active neuronal mechanisms. A continuous gradient from the injection site is produced by diffusion; this is excluded in HRP experiments by the complete lack of labelled elements between the injection site in the medulla and the labelled somata in PMKF.

Physiological results suggest that both structures described in the anatomical study are functionaly related to respiration. Bulbar fibers and terminals arising from PMKF are precisely located in that area where an inspiratory RBA is constantely recorded. Since this inspiratory RBA is resistant to L-glutamate applications, it is thought to result from the activity of fibers or terminals, but not from the activity of respiratory perikarya that can be recorded in the vicinity. Its location in a continuous elongated area extending from the hypoglossus to the ambiguus nucleus suggest that it involves axons arising from spinal or vagal ventral respiratory neurones (Merril, 1974; Kreuter et al., 1977) and fibers interconnecting the ventral and the dorsal groups of respiratory neurones (see Kalia, 1977). From our results, fibers and terminals from pontine neurones may also contribute to the inspiratory RBA.

Respiratory function of PMKF is supported by studies intended to localize the "pneumotaxic center" (Cohen, 1971; Bertrand, 1971). In our experiments lesions were made using kainic acid (Coyle et al., 1978). When injected in PMKF, it caused apneustic breathing. This result suggest that perikarya, in a position similar to those studied by anatomical method are involved in the pneumotaxic function. Anatomical controls, including optic and electron microscopy, are now in progress in order to evaluate directly the damage caused by Kainic acid applications.

It is thus likely that the present anatomical findings involve pathways functionnally implicated in respiration. Perikarya located in the PMKF are involved in the "pneumotaxic" function. They probably exert their effects via the demonstrated descending connections to the bulbar level and also possibly to the spinal level (Kalia, 1977). At the bulbar level, they project directly to a region that probably plays a crucial role in the central respiratory mechanisms. Interestingly, King and Knox (1977) and Kalia (1977) demonstrated connections in the reverse direction : PMKF receives direct ascending inputs from bulbar perikarya located in an area similar to that described above. This further emphasises the occurence of a close relationship between the bulbar and pontine structures implicated in respiration.

REFERENCES

Bertrand, F. and A. Hugelin (1971). Respiratory synchronizing function of nucleus parabrachialis medialis : Pneumotaxic mechanisms. J. Neurophysiol., 34, 189-207.

Cohen, M.I. (1971). Switching of the respiratory phases and evoked phrenic responses produced by rostral pontine electrical stimulation. J. Physiol.(Lond.) 217, 133-158.

Cowan, W.M., D.I. Gottlieb, A.E. Hendrickson, J.L. Price and T.A. Woolsey (1972). The autoradiographic demonstration of axonal connections in the central nervous system. Brain Res., 37, 21-51·.

Coyle, J.T., M.E. Molliver and M.J. Kuhar (1978). In situ injection of kainic acid : a new method for selectively lesioning neuronal cell bodies while sparing axons of passage. J. Comp. Neurol., 180, 301-313.

Denavit-Saubié, M., J. Champagnat and J.C. Velluti (1978). The central transmission of respiratory signals. This volume.

Denavit-Saubié, M. and D. Riche (1977). Descending input from the pneumotaxic system to the lateral respiratory nucleus of the medulla. An anatomical study with the horseradish peroxidase technique. Neurosci. Lett., 6, 121-126

Fries, W. and W. Zieglgänsberger (1974). A method to discriminate axonal from cell body activity and to analyse "silent cells". Exp. Brain Res., 21, 441-445.

Grafstein, B. (1969). Axonal transport; communication between soma and synapse. Advanc. Biochem. Psychopharmacol., I, 11-25

Graham, R.C., Jr., M.J. Karnovsky (1966). The early stages of absorption of injected horseradish peroxidase in the proximal tubule of mouse kidney : ultrastructural cytochemistry by a new technique. J. Histochem. Cytochem. 14, 291-302.

Kalia, M. (1977). Neuroanatomical organization of the respiratory centers. Fed. Proc., 36, 2405-2411.

King, G.W. and C.K. Knox (1977). Bulbo-pontine pathways possibly subversing respiration as studied with neuroanatomical tracing techniques. Proceedings of the International Union of Physiological Sciences, 13, 385.

Kreuter, F., D.W. Richter, H. Camerer and R. Senekowitsch (1977). Morphological and electrical description of medullary respiratory neurons of the cat. Pflügers Arch., 372, 7-16.

Lumsden, T. (1922). Observations on the respiratory centers in the cat. J.Physiol. (Lond.), 57, 153-160·.

Merrill, E.G. (1974). Finding a respiratory function for the medullary respiratory neurons, In : Essays on the nervous system, Clarendon Press, Oxford, pp 451-486.

ACKNOWLEDGEMENTS

The authors wish to thank B. GUIBERT and E. BOUDINOT for their technical assistance.
This study was supported by an A.T.P. from the D.G.R.S.T. n° 78.7.2776 and an A.T.P. from the I.N.S.E.R.M. n° 76.61

SHORT TERM EFFECTS OF BRAIN ELECTRIC STIMULATION ON THE RESPIRATORY RHYTHMIC ACTIVITY IN CATS

A. L. BIANCHI and M. BASSAL

*Laboratoire de Physiologie générale, Faculté des Sciences et Techniques St-Jérôme,
F 13397 Marseille Cedex 4, France*

ABSTRACT

The respiratory system can be considered as serving two major functions, metabolism and behavior. In the present paper, evidence is given to show how the higher nervous structures control the respiratory rhythmic activity in cats, together with a survey of the regions of the brain which might take part in the mechanisms regulating the behavioral respiratory function.

INTRODUCTION

Breathing is considered as an autonomic function the special feature of which is that it is entirely regulated by skeletal muscles which are under the control of both autonomic and voluntary components arising from separate structures in the central nervous system. The former is located in the medulla and pons, and the latter is located in higher brain structures. These two control systems interact to give rise to the final motor output which is as much determined by conscious and inconscious general sensory inputs as by chemical and pulmonary afferences. Thus, breathing is potentially a sensory-motor act, an idea already developed by Sears (1) a few years ago. This apparent ambiguity of the respiratory act has been emphasized during this symposium by Purves (2) who claimed that to understand how the automatic and behavioral components interact the essential prerequisite is to identify the respective pathways involved.

In the course of this paper, we will examine some aspects of these problems. More precisely, we will try to answer the following questions : 1°) What are the higher structures in the brain involved in the behavioral respiratory movements ? 2°) How do these structures drive the respiratory neurones at the medullary and spinal level ?

Our first approach was to apply brief electrical stimulation to various structures in the brain.

A wide variety of responses affecting the rhythm and depth of breathing result from electrical stimulation of the cerebral cortex or sub-cortical structures (Ref. 3 - 8). In these studies, it was found that different regions in the nervous system could be distinguished on the basis of specific respiratory effects, such as inspiratory or expiratory responses. But we think that the method of repetitive stimulation could give rise to indirect responses from structures which do not ne-

cessarily control the respiratory function under normal conditions. In more recent
work, it was possible to distinguish between immediate and delayed effects by the
use of short stimulus trains. Such a technique has been used by several workers to
stimulate the rostrolateral pons (ref. 9, 10), the limbic system (ref. 11, 12) and
the hypothalamus (ref. 13). In these latter studies, two major effects have been
elicited : 1 - inspiratory-facilitatory, obtained from dorsolateral points in the
rostral pons, limbic and hypothalamic regions ; 2 - expiratory-facilitatory, obtained from ventrolateral points in the rostral pons.

In our own studies, we have obtained similar responses at a number of sites in
the nervous system extending from the cerebral cortex to the pons. Moreover the
existence of paucisynaptic relations from these structures to the medullary and
spinal respiratory neurones has been shown by the fact that single or brief tetanic
stimulation can produce short latency bursts of potentials and depression of the
spontaneous discharge of phrenic, intercostal and laryngeal recurrent nerves or
medullary respiratory neurones.

METHODS

The experiments were performed on cats anaesthetized with chloralose (40-50 mg/kg)
or subjected to a low spinal section (level C7-T1) and given Nembutal (2 mg/kg/h) ;
this latter procedure together with bivagotomy minimized the sensory inputs to respiratory centres. Efferent activity of the phrenic nerve was recorded from roots
in the neck with bipolar electrodes on an ink-writer (Mingograph 800) or on an oscilloscope during stimulation of the brain with concentric bipolar stereotaxic e-
lectrodes. In some experiments the phrenic activity was recorded together with the
discharge of external and internal intercostal nerves (level T5-T6 and T8-T9 respectively) in animals with an intact spinal cord or with the inspiratory and expiratory discharge of distal twigs of the recurrent nerve dissected free from the
larynx. To record the unitary activity of the medullary respiratory neurones, we
used extracellular microelectrodes.

Stimuli consisting of rectangular pulses of 0.1 ms duration were delivered during a short period of 20-200 ms, at 300 Hz, at appropriate times during the respiratory cycles. Moreover, to examine the short-latency responses of the various
respiratory neurones, brief tetanic stimulation (2 or 3 pulses) were used. The evoked phrenic and intercostal potentials were processed on-line by an average-respon-
se computer (Didac 800, Intertechnique) and the response of the medullary neurones
were summed by dot-display.

RESULTS AND DISCUSSION

1° - There are two antagonist motor systems which interact reciprocally on the
respiratory neurones
One consist chiefly of the pyramidal and rubrospinal tracts and has been named the
lateral motor system. Brief stimulation (2 or 3 pulses) of these structures and of
the motor cortical area or orbital gyrus induced mainly a short latency inhibitory
response on the inspiratory bulbo-spinal neurones(IBSNs ; fig. 1) whereas a reciprocal excitatory response (latency 7-9 ms) was obtained on the expiratory bulbo-
spinal neurones (EBSNs ; fig. 2).

Another is made up of the reticulo-spinal, vestibulo-spinal, tecto-spinal pathways and has been named the *medial motor system*. Brief stimulation (2 or 3 pulses)
of these structures, of the primary sensory cortical areas and of the rostrolateral pons, limbic system and hypothalamus induced mainly a short-latency excitatory
response (8.3 ± 1.3 ms by stimulation of the mesencephalic reticular formation) on
the IBSNs (fig. 1) and reciprocally an inhibitory response on the EBSNs (fig. 2).

The situation at the spinal level is more complex because of the existence of an
interaction between the responses relayed at the medullary level and the responses
induced by direct pathways from these motor systems to the respiratory motoneurones (see the connection diagrams fig. 1 and 2). When stimulation was applied to
the *lateral motor system*, a direct response was obtained from phrenic or external
intercostal inspiratory motoneurones (fig. 1, the burst of potentials is drawn
with dotted-lines, latency 3-10 ms) together with an arrest of the spontaneous
discharge. When the *medial motor system* was stimulated only the external intercostal motoneurones responded with short latency facilitation, whereas the phrenic
nerve responded with bursts of longer latency (12-35 ms) which might be due to a
response relayed at the medullary level.

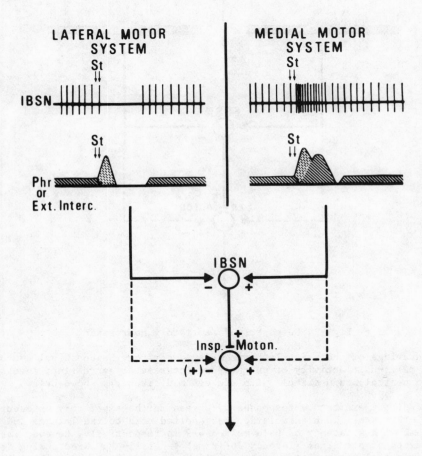

Fig. 1. Responses of inspiratory neurones

Schematic drawings of the unit discharge of an inspiratory bulbo-spinal neurone
(IBSN) and multi-unit activity of the phrenic or an intercostal nerve (Phr, Ext.
Interc.) in response to central brain stimuli with the assumed circuitry shown be-
low. The symbols + and - indicate excitatory and inhibitory synaptic connections.

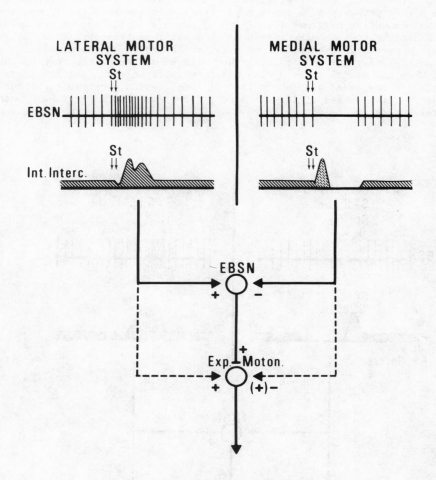

Fig. 2. Responses of expiratory neurones

Schematic drawings of the unit discharge of an expiratory bulbo-spinal neurone
(EBSN) and multi-unit activity of an internal intercostal nerve (Int. Interc.) in
response to central brain stimuli with the assumed circuitry shown below.

The same direct excitatory responses were seen in the expiratory motoneurones
(internal intercostal) when stimulation was applied both to the lateral and medial
motor systems with a latency of 6-14 ms and 4-9 ms respectively. However late excitatory bursts of potential (latency 16-18 ms) generally appeared during stimulation of the lateral motor system ; they could be changed into an inhibitory response by applying stimulation to the medial motor system (fig. 2).

As mentioned in the diagrams of fig. 1 and 2, we assumed that the early excitatory responses were the consequence of transmission in direct pathways to the respiratory motoneurones. These early excitatory responses could correspond to jerk
responses similar to those obtained from the somatic nerves during stimulation of
the cortical area (ref. 14). This latter possibility is indicated in the schema by

(+). The late excitatory bursts of potentials and part of the inhibitory responses were the consequence of transmission in pathways relayed at the medullary level. Similar results have been obtained during stimulation of the motor cortical area by Aminoff and Sears (15) for intercostal motoneurones, and by Colle and Massion (16) for phrenic motoneurones, but they did not describe late responses as Planche (17) did by stimulation of the primary sensory cortical areas.

2°) The "output" respiratory neurones are driven directly by the higher structures
We observed that the inspiratory interneurones, i.e. the inspiratory propriobulbar neurones (IPBNs) were always inhibited when stimulation was applied both to the lateral and medial motor systems. We have inferred from this that the "output" neurones (motoneurones and premotoneurones) are driven directly when the higher structures of the brain are controlling breathing while the interneurones belonging to the system which promotes their discharge are inhibited (fig. 3). Such a mechanism

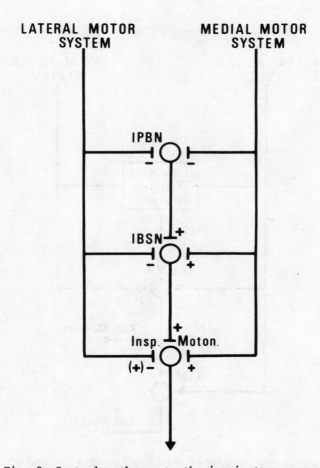

Fig. 3. Central pathways to the inspiratory neurones

Hypothetical schema which indicates how the central structures could drive the output neurones directly while the interneurones (inspiratory propriobulbar neurone , IPBN) are inhibited.

could be involved in the voluntary control of the laryngeal muscles. The higher structures in the brain give rise to an inhibition of the inspiratory laryngeal motoneurones (ILMs) and of the interneurones promoting their discharge (the inspiratory pattern generator) while the expiratory laryngeal motoneurones (ELMs) are facilitated ; the consequence of that being adduction of the vocal cords (fig. 4).

3°) <u>Respiratory effects lasting longer than the duration of stimulation are induced by higher structures</u>

We observed such respiratory effects when short stimulus trains (10-60 stimulus ; 300 c/s) were applied to a large number of structures in the central nervous system. Facilitation of inspiration together with switching from expiration to inspiration, was obtained by applying stimulation to the primary cortical areas, to the medial motor system and to the rostrolateral pons, limbic structures and hypothalamus, whereas facilitation of expiration together with switching from inspiration to expiration was obtained by applying stimulation to the motor cortical area and to the lateral motor system (fig. 5).

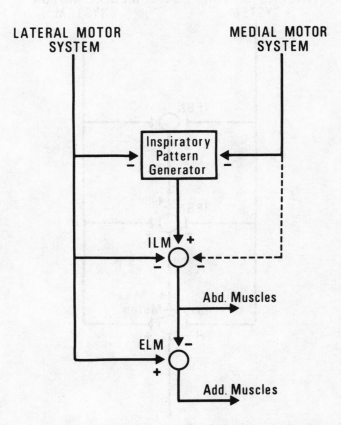

Fig. 4. Central pathways to the laryngeal motoneurones

Hypothetical schema showing how the higher structures could drive the laryngeal motoneurones during voluntary control. ILM : inspiratory laryngeal motoneurone; ELM : expiratory laryngeal motoneurone. (See also ref. 22).

In addition, when the stimulus trains were applied repetitively (1 to 5 trains/s), we obtained (fig. 5) : either 1) inspiratory bursts after each train by stimulation of the *medial motor system* and related structures (the inspiratory triggered bursts had a decreasing discharge pattern similar to that of polypneic respiration) ; or 2) expiratory apnea by stimulation of the *lateral motor system*.

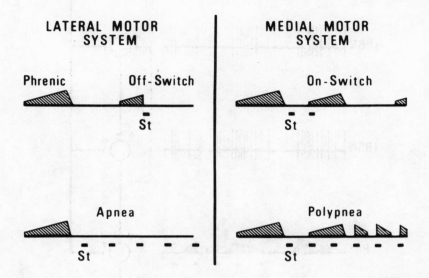

Fig. 5. Respiratory phase-switching triggered by central structures

These drawings show switching of the phrenic discharge by applying short trains of stimulation to the central structures.

It is of interest to note the similarity in the phase switching produced by sensory stimuli in the generation of respiration and locomotion. Such "triggered action" as termed by Bullock (18) appears to be determined by a central program and to have a stereotyped pattern.

The phenomenon of phase-switching by electrical stimulation was discussed by Cohen and Feldman (19) in the context of a general hypothesis of the origin of respiratory periodicity. They assumed that there is a continuous change in the activity level of the respiratory neurone population which is accompagnied by increasing activity in the "triggering systems" (see also ref. 20). Our aim is not to discuss the nature of these "triggering systems" which participate in the onset or termination of respiratory phases. However, it is of interest to note that the higher structures involve these "triggering actions" in the same way as the pneumotaxic system does. Thus, the respiratory synchronizing function is not strictly a function restricted to the nucleus parabrachialis medialis (ref. 9). Rather, switching on or switching-off the respiratory phases are apparently the basic mechanisms by which the higher structures take part in the control of behavioral aspects of respiratory activity. However, the nucleus parabrachialis appears to act as a crossway which receives afferent inputs from the vagus, laryngeal, brachial and lingual nerves as shown by Bertrand and Hugelin (ref. 9) as well as other inputs from the cerebral cortex (our own results, not published).

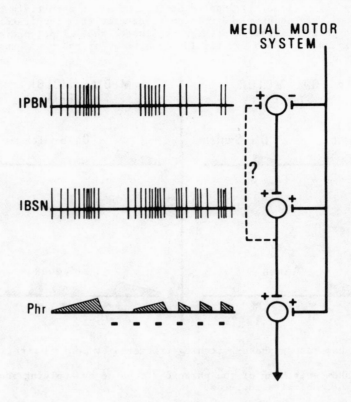

Fig. 6. Responses of the inspiratory neurones to central triggered actions

Unitary discharge of the medullary neurones (IPBN and IBSN) and multi-unit discharge of the phrenic nerve together with a hypothetical schema of the assumed connections.

4°) Triggered respiratory responses and polypnea

During a triggered respiratory response as in polypnea obtained by hypothalamic stimulation (ref. 13), the IBSNs are always the input neurones as we assumed above. However during such a triggered action the discharge of the IPBNs did not become completely silent although they were delayed and disorganized. From this we have tentatively inferred the relationships (connections) in fig. 6 to explain how higher structures trigger the respiratory system. In this we propose that the IPBNs are inhibited by the higher structures but facilitated by excitatory loops from the IBSNs.

5°) Summary of the connections

To summarize, we propose the schema in fig. 7. This diagram shows how the pathways which convey the automatic central respiratory drive to the respiratory neurones (see also ref. 21) could interact with the pathways which achieve the behavioral or postural control of respiratory movements. However this schema is relatively simple because the excitatory or inhibitory feed-back loops have been omitted. The actual connections are without doubt more complex.

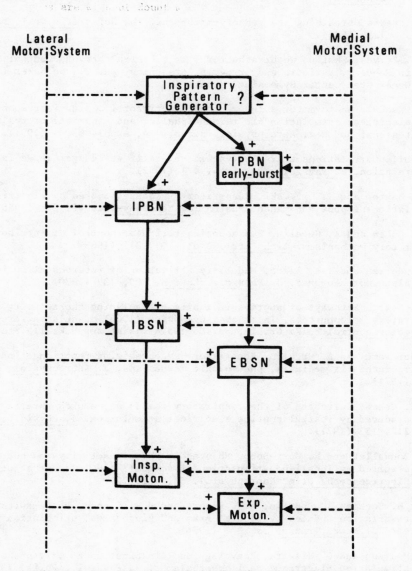

Fig. 7. Hypothetical schema of the assumed circuitry between the motor systems
        and the respiratory neurones

IPBN : inspiratory propriobulbar neurones
IBSN and EBSN : inspiratory and expiratory bulbo-spinal neurones.
The symbols + and − indicate the excitatory and the inhibitory synaptic connec-
tions.

REFERENCES

(1) T.A. Sears, Breathing : a sensory-motor act, The Scientific Basis Med. Ann.
     129 (1971).

(2) M.J. Purves, What do we breathe for ? In : Central Nervous Control Mechanisms
     in Regular, Periodic and Irregular Breathing. Ed. C. von Euler (1978)
     Wener-Gren Center Symposium, Stockholm.

(3) B.R. Kaada, Somato-motor autonomic and electrocortico-graphic responses to
     electrical stimulation of "rhinencephalic" and other structures in prima-
     tes, cat and dog, Acta physiol. scand. 24, suppl. 83, 1 (1951).

(4) P. Dell, Corrélations entre le système végétatif et le système de la vie de
     relation, J. Physiol., Paris 44, 471 (1952).

(5) D.W. Baxter and J. Olzewski, Respiratory responses evoked by electrical stimu-
     lation of pons and mesencephalon, J. Neurophysiol. 18, 276 (1955).

(6) M.I. Cohen and A. Hugelin, Suprapontine reticular control of intrinsic respi-
     ratory mechanisms, Arch. ital. Biol. 103, 317 (1965).

(7) P. Andersen and T.A. Sears, Medullary activation of intercostal fusimotor and
     alpha motoneurones, J. Physiol., London, 209, 739 (1970).

(8) T.A. Sears, Pathways of supra-spinal origin regulating the activity of respi-
     ratory motoneurones, In : Nobel Symposium (1966) Muscular afferents and
     motor control Ed R. Granit, pp 186-196 Almquist and Wiksell, Stockholm.

(9) F. Bertrand and A. Hugelin, Respiratory synchronizing function of nucleus pa-
     rabrachialis medialis, pneumotaxic mechanisms, J. Neurophysiol. 34, 189
     (1971).

(10) M.I. Cohen, Switching of the respiratory phases and evoked phrenic responses
     produced by rostral pontine electrical stimulation, J. Physiol., London,
     217, 133 (1971).

(11) M. Bonvallet and E. Gary-Bobo, Changes in phrenic activity and heart rate
     elicited by localized stimulation of amygdala and adjacent structures.,
     Electroenceph. Clin. Neurophysiol. 32, 1 (1972).

(12) Ch. H. Hockman, J. Duffin, A.M. Rupert and B.R. Vachon, Phase-switching of
     respiration induced by central gray and hippocampal stimulation in the
     cat, J. Neur. Transm. 35, 327 (1974).

(13) R. Monteau and G. Hilaire, Recyclage de l'inspiration et polypnée obtenue par
     stimulation électrique de l'hypothalamus, J. Physiol., Paris, 73, 1057
     (1977).

(14) P. Ascher and D. Jassik-Gerschenfeld, Modalités d'obtention de décharges
     périphériques par stimulation corticale chez le chat, J. Physiol., Paris,
     52, 8 (1960).

(15) M.F. Aminoff and T.A. Sears, Spinal integration of segmental, cortical and
     breathing inputs to thoracic respiratory motoneurones, J. Physiol., London
     215, 557 (1971).

(16) J. Colle and J. Massion, Effet de la stimulation du cortex moteur sur l'activité électrique des nerfs phréniques et médians, Arch. int. Physiol. 66, 496 (1958).

(17) D. Planche, Effets de la stimulation du cortex cérébral sur l'activité du nerf phrénique, J. Physiol., Paris, 65, 31 (1972).

(18) T.H. Bullock, The origin of patterned nervous discharge, Behaviour 17, 48 (1961).

(19) M.I. Cohen and J.L. Feldman, Models of respiratory phase-switching, Feder. Proc. 36, 2367 (1977).

(20) R.J.Wyman, Neural generation of the breathing rhythm, Ann. Rev. Physiol. 39, 417 (1977).

(21) E.G. Merrill, Finding a respiratory function for the medullary respiratory neurons. In : Essays on the Nervous System, ed. R. Bellairs and E.G. Gray (1974) pp 451-486 Clarendon Press Oxford.

(22) J.C. Barillot and M. Dussardier, Activité des motoneurones laryngés expiratoires, J. Physiol., Paris, 72, 311-343 (1976).

ANALOGIES BETWEEN PATTERN GENERATION IN LOCOMOTION AND BREATHING

S. GRILLNER

Department of Physiology III, Karolinska Institutet, Lidingövägen 1,
S-114 33 Stockholm, Sweden

Sten Grillner
Department of Physiology III, Karolinska Institutet,
Lidingövägen 1, S-114 33 Stockholm, Sweden

The neural control of locomotion or respiration can conceptually be divided into three different parts (1) the generation of the basic motor synergy i.e. the stereotype body and trunk movements characteristic of locomotion or respiration (2) the adaptation of these movements to the environment or to other motor demands. During walking we often turn or jump aside and one step is rarely exactly alike another; in respiration the movements change with body position but also with speech or swallowing etc. (3) In both cases the equilibrium control must be adequately dealt with. The projection of the center of gravity should be kept stable between the points of support. In respiration for instance, hip movements act to compensate the movement of the center of gravity that would result from the inspiratory chest movements themselves (ref. 11).

Although it may seem surprising, at first sight, the neural generation of "automatic breathing" and the "basic locomotor synergy" have striking similarities in their control structure (ref. 6, 7). Both systems are controlled by a central pattern generator (CPG). This is a group of neurones, connected in such a way that they can produce the repetitive activation of the different muscles taking part in the behavior without peripheral feedback.

The respiratory CPG can thus, deprived of all afferent inflow generate bursting activity but only at one given frequency (ref. 3, 4, 17). Changes in the tonic level of CO_2 changes the amplitude, that is the degree of activation of different muscles (depth of the breath). Changes in temperature modifies, however, the frequency of the CPG. Afferent inflow from the Hering Breuer reflex will normally, however, exert a direct control of the central pattern generator itself. The time in the cycle, and the degree of expansion of the chest will decide when the inspiration will be terminated ("off switch"). The duration of the expiration may also be reflexly influenced.

Spinal CPGs for locomotion exist, one set for each limb. Their

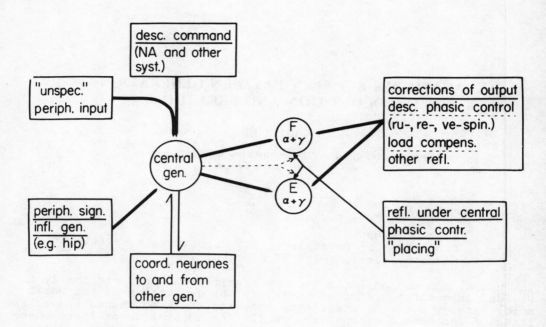

Fig. 1. Schematical representation of different components in the
control system for locomotion

The central pattern generator (centre) can be driven by different
descending command systems. It is implicated that noradrenergic
systems (NA) may be of importance in this context but also other
systems are inferred. Peripheral signals influence the central
pattern generator in a way resembling that of the "Hering Breuer
reflex", although other well defined reflex effects also occur. The
coordination between the different limbs and presumably also the
muscles of the trunk are coordinated through the interaction between
the central pattern generators. Particular "coordinating neurones"
with "efference copy signals" are thought to provide the basis for
this coordination. The central generator drives both alfa and gamma
motoneurones to both flexor (F) and extensor (E) motoneurones. In
fact the hindlimb muscles of the cat should be subdivided into more
than two functional groups with different central commands (at least
4). In addition the central pattern generator exerts a phasic control
of different reflex pathways in the stepcycle. A given pathway may be
open in only one phase of the movement, being closed in the remaining
parts. The final motor output is also controlled by phasic descending
signals from "the higher centres" such as rubro-, reticulo-, and
vestibulospinal pathways (from Grillner 1975, ref. 6).

activity can be driven by a tonic descending inflow and the pattern
generators can thus be made to change their frequency by <u>tonic</u> neural
signals. The amplitude of the output signals increase to some extent
with frequency. The CPG provides the output to the individual muscles
assuring an appropriate timing. Both respiration and locomotion exhibit α - γ -linkage (ref. 1, 3, 16).

However, a very effective reflex overlay acting on the CPG also
exists. Thus, the transition from support to swing will be prevented
if the limb is stopped in mid-support (ref. 9). If the limb is
brought backwards to a hip position close to that in which the
support phase is terminated normally, this will by itself contribute
to the initiation of active flexion (c.f. the control of inspiration
in the Hering Breuer reflex). If the load on the extensors are high
as during mid-support this factor will in itself contribute to a
maintained extensor activity (ref. 14).

In both respiration and locomotion, continuous activity of the CPGs
can be recorded if the animals are kept motionless by curarisation
(ref. 2, 3). In both cases a chest, or a limb movement similar to
the natural movement can be artificially produced. This movement may
be different from that which should have resulted from the resting
activity of the CPG. In both cases the CPG bursting can be entrained
by the peripheral movement. In such a way that the efferent bursts
occur at the same place in the movement cycle, as they would have
occurred during an actively induced movement. In respiration this
may be explained by the Hering Breuer reflex terminating the inspiration; in locomotion partially to the hip position approaching maximal
extension (i.e. a position dependent, negative feedback). An analogous
position dependent mechanism operates at maximal flexion (ref. 2).
It turns out that the cat limb also has an additional mechanism i.e.
a directional sensitivity reinforcing the ongoing movement (i.e. a
positive feedback). These reflexes will in the normal situation
effectively adapt the motor output to the actual mechanical situation
in each step.

The mechanism of the bursting i.e. the mode of operation of the CPG
is, however, unknown. In locomotion, flexor and extensor activity is
mutually exclusive (ref. c.f. 13) but at least four different output
patterns exist (ref. 8, 10). It is striking that most of the different hypotheses, trying to explain the CPG, is common to respiration
and locomotion. It may be very appropriate to compare these systems
to simple invertebrate networks in which a redundant number of
bursting mechanisms have been revealed as in the stomatogastric
system (ref. 12, 15) or in the leech (ref. 5).

REFERENCES

(1)   P. Andersen and T. A. Sears, Medullary activation of intercostal
      fusimotor and alpha motoneurones, <u>J. Physiol</u>., 209, 739-755
      (1970).

(2)   O. Andersson, S. Grillner, M. Lindquist and M. Zomlefer, Peri-
      pheral control of the spinal pattern generators for locomotion
      in cat, <u>Brain Research</u>, 150, 625-630 (1978).

(3)   G. W. Bradley, C. v. Euler, I. Marttila and B. Roos, A model of
      the central and reflex inhibition of inspiration in the cat,

Biol. Cybernetics, 19, 105-115 (1975).

(4) F. J. Clark and C. v. Euler, On the regulation of depth and rate
    of breathing, J. Physiol., 222, 267-295 (1972).

(5) W. O. v. Friesen, M. Poon, G. S. Stent, Neuronal control of
    swimming in the medicinal leech IV. Identification of a net-
    work of oscillatory interneurones, J. Exp. Biol., (1978) (in
    press).

(6) S. Grillner, Locomotion in vertebrates: central mechanisms and
    reflex interaction, Physiol. Rev., 55, 247-304 (1975).

(7) S. Grillner, On the neural control of movement - a comparison
    of different basic rhythmic behaviors. In Dahlem Workshop
    on Function and Formation of Neural Systems, Ed. G. S. Stent,
    Berlin, 197-224 (1977).

(8) S. Grillner, Control of locomotion in bipedes, tetrapodes and
    fish. In APS Handbook on "Motor Control", Ed. V. Brooks
    (in press)

(9) S. Grillner and S. Rossignol, On the initiation of the swing
    phase of locomotion in chronic spinal cats, Brain Research,
    146, 269-277 (1978).

(10) S. Grillner and P. Zangger, On the central generation of loco-
     motion in the low spinal cat, Exp. Br. Res. (in press).

(11) V. S. Gurfinkel and M. L. Shik, The control of posture and
     locomotion. In "Motor Control", Eds. A. Gydikov, N. Tankov
     and D. Kosarov, Plenum Press, New York, 217-234 (1973).

(12) D. F. Russel and D. K. Hartline, Bursting neural networks: A
     reexamination, Science, 200, 453-456 (1978).

(13) E. Jankowska, M. G. M. Jukes, S. Lund and A. Lundberg, The
     effect of DOPA on the spinal cord. 5. Reciprocal organization
     to alpha motoneurones of flexors and extensors, Acta physiol.
     scand., 70, 369-388 (1967a)

(14) K. G. Pearson and J. Duysens, Function of segmental reflexes
     in the control of stepping in cockroaches and cats. In
     Neural Control of Locomotion, Eds. R. Herman, S. Grillner,
     P. Stein and D. Stuart, Plenum Press, New York, 519-538
     (1976).

(15) I. Selverston, Neuronal mechanisms for rhythmic motor pattern
     generation in a simple system. In Neural Control of Locomotion,
     Eds. R. Herman, S. Grillner, P. Stein and D. Stuart, Plenum
     Press, New York, 377-399 (1976).

(16) A. Sjöström and P. Zangger, Muscle spindle control during loco-
     motor movements generated by the deafferented spinal cord,
     Acta physiol. scand., 97, 281-291 (1976).

(17) R. J. Wyman, Neural generation of the breathing rhythm, Ann.
     Rev. Physiol., 39, 417-448 (1977).

SESSION II

GENERATION AND REGULATION OF PATTERN OF BREATHING

B. Developmental Aspects

DIFFERENCES AND SIMILARITIES IN THE CONTROL OF BREATHING PATTERN IN THE ADULT AND NEONATE

T. TRIPPENBACH, R. ZINMAN, R. MOZES and L. M. MURPHY

McGill University, Department of Physiology, Montreal, Canada

Data in the literature suggest that control of breathing differs in many ways between newborns and adults. Premature infants have an irregular respiratory pattern and frequently experience repeated and prolonged apneic episodes. Respiration becomes more regular and the frequency of apneic episodes diminishes with age (Refs. 1,2). Although the development of all the areas of the central nervous system is simultaneous, some areas develop more rapidly than others. Thus, apparent respiratory reflexes in the newborn may be different from those known in the adult. The responses to chemical drive (Refs. 3,4,5,6,7,8,9), to stimulation of the superior laryngeal nerve (Refs. 10,11,12,13,14), to stimulation of the bronchial mucosa (Ref. 15), and to pentobarbital anaesthesia (Refs. 16,17) have been shown to differ between newborns and adults. However, relatively little emphasis has been given to the developmental changes occurring in the control mechanisms of breathing. Thus, our recent study on kittens and rabbit pups was directed towards the early developmental period including the first twenty-one days of life. The aim of our investigation was to define developmental changes in both the central and reflex controls of breathing.

The animals, anaesthetized intraperitoneally (i.p.) with 20 mg/kg pentobarbital and tracheostomized, breathed an enriched oxygen mixture (50% O_2, balance N_2). The C_5 root of the phrenic nerve was separated from the surrounding tissue, and when necessary it was cut and desheathed. Body temperature was maintained at about 37^OC.

Pentobarbital Effects on Timing Parameters

In Fig. 1 examples of 'integrated' phrenic activity monitored from 5, 13 and 19 day-old kittens illustrate pentobarbital effects on the respiratory pattern during the early developmental period of the animals. Airway occlusion at FRC was maintained throughout the time interval between the arrows. With vagal volume-related feedback intact, during control conditions (obtained 30 mins after the initial dose of pentobarbital, panels A), respiratory frequency decreased with age. This effect is similar to the developmental change in respiratory frequency seen in unanaesthetized newborn rabbits (Ref. 19) and kittens (Ref. 8). Fifteen minutes following an additional dose of 10 mg/kg (i.p.) of pentobarbital (panels B) an opposite response was observed: the younger the animal, the lower was the respiratory frequency (Refs. 17,19). In the youngest kitten, the pentobarbital effect on respiratory rate was due to a marked prolongation of expiration since inspiration did not change. With increasing age of the kittens, the prolongation of expiration by pentobarbital anaesthesia decreased whereas inspiration was increasingly prolonged by the anaesthetic. On the 19th day of life, the additional dose

313

of pentobarbital produced a concomitant prolongation of both inspiration and expiration. The latter is a typical response to pentobarbital in the adult cat
(Ref. 20,21).

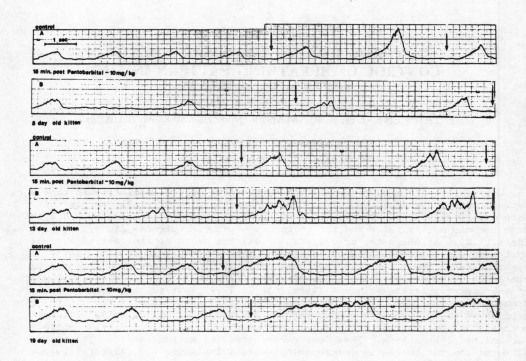

Fig.1. Examples of the records of 'integrated' phrenic activity
taken from 5, 13 and 19 day-old kittens. Control was obtained
30 mins after the initial dose of 20 mg/kg of pentobarbital (i.p.)
(panels A). Panels B illustrate the records taken 15 mins after
an additional dose of pentobarbital (i.p.). The time interval
during which airway occlusion at the end expiratory level (FRC)
was maintained is indicated between the arrows.

In adult cats with vagi cut, deep pentobarbital anaesthesia is characterized
by an apneustic breathing pattern (Refs. 21,22,23). However, in newborn kittens
up to the 18th day of life under deep pentobarbital anaesthesia and without vagal
volume-related feedback, the apneustic pattern of breathing cannot be recorded.
Instead, during airway occlusion at FRC there is either no change in time parameters, as in the 5 day-old kittens presented in Fig. 1, or the changes are more
related to expiratory time (T_E) than to inspiratory time (T_I) (Fig. 2). In older
kittens without phasic vagal input, the prolongation of inspiration caused by
pentobarbital increases, while the prolongation of expiration decreases. Finally,
by the 19th day of life, the changes in T_I and T_E are similar to those observed in
the adult cat: a long apneustic inspiratory effort is followed by a relatively
short expiration (Ref. 24).

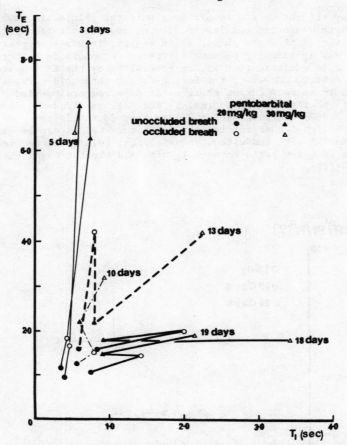

Fig. 2. The relationship between expiratory time (T_E) and
inspiratory time (T_I) obtained: 30 mins after the initial dose
of 20 mg/kg of pentobarbital (i.p.) with (●) and without (o)
vagal volume-related feedback; 15 mins after an additional dose
of 10 mg/kg of pentobarbital (i.p.) with (▲) and without (△)
vagal volume-related feedback. Ages of the 6 kittens used in
this plot are indicated in the figure.

Hering-Breuer Inspiratory-Inhibitory Reflex

Prolongation of T_I during airway occlusion at FRC is related to the withdrawal
of the Hering-Breuer inspiratory-inhibitory reflex mediated by slowly adapting
pulmonary stretch receptors (Ref. 25). The character of the activity and the
firing frequency of vagal stretch receptors in newborns change with development.
In 1 to 3 day-old kittens, only "high threshold" vagal stretch receptors firing
strictly during the inspiratory phase have been found. In 7 to 10 day-old kittens,
both "low threshold" and "high threshold" pulmonary stretch receptors have been
described. Although the receptors have been seen to fire with low frequency at
birth, they have been observed to fire continuously in response to maintained distention of the lungs (Ref. 8).

The role of the pulmonary stretch receptors in breathing can be established by

studying vagotomy effects on the respiratory pattern. Since, in newborns immediately after birth, vagotomy results in slowing down respiration partly due to a
prolongation of the inspiratory phase, as in adults, it has been postulated that
the role of the slowly adapting pulmonary stretch receptors in newborns is similar
to that described in adults: that is, to control T_I by the Hering-Breuer inspiratory-inhibitory reflex. However, the Hering-Breuer threshold curve (Ref. 26) has
not been studied in animals during their early developmental period. When phasic
vagal feedback is abolished in newborns, T_I and peak amplitude of 'integrated'
phrenic activity (PHR) increase (Ref. 27) as they do in adults. Thus, the
strength of the Hering-Breuer inspiratory-inhibitory reflex can be estimated from
the ratio between PHR with and without phasic vagal volume-related feedback (PHR^O/
PHR^C) as well as from the ratio between T_I with and without vagal phasic volume-
related input (T_I^O/T_I^C).

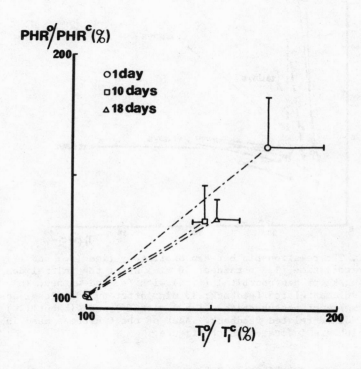

Fig.3. To illustrate the effects of the Hering-Breuer
inspiratory-inhibitory reflex on peak amplitude of the
'integrated' phrenic activity and inspiratory time in three
kittens. Their ages are given in the figure. The data are
presented as percent changes from the control values (100%)
obtained before airway occlusion at FRC. For further explanation see text.

It is very difficult to assess the strength of the Hering-Breuer inspiratory-
inhibitory reflex in the pentobarbital anaesthetized newborn kittens, since an
overdose of the anaesthetic may completely abolish this reflex (see Fig. 1) or
cause a gasp-like pattern of breathing. The latter observation may suggest that
vagal afferentation is of great importance in maintaining the semi-regular pattern

of respiration present in kittens during their early developmental period. On the other hand, in kittens during the second and the third week of life, similar to adult animals (Ref. 28), an overdose of pentobarbital augments the Hering-Breuer inspiratory-inhibitory reflex.

An attempt was made to evaluate the Hering-Breuer inspiratory reflex during postnatal development in kittens under light pentobarbital anaesthesia, using the two estimates defined above (see Fig. 3). As long as anaesthesia is light enough so as not to produce: 1) a gasp-like pattern of breathing or loss of the Hering-Breuer inspiratory-inhibitory reflex during the first week of life, or 2) apneusis in kittens of the third week of life, then in the absence of vagal volume-related feedback in newborn kittens (1 to 21 days old) the greatest increases in both PHR and in T_I occur in the 1 day-old animals. The latter indicates that the Hering-Breuer reflex decreases in strength with maturation. Similarly, the effect of vagotomy on respiratory frequency has been described as being greater in the younger animals (Refs. 8,10). Changes in the strength of the Hering-Breuer inspiratory reflex have also been found in newborn babies. At a gestational age of 32 weeks, the Hering-Breuer reflex is very weak and the strength of the reflex gradually increases until 32-38 weeks of life and then decreases (Ref. 30) until almost abolished by adulthood (Refs. 31,32). This decline in strength of the Hering-Breuer reflex after 32-38 weeks of life may be explained by the fact that other reflexes, such as those from the thoracic wall, are becoming relatively more important (Refs. 30,33,34).

Hering-Breuer Expiratory Promoting Reflex

The Hering-Breuer expiratory promoting reflex is present at birth in newborn babies (Ref. 35) and animals (Refs. 9,36). In newborn lambs, lung inflation causes an inhibition of the inspiratory medullary neurons while the expiratory medullary neurons fire tonically (Ref. 27). This response can be compared to a similar observation made in adult animals (Refs. 37,38). In kittens and rabbit pups lightly anaesthetized with pentobarbital, the Hering-Breuer expiratory promoting reflex is strong and the characteristics of this reflex are the same as in adult cats: the greater the respiratory frequency, the stronger is the reflex (Ref. 39). Fig. 4 illustrates the expiratory reflex prolongation (T_E^L/T_E^C) in 2 to 4 day-old rabbit pups obtained by airway occlusion at the end of inspiration. The same qualitative results were obtained in newborn kittens of the same age.

Because of the differences in sensitivity to pentobarbital anaesthesia during the early developmental period, the response to airway occlusion at the end of inspiration may be reversed by the anaesthetic, such that the lower the respiratory frequency, the stronger is the reflex (Ref. 36). This result may not only be related to a different pentobarbital effect in younger animals but may also be due to concomitant decrease in chemical sensitivity caused by the anaesthetic.

Hering-Breuer Deflation Reflex

Pulmonary deflation sensitive receptors and their role in the control of the respiratory pattern have not been systematically investigated in either newborn animals or in babies. However, sighs or "augmented breaths," which are probably mediated by the same receptors (Ref. 40), are very common in newborn infants, rabbits and kittens. In kittens during the first week of life, sighs frequently occur when the airway is occluded at FRC (see Fig. 1). In newborn lambs, the frequency of sighs decreases with increasing body size (Ref. 41).

There are controversial data in the literature about the effect of lung deflation in newborn. It has been claimed that in kittens younger than three weeks, the deflation reflex cannot be provoked (Ref. 42). It has also been impossible to elicit this reflex in newborn babies (Ref. 43). However, direct stimulation of the

bronchial mucosa in infants whose gestational age is greater than 35 weeks, results
in a consistent increase in inspiratory effort usually followed by apnoea. In the
younger infants, this response is absent (Ref. 15).

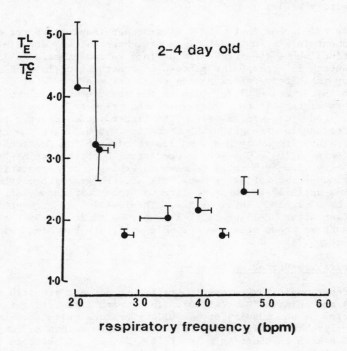

Fig.4. Reflex prolongation of expiration expressed in relative
terms in response to airway occlusion at end inspiration in 8
rabbit pups aged from 2 to 4 days, as a function of the respiratory frequency. Each point represents the mean value obtained
from at least 5 manoeuvres (± SD) in each animal.

In newborn sheep, the central effect of lung deflation is variable. The most
common effect is a prolongation of the discharges of inspiratory neurons, and
either no change or a reduction in the respiratory frequency (Ref. 27). In newborn rabbits the deflation reflex was observed immediately after birth (Refs. 29,
36). In a 2 hour-old monkey anaesthetized with 1% halothane (Fig. 5, Bryan and
Trippenbach, unpublished observations) and in lightly pentobarbital anaesthetized
newborn kittens, the deflation reflex was found to be very powerful (Ref. 44).
An example of the response to lung deflation in a 2 day-old kitten is illustrated
in Fig.6. Deflation was produced by applying a negative pressure of about -5 cm
H_2O to the tracheal cannula. The deflation reflex shown in this figure is similar
to that observed in the newborn monkey and also to that described for adult cats
(Ref. 32), that is, a prolongation of inspiration, a shortening of expiration, an
increase in respiratory frequency, and an augmentation in phrenic activity.
Phrenic activity persisted throughout T_E as is indicated in the figure by the upward shift in the baseline of the 'integrated' phrenic activity. In our study
on newborn kittens (1 to 21 days old), all the lightly pentobarbital anaesthetized
animals possessed a typical "mature" (adult-like) response to lung deflation.
However, the reflex was drastically influenced by the level of pentobarbital anesthesia. Thus, besides this typical adult response to lung deflation, other

2 hour old monkey

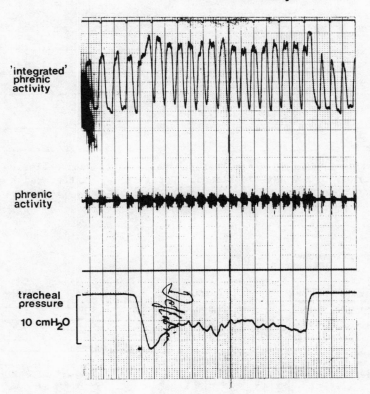

'integrated' phrenic activity

phrenic activity

tracheal pressure

10 cmH$_2$O

Fig.5. To illustrate the effect of lung deflation in a 2 hour-old monkey. Upper trace: 'integrated' phrenic activity; middle trace: phrenic activity before processing; lower trace: tracheal pressure. The paper speed indicated at the top of the figure is 1 cm/sec. Augmentation of phrenic activity, prolongation of inspiration, shortening of expiration, and increase in respiratory frequency are shown.

changes in the respiratory pattern were observed. These are illustrated in Fig.7. Examples of 'integrated' phrenic activity were taken from two kittens: 3 and 5 days old, 30 mins after an initial dose of 20 mg/kg of pentobarbital, i.p. (panels A and B), and 15 mins after an additional dose of 10 mg/kg of the anaesthetic, i.p. (panels C and D). The ratio between T_I and T_E (T_I/T_E) given with ± SD in the table to the left of the tracings, provides an index of the depth of anaesthesia: the higher the ratio, the lower the anaesthetic level. Type 1 of the response was obtained when the T_I/T_E ratio was the highest and was characterized by a shortening of both T_I and T_E. Changes in T_E were always greater than changes in T_I. Phrenic activity was augmented and was present during expiration. The latter was seen as an upward shift in the baseline of the 'integrated' phrenic activity. This type of response was also obtained in newborn rabbits during the first week of life. When T_I/T_E was slightly lower than the T_I/T_E ratio for Type 1, the adult type of response to lung deflation (Type 2 responses) was recorded. This was distinguished

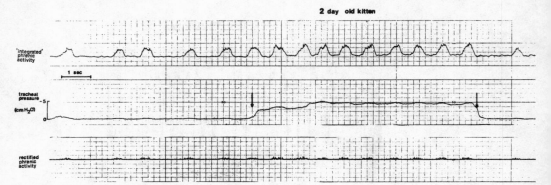

Fig. 6. An example of the "mature" response to lung deflation recorded in a 2 day-old kitten. Upper trace: 'integrated' phrenic activity; middle trace: tracheal pressure, lower trace: rectified phrenic activity.

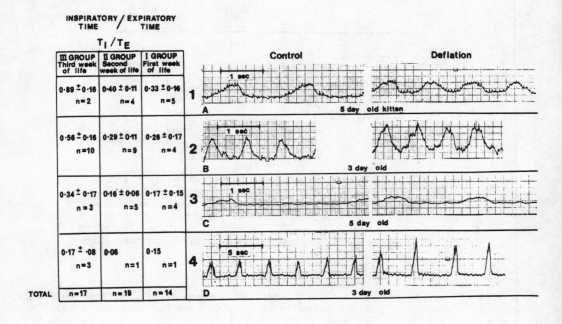

III GROUP Third week of life	II GROUP Second week of life	I GROUP First week of life		
0.89 ± 0.16 n=2	0.40 ± 0.11 n=4	0.33 ± 0.16 n=5	**1** A	
0.56 ± 0.16 n=10	0.29 ± 0.11 n=9	0.26 ± 0.17 n=4	**2** B	
0.34 ± 0.17 n=3	0.16 ± 0.06 n=5	0.17 ± 0.15 n=4	**3** C	
$0.17 \pm .08$ n=3	0.06 n=1	0.15 n=1	**4** D	
TOTAL n=17	n=19	n=14		

Fig.7. To illustrate four types of the responses to lung deflation in relation to the depth of anaesthesia. Each T_I/T_E value is a mean ($\pm$ SD); n is equal to the number of individual responses. For further explanation see text.

by a prolongation of T_I, a shortening of T_E, and an augmentation of phrenic activity during inspiration as well as the presence of phrenic activity during expiration. In animals highly sensitive to pentobarbital or in others after an additional dose of the anaesthetic, the Type 3 response to lung deflation was obtained. In this type of response, there was no change in either T_I or in phrenic activity. However, T_E was significantly shortened. When the anaesthetic caused a further decrease in the T_I/T_E ratio, the Type 4 response was observed. The latter was typified by a decrease in respiratory frequency due to a prolongation of T_E with no change in T_I, but with an augmentation of phrenic activity. Therefore, our results may explain the lack of success in producing the "mature" deflation reflex in the one week old kittens of Duron and Marlot (Ref. 42). Thus, interpretation of the results obtained in studies with anaesthetized newborns necessitates taking into account the sensitivity to the anaesthetic.

The presence of the deflation reflex in animals immediately after birth may have important clinical implications. For example, in premature babies, contraction of the diaphragm during inspiration pulls the chest wall inwards, especially during active sleep (Ref. 44). This can lead to partial deflation of the lungs, and hence excitation of the deflation sensitive receptors. Through this reflex, central respiratory rhythmicity may be disrupted. Thus, in premature infants, the information from deflation sensitive receptors may be one of the sources producing an irregular pattern of breathing (see also Ref. 15), especially during active sleep, when the distortion of the ribcage is most noticeable. The presence of "sighs" during airway occlusion in newborn kittens in their first week of life and a shortening of T_I during airway occlusion in an infant after a complete lesion of the spinal cord at the cervical level (Ref. 45) may be both caused by a similar stimulation of deflation sensitive receptors.

In summary, pentobarbital anaesthesia in newborn kittens has different effects on the respiratory pattern from those known in adult cats. While deepening pentobarbital anaesthesia produces concomitant prolongation of both T_I and T_E in the adult cat, in kittens immediately after birth, T_I is little affected and T_E is markedly prolonged. While deepening pentobarbital anaesthesia in the adult cat without vagal input results in an inhibition of the expiratory medullary units in the presence of tonic activity of the inspiratory units (Ref. 23), the prolonged T_E and short T_I in the deeply pentobarbital anaesthetized newborn kitten may indicate potentiation of expiratory units as an inhibition of the inspiratory neurons. This may indicate a different functional organization of the respiratory medullary network during the early developmental period.

The depressing action of the pentobarbital might arise from withdrawal of background excitation (Ref. 46) and activation of GABA receptors (Ref. 47). GABA is thought to be a transmitter involved both in pre- and postsynaptic inhibitions at the supraspinal level (Ref. 48). The depressant action of GABA has been described on both medullary respiratory and non-respiratory neurons in the vicinity of the nucleus ambiguus. The hyperpolarization by GABA has a greater effect on the non-respiratory neurons than on the respiratory neurons (Ref. 49). Thus, when pentobarbital is present, the number of active respiratory neurons and the reticular system neurons decrease (Ref. 50). In the immature brain with less dendritic synapses (Ref. 51), less myelinated fibres (Ref. 52), less mitchondria (Ref. 53) and lower secretion rates of transmitters (Ref. 54), the inhibition mediated through the GABA mechanism may be augmented. In other words, sensitivity to the anaesthetic would be greater during the early postnatal period. The inhibitory effect on the generation of central inspiratory activity is demonstrated by a decrease in both PHR and rate of rise of 'integrated' phrenic activity in the 10 day-old kitten. However, in the 19 day-old kitten, the same additional dose of the anaesthetic produced a slight increase in PHR probably due to a decrease in ventilation (see Fig. 8). On the other hand, the gasp-like pattern of breathing observed so often in the pentobarbital anaesthetized newborn kittens may reflect a withdrawal of background excitation by pentobarbital. It has been postulated that in the immature brain with lack of integrative abilities, all the neurons, including those involved in respiration need the combined input of respiratory and all other sensory stimuli to sustain respiration (Ref. 55). Pentobarbital, as a competitive blocker of GABA uptake, would decrease facilitation from higher structures of the central nervous system. The prolongation of the unitary postsynaptic inhibition would lead to more effective summation of repetitive inhibitory actions (Ref. 56). In lamb foetus devoid of respiratory-like movements, expiratory medullary neurons are active tonically and become phasic during changes in tracheal pressure (Ref. 27). Thus, if inhibition of the medullary respiratory complex from the higher structures (Ref. 52) persists beyond the gestational period, this intrinsic inhibition could be potentiated by pentobarbital during the early postnatal age. Therefore, the activity of the inspiratory neurons would be depressed and that of the expiratory neurons augmented. This "paradoxical" effect of pentobarbital is greater in the youngest newborns.

In conclusion, in newborns, vagal respiratory reflexes are similar to those known in adult animals, and are present immediately after birth. They can be abolished or reversed by use of pentobarbital anaesthesia. The different degrees of sensitivity to this anaesthetic indicate an immaturity of the functional organization of the inspiratory 'off-switch' mechanism in the animals during the first two weeks of life. The fact that bilateral lesion of the site of the pneumotaxic mechanism (Refs. 58,61) or deep pentobarbital anaesthesia does not produce apneusis in newborns before the third week of life without vagal input, suggests that the inspiratory 'off-switch' mechanism during the early developmental period is lacking the facilitatory influence from the pneumotaxic mechanism, which has been described in adult cats (Refs. 24,59). On the other hand, prolongation of T_E both by the lesion and by pentobarbital may indicate that the mechanisms controlling T_E are deprived of their integrative abilities when facilitation from the pneumotaxic mechanism and other sites of the central nervous system is withdrawn. By the 18th day of life, the role of the pneumotaxic mechanism seems to be similar to that known in the adult. The hypothesis of the functional reorganization of the central respiratory control system may explain the fact that in premature babies, respiration is always arrested during expiration (premature apnoea), and in infants with "breath holding" spells, respiration is always arrested during inspiration. Finally it appears that the changes in functional organization of the respiratory rhythm generator are related to increasing integrative abilities of the whole central nervous system during maturation.

ACKNOWLEDGEMENT

    Dr. Trippenbach wishes to thank Prof.A.C. Bryan for inviting her to cooperate in the experiments on monkeys in the Hospital for Sick Children in Toronto, Ontario. The authors also wish to thank Mrs. P. Bynoe for secretarial help and Mr. Gregory Trippenbach for preparing the illustrations. This research was supported by the Medical Research Council of Canada.

REFERENCES

1. Dreyfus-Brisac, C. Ontogenesis of sleep in human prematures, after 32 weeks of conceptional age, Develop. Psychobiol.3, 91 (1970).

2. Parmelee, A.M., E. Stern and M.A. Morris. Maturation of respiration in prematures and young infants, Neuropaediatric.3, 294 (1972).

3. Mott, J.C. The ability of young mammals to withstand total oxygen lack. Brit. Med. Bull. 17, 144 (1961).

4. Stahlman, M. Ventilation control in newborn. Am. J. Dis. Childh.101,216 (1961).

5. Avery, M.E., V. Chernick, R.E. Dutton and S. Permutt. Ventilatory responses to inspired carbon dioxide in infants and adults, J. Appl. Physiol. 18, 895 (1963).

6. Cross, K.W. (1964) Respiratory Responses of the Neonate to Changes of Oxygen Tension. Oxygen in the Animals Organism, Pergamon Press, Oxford-Frankfurt.

7. Godfrey, S. Respiratory and cardiovascular changes during asphyxia and resuscitation of foetal and newborn rabbits, Q. J. Exp. Physiol. 53, 97 (1968).

8. Schwieler, G.H. Respiratory regulation during postnatal development in cats and rabbits and some of its morphological substrate, Acta Physiol.Scand. (suppl.) 304, 72 (1968).

9. Johnson, P. Airway reflexes and chemoreception during development, XXVll International Congress of Physiological Sciences, Paris, July, 12, 328 (1977).

10. Wealthall, S.R. (1976). Factors resulting in a failure to interrupt apnea. Development of Upper Respiratory Anatomy and Function: Implications for Sudden Infants Death Syndrome. U.S. Government Priting Office, Washington, pp.212-228.

11. Downing, S.E., and J.C. Lee. Laryngeal chemosensitivity, a possible mechanism for sudden infant death, Pediatrics. 55, 640 (1975).

12. Johnson, P., D. Salisbury and A.T. Storey (1976). Apnea induced by stimulation of sensory receptors in the larynx. Development of Upper Respiratory Anatomy and Function: Implications for Sudden Infant Death Syndrome. U.S. Government Printing Office, Washington, pp.160-178.

13. Miller, A.J., and C.R. Dunmire. Characterization of the postnatal development of superior laryngeal nerve fibres in the postnatal kittens, J. Neurobiol. 7, 483 (1976).

14. Storey, A.T., and P. Johnson (1976). Laryngeal receptors inviting apnea. Development of Upper Respiratory Anatomy and Function: Implications for Sudden Infant Death Syndrome. U.S. Government Printing Office, Washington, pp.184-198.

15. Fleming, P.J., A.C. Bryan and M.H. Bryan. Functional immaturity of pulmonary irritant receptors and apnea in newborn preterm infants, Pediatrics. 61, 515 (1978).

16. Goldberg, M.S., and Milic-Emili. Effect of sodium pentobarbital on respiratory control in newborn rabbits, J. Appl. Physiol. 42, 845 (1977).

17. Marlot, D. and B. Duron. Extrapulmonary afferents and respiratory activity in the newborn kitten, Bul. Eur. Physiol. Resp. 12, 94P (1976).

18. Wyszogrodski, I., B.T. Thach and J. Milic-Emili. Maturation of respiratory control in unanesthetized newborn rabbits, J. Appl. Physiol.: Respirat. Environ. Exercise Physiol. 44, 304 (1978).

19. Zinman, R., T.Trippenbach. Developmental changes in ventilatory parameters of anesthetized newborn rabbit, Can. Fed. Biol. Soc. 21, 21 (1978).

20. Gautier, H. Pattern of breathing during hypoxia or hypercapnia of the awake or anesthetized cat, Respir. Physiol. 27, 193 (1976).

21. Murphy, L.M. The effect of sodium pentobarbital on the control of breathing in cats. Ph.D. Thesis, 1977.

22. Webber, C.C., and C.N. Peiss. Barbiturate-induced apneusis in the cat
    (Abstract) Physiologist 12, 299 (1972).

23. Robson, J.G., M.A. Houseley, O.H. Solis-Quiroga. The mechanism of respira-
    tory arrest with sodium pentobarbital and sodium thiopental, Ann. N.Y. Acad.
    Sci. 109, 494 (1963).

24. Euler, C.v., I. Marttila, J.E. Remmers and T. Trippenbach. Effects of lesion
    in the parabrachial nucleus on the mechanisms for central and reflex termina-
    tion of inspiration in cat, Acta Physiol. Scand. 96, 324 (1976).

25. Adrian, E.D. Afferent impulses in the vagus and their effect on respiration,
    J. Physiol (London) 79, 332 (1933).

26. Clark, F.J., and C.v. Euler. On the regulation of depth and rate of breathing,
    J. Physiol (London) 222,267 (1972).

27. Bystrzycka, E., B.S. Nail and M.J. Purves. Central and peripheral neural
    respiratory activity in the mature sheep foetus and newborn lamb, Resp.
    Physiol. 25, 199 (1975).

28. Sant'Ambrogio, G., and J.G. Widdicombe. Respiratory reflexes acting on the
    diaphragm and inspiratory intercostal muscles of the rabbit, J. Physiol.
    (London) 180, 766 (1965).

29. Dawes, G.S. and J.C. Mott. Reflex respiratory activity in the newborn rabbit.
    J. Physiol.(London) 145, 85 (1959).

30. Bodegard, G., G.H.Schwieler, S., Skoglund and R. Zetterstrom. Control of
    respiration in newborn babies I. The development of the Hering-Breuer in-
    flation reflex, Acta Paediat. Scand. 58, 567 (1969).

31. Guz, A., M.I.M. Noble, D. Trenchard, H.L. Cochrane and A.R. Makey. Studies
    on the vagus nerves in man: Their role in respiratory control, Clin. Sci.
    27, 293 (1964).

32. Widdicombe, J.G. Respiratory reflexes. Handbook of Physiology. Amer.
    Physiol. Soc. Washington (1964).

33. Bodegard, G., and G.H. Schwieler. Control of respiration in newborn babies
    II. The development of the thoracic reflex response to an added respiratory
    load, Acta Paediat. Scand. 60, 181 (1971).

34. Olinsky, A., M.H. Bryan and A.C. Bryan. Response of newborn infants to added
    respiratory loads, J. Appl. Physiol. 37, 190 (1974).

35. Cross, K.W., M. Klaus, W.H. Tooley and K. Weiser. The response of the new-
    born baby to inflation of the lungs, J. Physiol. (London) 151, 551 (1960).

36. Trippenbach, T., R. Zinman and J. Milic-Emili. Caffeine effects on central
    and reflex control of respiration in newborn rabbits. (Manuscript in prepara-
    tion).

37. Wang, S.C., and S.H. Ngai. General organisation of central respiratory
    mechanisms. Respiration. Handbook of Physiology 1, 487 (1964).

38. Bystrzycka, E., H. Gromysz and A. Huszczuk. Functional organisation of the
    brain stem respiratory neurons. Acta Physiol.Pol. (suppl.) 2, 299 (1971).

39. Euler, C.v., and T. Trippenbach. Temperature effects on the inflation reflex
     during expiratory time in cat, Acta Physiol. Scand. 96, 338 (1976).

40. Hughes, D.T.D., H.R. Parker and I.V. Williams. The response of foetal sheep
     and lambs to pulmonary inflation. J. Physiol.(London) 189, 177 (1967).

41. Knowlton, G.C. and M.G. Larrabee. A unitary analysis of pulmonary volume
     receptors, Am. J. Physiol. 147, 100 (1957).

42. Duron, B. and D. Marlot. Hering-Breuer reflex during postnatal development,
     Bul. Eur. Physiol. Resp. 12, 94P (1976).

43. Bryan, A.C., M.H. Bryan, S.M.L. Kirkpatrick and R.L. Knill. The use of air-
     way occlusion in infants, Chest. 70, 142 (1976).

44. Trippenbach, T. and R. Zinman. Deflation reflex in newborn animals, Can. Fed.
     Soc. 21, 22 (1978).

45. Thach, B.T., I.F. Abroms, I.D. Frantz III, A. Sotrel, E.N. Bruce and
     M.D. Goldman. REM sleep breathing pattern without intercostal muscle (IM)
     influence, Fed. Proc. 36, 445 (1977) (Abstract).

46. Gordon, M., F.J. Rubin and P. Strata. The effect of pentobarbital on the
     activity evoked in cerebellum cortex, Exp. Brain Res. 17, 50 (1973).

47. Nicoll, R.A. Pentobarbital: action on frog motoneurons, Brain Res. 96, 119
     (1975).

48. Hosli, L., A.K. Tebecis and N. Fillias. Effects of glycine beta alamine and
     GABA and their interaction with strychmine on brain stem neurons, Brain Res.
     16, 293 (1969).

49. M. Denant-Saubié and J. Champagnat. The effect of some depressing amino
     acids on bulbar respiratory and non-respiratory neurons, Brain Res. 97, 356
     (1975).

50. Bertrand, F., D. Caille, J.F. Vibert. Quantitative effects of anesthesia on
     bubo-pontine respiratory unit populations, Bul. Eur. Physiol. Resp. 12, 70P
     (1976).

51. Changeux, J.P., and A.Danchin. Selective stabilization of developing synapses
     as a mechanism for the specification of neuronal networks, Nature 269, 705
     (1976).

52. Skoglund, S., and C. Romero. Postnatal growth of spinal nerves and roots.
     A morphological study in the cat with physiological correlations. Acta
     Physiol. Scand. 66, 260 (1965) (suppl.).

53. Samson, F.E., W.M. Balfour and R.J. Jacobs. Mitochondrial changes in de-
     veloping rat brain, Amer. J. Physiol. 199, 693 (1960).

54. Jones, C.T., and R.O. Robinson. Plasma catecholamines in foetal and adult
     sheep, J. Physiol. 248, 15 (1975).

55. Schulte, F.J., and U. Jurgens. Apnoen bei reifen und unrei en Neugeborchen.
     Mschr. Kinderheill. 117, 595 (1969).

56. Nicoll, R. A., J. C. Eccles, T. Oshima and F. Rubia. Prolongation of hippo-
     campal inhibitory postsynaptic potentials by barbiturates, Nature 258,625 (1975).

57. Barcroft, J., and M.J. Karvonen. The action of CO_2 and cyanide on fetal res-
     piratory movements. The development of chemoreflex function in the sheep,
     J. Physiol.(London) 107, 153 (1948).

58. B. Duron and D. Marlot (1978). Some aspects on the central and reflex control
     mechanisms of breathing in newborn kitten. Wenner-Gren Center Symposium.
     Central Nervous Control Mechanisms in Regular Periodic and Irregular Breathing
     (Physiological and clinical aspects in the adult and prenatal states) Pergamon
     Press, Oxford.

59. Cohen, M.I. Switching of the respiratory phases and evoked phrenic responses
     produced by rostral pontine electrical stimulation. J. Physiol.(London)
     217, 133 (1971).

Discussion after the next paper.

POSTNATAL EVOLUTION OF INSPIRATORY
ACTIVITY IN THE KITTEN

B. DURON and D. MARLOT

Laboratoire de Neurophysiologie, U.E.R. de Médecine, 12 rue Frédéric Petit,
80036 Amiens Cédex, France

INTRODUCTION

The study of respiratory nervous control maturation implies, a priori, determining real differences between respiratory function of the newborn at birth and that of the adult animal. It is then necessary to systematically study week after week the postnatal evolution of the differences observed.

The most profound analysis of the mechanisms and of their maturation is made difficult because of the numerous unanswered problems still remaining in the adult animal. Given the little information we presently have about respiratory control in the newborn animal, it is practically indispensable to approach answering any given question by different and complementary methods. Therefore, this methodology means multiplying the experimental series, which considerably delays the interpretations.

Among the most interesting facts that we have observed during these last years, the most important seems to be the relative lack of inspiratory activity of the kitten whether in eupnea (1) or in the course of pulmonary reflexes (2).

In the present work, we will report various experimental results illustrating this fact and enabling us to orient an interpretation.

MATERIAL AND METHODS

With the exception of the study of the phrenic motor unit discharges performed only on the animal anaesthetized with Nembutal (30 mg kg I.P.), all the results have been obtained both on the anaesthetized animal and on the decerebrated preparation by transcollicular section of the brain stem.

Each experimental series has been performed on newborn kittens and then on group aged respectivelly 1, 2, 3, 4 weeks. A minimum of 10 kittens constitutes the experimental material of each group.

In these conditions, we have studied the effect, on the inspiratory activity of the occlusion of the tracheal canula at the end of inspiration or at the end of expiration. Secondly, we have analyzed the consequences of bivagotomy and finally, the results of pontine section performed at the level of the presumed pneumotaxic center. In order, to compare the results obtained in this latter series,

the pontine section was preceded by a transcolliculary decerebration in the anaesthetized animals.

The inspiratory activity was picked up by electrodes implanted either in the diaphragm or in the second latero-sternal interchondral muscle. This latter technique avoids opening the abdomen and the risk of provoking a pneumothorax.

RESULTS

Postnatal evolution of inspiratory activity

The duration of inspiratory time (T.I.) progressively augments in absolute value
during the postnatal period whether in the anaesthetized animal or in the decerebrated animal. In the first case the duration of T.I. goes from 0,7 sec to 1 sec
during the first four weeks of postnatal life.

In the decerebrated animal, we note an analogous variation but the T.I. values at
birth are much lower and are on the order of 0.2 sec. The essential difference
between the two types of preparations is due to the much longer expiratory time
(T.E.) in the anaesthetized cat than in the decerebrated animal.

The analysis of the phrenic motor unit discharges (fig. 1) clearly objectivies
these first results, at birth the average duration of discharges does not exceed
500 ms.

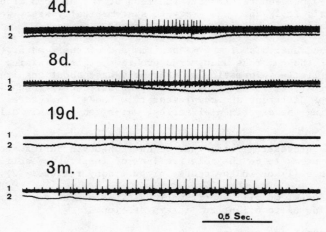

Fig. 1 Phrenic motor units in kittens between the age of 4
days to 3 months (anaesthetized with nembutal)
1 : Phrenic motor unit ; 2 : Oesophageal pressure

Progressively, during development, this period lengthens at the same time as the
discharge pattern changes (fig. 2). At birth, in regard to early inspiratory motor units (3), we observe a very rapid increase in discharge frequency which reaches values neighboring 60 Hz, very clearly superior to those found in the adult
animal. The stop of discharge is brutal, suggesting the intervention of powerful
inhibitory mechanisms. We have not actually studied the relative proportion of
early and late phrenic motor units.

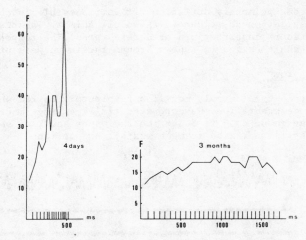

Fig. 2 Frequence histograms of 2 phrenic motor units in 2
        kittens (anaesthetized with nembutal)
        Ordinate : frequency in Hz ; Abscissa : time in ms.

Postnatal evolution of Hering-Breuer reflexes

Under anaesthesia or after decerebration occlusion of the tracheal canula at the
end of inspiration, provokes a powerful and often long lasting inhibition of inspiratory activity (fig. 3). Inversely, tracheal occlusion during expiration provokes a reinforcement of inspiration characterized by a prolongation of T.I. (fig. 3).
Nevertheless, inspiratory activity stimulated in this way is very quickly inhibited.

5 DAYS

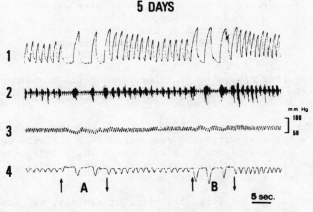

Fig. 3 Effects of occlusion of the trachea in a 5 day old
        decerebrated kitten
        A : tracheal occlusion at the end of inspiration
        B : tracheal occlusion at the end of expiration
        1 : electrical integrated activity of the 2nd inter-
            chondral muscle
        2 : E.M.G. of the 2nd interchondral muscle
        3 : arterial pressure
        4 : oesophageal pressure
Note in B the predominance of expiratory reinforcement.

When we make strong pulmonary deflations it is impossible to obtain a tonic reinforcement of inspiration as we can in the adult animal. The results are identical
whether the kitten is anaesthetized or decerebrated. The response similar to that
obtained in the adult begins to appear around the third week of postnatal life.

Effects of bivagotomy

Cervical bivagotomy considerably modifies respiratory rhythm whether under anaesthesia or after decerebration. We note essentially a very important prolongation
of T.E. which can go up to 4 to 5 sec. On the other hand, as shown in fig. 4, inspiratory activity is increased in much weather proportions.

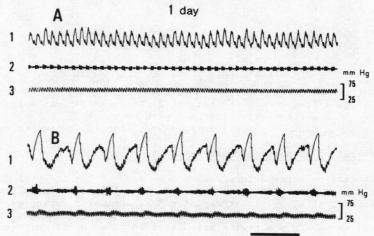

Fig. 4 Effects of bivagotomy on respiratory activity in a
       1 day old decerebrated kitten
       A : control ; B : after bivagotomy ; 1 : electrical
       integrated activity of the 2nd interchondral muscle ;
       2 : E.M.G. of the 2nd interchondral muscle ; 3 : ar-
       terial pressure ; Scale : 5 s.
Note after bivagotomy the important reinforcement of expiration which becomes active, and the moderated reinforcement of inspiratory activity.

Not only does T.E. lengthen, but an electrical activity in the expiratory muscle
appears. We have not systematically researched this activity but it is present in
every case where we have placed an electrode in the interchondral muscle sufficiently deep so that it can simultaneously pick up the activity of the triangularis
sterni muscle which is an expiratory muscle.

During the postnatal period (fig. 5), after bivagotomy, we observe a progressive
prolongation of T.I. and a concomitant shortening of T.E. It is interesting to note that the total duration of the respiratory cycle remains relatively constant
after section of the two vagus nerves no matter how old the animal is. Nevertheless,
fluctuations exist in one day old kitten that are too important for us to give relative average values at present.

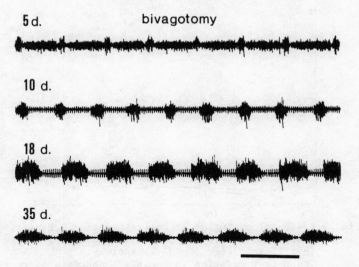

Fig. 5 Respiratory effects of bivagotomy during postnatal
       development
       E.M.G. of the 2nd interchondral muscle in decerebra-
       ted bivagotomized kittens between the ages of 5 and
       35 days. Scale : 5 s.

Figures 6 and 7 resume the postnatal evolution of respiratory frequency and of the
duration of T.I. and T.E. before and after bivagotomy in the decerebrated animal.

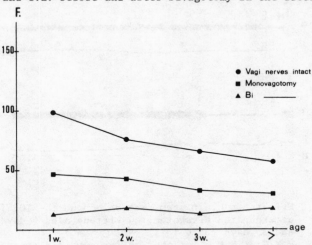

Fig. 6 Postnatal evolution of respiratory frequency in de-
       cerebrated kittens before bivagotomy (black dots),
       after monovagotomy (black squares) and after biva-
       gotomy (black triangles).
       Ordinate : frequence in cycles/mn ; Abscissa : age
       in weeks.

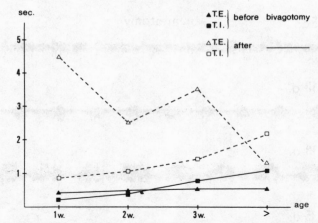

Fig. 7 Postnatal evolution of expiratory time T.E. (triangles) and inspiratory time T.I. (squares), before
(black) and after (open) bivagotomy.
Ordinate : duration in seconds ; Abscissa : age in
weeks.

Effects of pontine section at the level of the pneumotaxic center (fig. 8)

In the decerebrated unanaesthetized animal with intact vagus nerves, a section performed behind the posterior colliculi basically prolongs T.E. Under anaesthesia,
this prolongation is sometimes very important.

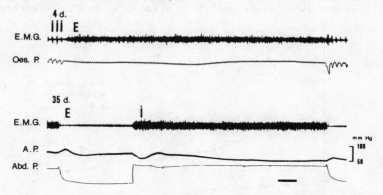

Fig. 8 Effects of brain stem section behind the TQP in 2
decerebrated bivagotomized kittens aged 4 days (4 d.)
and 35 days (35 d.)
E.M.G. : E.M.G. of the 2nd interchondral muscle
Oes.P. : oesophageal pressure
A.P.   : arterial pressure
Abd.P. : abdominal pressure
I : inspiration ; E : expiration ; Scale : 5 s.
Above : expiratory apnea of long duration
Below : inspiratory apnea of long duration

The same sections performed after bivagotomy provoke very long expiratory apneas
often with the appearance of an electrical activity on the expiratory muscles.

In these conditions we have never observed any apneusis during the first two weeks of postnatal life. Progressively, around the third, fourth week, the effect of the trans-pontic section inverses and provokes the appearance of classic apneustic attacks (fig. 8).

DISCUSSION

As have already observed in the animal (4) (5) (6) (7) and in man (8), our results indicate that the vagal system plays an important role in the control of the kitten respiration.

There seems to be unanimity concerning the powerful inhibition of inspiration, that we observe in the newborn, following the stimulation of the pulmonary stretch receptors. Nevertheless, it would be useful to clarify this point on the basis of a careful quantitative study of the stimulus-response relationship. The interpretation of results concerning pulmonary deflation on inspiratory activity is more difficult. Generally inspiratory reinforcement following a pulmonary deflation is much weaker in the newborn kitten than in the adult animal. This fact is very clear during strong deflation. If with ADRIAN (9) we agree that the inspiratory reflex reinforcement following pulmonary deflation is linked to the withdrawal of the discharge of low treshold pulmonary stretch receptors we can make in the kitten the following hypotheses : 1. Pulmonary deflation does not put all low treshold pulmonary stretch receptors at rest ;
2. The central generator mechanism of the CIA are less developed than in the adult.

The study of the electrical activity of the vagus nerve during deflation (10), doesn't allow us to sustain the first hypothesis. On the other hand, the second seems to be more likely. However, as PAINTAL (11) stresses, there remains an ambiguity in the litterature concerning the existence in the adult animal of bronchopulmonary receptors with slow adaptation, sensitive to deflation and susceptible of having a central excitatory action. If the existence of such a receptor category was really proven in the adult animal, our results obtained from the kitten could be due to a functional immaturity of the latter analogous to KALIA's demonstration for J receptors (12).

Moreover, the results observed after bivagotomy show an increase of T.I. during the postnatal period. Nevertheless, because this prolongation takes place to the detriment of the T.E., the respiratory cycle remains rather constant. Thus central mechanisms participating in the genesis of respiratory rhythm in the kitten seem to be similar to those involved in the adult cat, but mechanisms which maintain inspiratory activity are deficient.

Our results obtained after section of the brain-stem behind the posterior colliculi, indicate that, after bivagotomy, the pneumotaxic system certainly plays a role in the genesis of respiratory rhythm, contrary to what COOMBS and PIKE (13) have indicated. Nevertheless, the impossibility of obtaining apneustic attacks confirms the deficiency of mechanisms responsible for maintaining inspiratory activity.

The facility with which a predominant expiration appears in the young kitten seems to result in mechanisms causing a predominant activation in all of the flexor muscles (14) in the first weeks of postnatal life. Progressively during development diffused expiratory control loes its importance while, simultaneously, generator mechanisms of inspiratory activity develop.

Our hypothesis according to the model presented are resumed in figure 9. Thus the reticular excitatory system (RES) would facilitate the central expiratory activity (C.E.A.) and the spinal reflexes by the pathway of flexor reflex afferences (FRA).

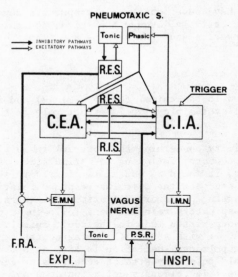

Fig. 9 Schema resuming our hypothesis
   E.M.N. : expiratory motor-neurones
   I.M.N. : inspiratory motor-neurones
   EXPI   : expiration ; INSPI : inspiration
   (See text for explanation).

This activation is very important in the decerebrated animal. Expiration puts the pulmonary stretch receptors (PSR) to rest thus permitting the central inspiratory activity (CIA) to manifest. Immediate and powerful activation through inspiration of PSR causes an almost immediate inhibition of the inspiratory center via the vagus nerve. Thus the high respiratory frequency in decerebrated animals can be explained as well as the increase of respiratory frequency following cutaneous stimulations (10). The pneumotaxic system could exert a tonic inhibition of the excitatory reticular formation. It is possible to think that a similar tonic inhibition of vagal origin is driven by the intermediary of the bulbar reticular inhibitory system (R.I.S.) (15) (16).

The trans-pontic section associated with bivagotomy frees the reticulary system, the activation of the flexors and the expiratory command. Nevertheless, in these conditions, the advent of some inspiratory movements linked probably to the activation of the inspiratory center by chemosensitive stimulations, makes us consider the possibility of an intercentral reciprocal inhibition between CIA and CEA.

REFERENCES

1. D. Marlot and B. Duron, Cutaneous stimulations and spontaneous respiratory activity in the newborn kitten. In Respiratory Centres and Afferent System, I.N.S.E.R.M. Symp. B. Duron ed., Amiens, 273-279 (1976).

2. B. Duron et D. Marlot, Evolution des réflexes d'Hering-Breuer au cours de la période néonatale chez le chaton. In Respiratory Centres and Afferent System, I.N.S.E.R.M. Symp. B. Duron éd., Amiens, 281-286 (1976).

3. G. Hilaire, R. Monteau et M. Dussardier, Modalités du recrutement des motoneurones phréniques. J. Physiol. (Paris), 64, 457-478 (1972).

4. G.S. Dawes and J.C. Mott, Reflex respiratory activity in the newborn rabbit. J. Physiol. (Lond.), 145, 85-97 (1959).

5. G.S. Dawes, H.N. Jacobson, J.C. Mott and H.J. Shelley, Some observations of fetal and newborn rhesus monkeys. J. Physiol. (Lond.), 152, 271-298 (1960).

6. D.T.D. Hughes, H.R. Parker and J.V. Williams, The response of foetal sheep and lambs to pulmonary inflation. J. Physiol. (Lond.), 189, 177-187 (1967).

7. G.H. Schwieler, Respiratory regulation during postnatal development in cats and rabbits and some of its morphological substrate. Acta Physiol. Scand. Suppl. 304 (1968).

8. K.W. Cross, M. Klaus, W.H. Tooley and K. Weisser, The response of the newborn baby to inflation of the lung. J. Physiol. (Lond.), 51, 551-565 (1960).

9. E.D. Adrian, Afferent impulses in the vagus and their effect on respiration. J. Physiol. (Lond.), 79, 332-358 (1933).

10. D. Marlot, Recherches sur le contrôle nerveux de la respiration chez le chaton. Thèse 3ème cycle, Université de Paris VI, 242 p. (1976).

11. A.S. Paintal, Vagal sensory receptors and their reflex effects. Physiol. Rev. 53, 159-227 (1973).

12. M. Kalia, Visceral and somatic reflexes produced by J pulmonary receptors in newborn kittens. J. Appl. Physiol. 41, 1-6 (1976).

13. H.S. Coombs and F.H. Pike, The nervous control of respiration in kittens. Am. J. Physiol. 95, 681-693 (1930).

14. S. Skoglund, On the postnatal development of postural mechanisms as revealed by electromyography and myography in decerebrate kittens. Acta Physiol. Scand. 49, 299-317 (1960).

15. P. Dell et Y. Padel, Endormissement rapide provoqué par la stimulation sélective d'afférences vagales chez le chat. Rev. Neurol. 111, 381 (1964)

16. P. Dell, Afferences baroceptives, phases de synchronisation corticale et sommeil. Arch. Ital. Biol. 111, 553-563 (1973).

DISCUSSION

of the papers by Trippenbach et al. and by Duron and Marlot

The apparent discrepancies between some of the results of Trippenbach
et al. and by Duron and Marlot were discussed especially those concerning the inspiratory activity and the reflex facilitation of CIA
by lung deflations. One possible reason for some of these discrepancies would seem to reside in the fact that Duron used considerably
deeper levels of anaesthesia in his pentobarbital animals (30 mg/kg
bwt as compared to 20 mg/kg bwt in the work of Trippenbach et al.).
However, this would not explain the difficulty encountered by Duron
to evoke prominent lung deflation reflex in the decerebrate newborn
kitten.

With respect to the summarizing model presented by Duron it was
recalled that the previous discussion on the role of reciprocal
inhibition had born out that there does not seem to exist any reciprocal inhibition between those neural populations denoted CEA and
CIA (see Discussion after the papers by Richter et al. and by
Merrill, p. 254, this volume). This would seem to invalidate an
important hypothesis incorporated in this model.

COMPARATIVE ASPECTS OF THE CONTROL OF BREATHING DURING DEVELOPMENT

P. JOHNSON

Nuffield Institute for Medical Research, University of Oxford, U.K.

An accurate description of the development of the regulation of breathing is only now starting to be completed. Considering the time and level of effort that has been invested in studying the regulation of breathing, the reasons for this apparent delay in defining the developmental factors involved are of more than academic interest.

Longitudinal studies of sufficient length and frequency during development in any one species are rare. Their incompleteness have probably led to the spurious comparisons made between the species and until recently have offered little to clinical practice.

The clinical situation itself completely revolves around the premature human infant and most of the neonatal data on the control of breathing in the human is gained from this biological anomaly which has little parallel in other species. In fact the human premature could be viewed as a product of unnatural selection. The ethical need for non-invasive and thus usually non-quantitative measurement has been a further major restriction in the value of this data.

Conventional investigative procedures developed in adult mammals, invariably anaesthetised, have been systematically applied to the newborn. It is small wonder that the chemoreceptor drive to respiration has gained a pre-eminence amongst the factors considered to regulate breathing (Ref. 1). When examined in this way the newborn has been viewed as defective or deficient in respiratory drive (Ref. 2,3). Indeed the absence of response to hypoxaemia and the transient response to hypercapnia observed in some species and premature man (Ref. 4), should make one marvel at their very survival; if the chemical drive to breathing is so important. The conventional approach to respiratory physiology employing anaesthesia and the isolation of portions of the respiratory system, both central and peripheral, has repeatedly underated the contribution of respiratory factors other than the lung and the chemoreceptors, to respiratory drive. The influence of behavioural state has received very little attention until recently (Ref. 5), and even then substantially in the hands of sleep physiologists.

Since a number of these factors still confuse the understanding of the regulation of breathing during development, this paper will examine evidence in support of the view that experimental data has to be shown to be of functional significance in the intact animal in order for its relevance to be properly assessed. This approach coincides with the emphasis of the conference being placed on concept and hypothesis.

Chronic longitudinal studies

As recently as 1968 Schweiler (6), in one of the most comprehensive
developmental studies of respiratory regulation, suggested the limitations of
acute studies conducted under anaesthesia in quantifying changes that occur with
age. Anaesthetic agents have been shown to 'reverse' reflex responses in conventional acute studies on respiratory control in the adult (Ref. 7). However
recent studies on chronically monitored developing mammals have provided an
appreciation for the functional significance of the changes that occur with age.

Two aspects will be emphasised. Firstly that physiological variables do not
simply change in a progressive manner from neonatal to adult life as befits the
current text-book description. Secondly that the timing of birth is an accident
with regard to the relative organisation of respiratory control as observed
between species. It appears that the regulation of breathing is not a limiting
factor in survival in most naturally reproducing species and yet the range of
maturation of the respiratory system at birth is enormous. While little is known
of the respiratory regulation in the marsupial, the rabbit and kitten at one end
through to the lamb and the guinea pig at the other are species which all breed
successfully yet have been shown to have anatomic and functional differences at birth
which often exceed those generally considered to span the period from neonatal
to adult life. These differences range from no gamma innervation of intercostal
muscles, a greatly reduced myelination of vagal fibres (Ref. 6) to apparently
absent or diminished ventilatory responses to hypoxia and hypercapnia (Ref. 4);
to the more recent observation on the differences between sleep state, notably
REM and non-REM (Ref. 3).

This view is illustrated by examining in some detail the changes observed in the
lamb, continuously recorded through fetal, neonatal and infant life. Maloney (9),
recording the diaphragm EMG, has shown that the fetal lamb breathed irregularly,
often rapidly, but almost continuously from 60 days (0.4 gestational age) to
approximately 105-110 days (0.73 gestational age). The breathing gradually
became episodic after this time, most of the breathing activity being related
to low voltage de-synchronised ECOG activity and rapid-eye movements. We have
observed that most of this breathing activity after 115 days gestational age
is diaphragmatic with only occasional phasic involvement of intercostal or
adductor (expiratory) laryngeal muscles. The differentiation of the electrocorticogram into high voltage slow-wave and low-voltage de-synchronised epochs
occur soon afterwards and is a feature of the last quarter of fetal life in
this species. The detailed characteristics of fetal breathing appear elsewhere
in this volume. However, of particular relevance to breathing after birth are
three facts.

Firstly is the absence of continuous breathing movements in the high voltage
electrocortical state. Moreover the inability to stimulate sustained breathing
activity in the normal fetus while in this state (Ref. 10) suggests an actively
inhibited state. A paradox appears to exist here in that after birth and in
adult life, it is in the REM state that a relative insensitivity to some respiratory stimuli occurs, while in non-REM sleep an increased dependence on peripheral
sensory input exists. Secondly, the breathing movements occurring in REM sleep
are chiefly diaphragmatic and are very similar to those observed in rapid-eye-
movement sleep after birth in this species (Ref. 3,11). Detailed information
of the activity of the respiratory muscles prior to differentiation of the
electrocorticogram has not yet been described. Thirdly the fetal response to
experimentally induced hypoxaemia is apnoea.

After birth   the lamb, which has already established a definitive rest-activity cycle in fetal life (Ref. 12,13), continues with this cycle only changing the epoch length and the proportion of time awake with little further change until after weaning. It is important to emphasise that this data was collected by radio-telemetric techniques from free-ranging lambs growing up with their ewes. However, the respiratory frequency after birth did not simply decline but actually increased both in REM and non-REM sleep before declining to adult values (Fig. 1).

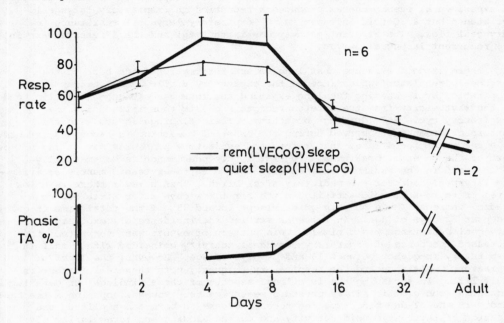

Fig. 1. The mean respiratory rates sampled every minute throughout 8 hr recording periods at each age is shown in quiet sleep and REM sleep. There was a significant rise and then a fall in frequency in both sleep states. A variable amount of thyro-arytenoid activity occurs at birth, and then there is a progressive rise in expiratory laryngeal activity to 32 days of age; but only in quiet sleep. Expiratory braking does not occur in REM. This activity is rarely seen in the adult animal.

This suggests changes in regulatory mechanisms which peak after birth. However, the changes in non-REM sleep were greater both at the zenith and nadir and more important perhaps was the association with upper airway (laryngeal) expiratory activity. The details of the relationship between expiratory laryngeal activity and respiration have already been described (Ref. 14). However, some points are relevant here.

The large inspiratory efforts, up to 80 cm of water, that usually accompany the onset of respiration as the lung fluid is both exuded and absorbed, have received much attention (Ref. 15). Some authors believe that fetal lung volume (FRC) equates with the neonatal lung volume (Ref. 16). However, it has been shown recently that the onset of respiration may simply ensue smoothly and

rhythmically, effectively exchanging air with only modest inspiratory efforts
(Ref. 17). The same authors demonstrate equally large positive intra-thoracic
pressures on expiration but did not comment on the possible significance of
these lung-distending efforts. It has been demonstrated in hyaline membrane
disease in the human premature, where FRC is diminished, that the characteristic
expiratory grunt was beneficial in assisting gas exchange (Ref. 18). Consistent
with this was Widdicombe's (19) finding that a reduction in FRC by the use of
an experimental pneumo-thorax produced a reduction in inspiratory laryngeal
resistance but a 10-fold increase in the expiratory laryngeal resistance to
laryngeal flow. The afferent pathway was in the vagi and the efferents were in
the recurrent laryngeal nerves.

Thus there is good evidence that lung volume information feeds back to the
laryngeal 'regulator' which impedes the expiratory airflow and enhances
respiration by 1) keeping the lung expanded and thus gas exchange effective, and
2) the rhythmicity from the stretch receptors phasic thus influencing the
respiratory cycle and 'driving' breathing. These findings accord with the
pattern of breathing observed during the onset of breathing in lambs and infants.
As already mentioned large inspiratory and expiratory pressures may or may not be
part of the onset of breathing. In Fig. 1 this phenomenon is schematically
represented in the variable incidence of phasic thyro-arytenoid muscle activity -
the laryngeal adductor - immediately after birth. Then however there is a low
level of thyro-arytenoid activity in the first few days after birth before a
gradual increase (note only in quiet sleep) toward 95% of the total time in quiet
sleep at 32 days of age. In two ewes studied the incidence of expiratory
laryngeal resistance was minimal. This pattern of events was unexpected; the
increased incidence of expiratory laryngeal activity coincided with a fall in
respiratory frequency between 16 and 32 days of age. However, the level of
expiratory resistance and the respiratory frequency both then fell further in
adult life. In stressing the functional aspects of these findings our data lacks
sequential sub-glottic airway pressure measurements. However, opening a tracheal
window in the 32-day-old lambs led to an increase in both the amplitude and
duration of thyro-arytenoid activity and marked slowing and irregularity of
respiratory frequency again only during quiet sleep (Fig. 2a & b). The breathing
pattern during REM sleep is unaffected. In the ewe there was no discernible
effect of such a manoeuvre which was consistent with the finding of little or no
spontaneous TA expiratory activity during quiet sleep. There is then an age-
related dependence on expiratory laryngeal resistence to airflow. The reason for
the lack of thyro-arytenoid activity in the first few days after birth has not
yet been investigated. It is known that the lung becomes more compliant with age
and thus at higher respiratory rates shortly after birth the tendency to lung
collapse would be less. It could follow that laryngeal expiratory resistence is
unnecessary in this situation. The ewe has a more rigid rib-cage which would
resist collapse even with the airway open. Indeed negative pressures of 15 cm
H_2O applied to the tracheotomy in the ewes was necessary before any significant
change in expiratory laryngeal activity or respiratory frequency occurred.

It seemed unlikely that the stage of maturation e.g. myelination of vagal pathways, was responsible in this species for these changes, but rather that the
mechanical state of the lungs and the chest wall was the determining factor. If
this proves to be the case then the evidence for the disappearance of the Hering
Breuer reflexes with age (Ref. 20) elicited by a technique producing a constant
stimulus, e.g. airway inflation or deflation, must be questionable. Of course
the central organisation would also be expected to change in response to the new
air-breathing state. Thus the regulation of breathing during post-natal
development depends heavily on respiratory afferents, such as those from the
lungs and larynx, which change with age though not simply in an incremental or
decremental fashion. The actual sequence of events would be expected to depend

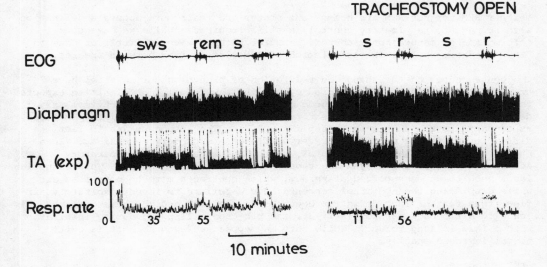

Fig. 2a. A typical recording period is shown (left) in a
33-day-old lamb which shows the cycling sleep state. The
thyro-arytenoid muscle was always active in quiet sleep at
this age. When a tracheal window is opened (right) a large
increase in degree of laryngeal constriction occurred with
a fall in respiratory frequency (35 to 11). However the
pattern of breathing was unaffected in REM sleep.

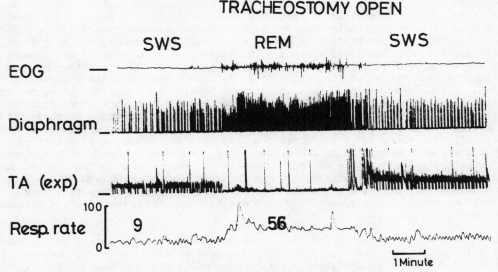

Fig. 2b. Is a faster record with the tracheotomy open and
shows the striking loss of rhythm and frequency in quiet
sleep.

on the relative maturation of the particular species at birth and its future life-
style.

Neither REM nor non-REM are homogenous states and their more accurate definition
with respect to respiratory control is still required. While we have some
information on maturational changes in quiet sleep, there is little or none in
REM. Furthermore, the characteristics of REM sleep differ between species.

The consequences of the change in regulation of breathing during sleep have
aroused much interest. The tutored eye of the physiologist or clinician expects
rhythmicity as an indication of good control. This has led to such terms as
depressed, deficient or defective responses to respiratory stimuli in REM sleep,
as compared to those in quiet sleep (Ref. 2,3). The responses are in fact
different, as is the evidence for very different regulatory mechanisms. In a
number of species phasic intercostal, rectus abdominus and the expiratory
adductor muscle of the larynx are reduced or absent in REM sleep. This situation
leads both to an unsupported diaphragm, which contracts more to move less air
while displacing the abdominal contents, and a failure to impede expiratory airflow; thus further lung deflation occurs. In the lamb and the human infant, this
leads to a rib-cage paradox (Ref. 3); the rib-cage collapsing during inspiration
with a fall in lung volume. While this may appear unfavourable it is quite
normal in these species.

Acute studies

While awaiting more detail from chronic studies, results of some acute studies
on the interactions between peripheral and central respiratory reflexes are
relevant here.

Lung distension, sleep state and anaesthesia. In five lambs aged between 11 and
43 days with a tracheostomy and under sedative levels of anaesthesia, the end-
expired airway pressure was raised by 10 and then 20 cm H_2O for periods of three
minutes. The response was an initial slowing of breathing followed by a gradual
increase in respiratory frequency to a level above control. Thus a stimulation
of breathing, by maintaining a sustained distending pressure on the lung, was
achieved with no significant change in blood gases; indeed often a fall in (Fig. 3)
arterial PCO_2 was observed. The reflex abolition of expiratory thyro-arytenoid
activity has been described already. Thus sustained distension of the lung, with
an increased FRC, stimulated breathing and appeared to conflict with published
data in anaesthetised adult mammals (Ref. 21). However, when the anaesthetic
level in the lambs was increased to surgical levels, i.e. in order to record from
single vagal fibres, an increase in pressure then reduced respiratory frequency.
In such a study a pulmonary stretch receptor is seen to discharge in phase with
the trans-pleural pressure gradient (Fig. 4). When the trans-pleural pressure was high
as initially, there was a sustained discharge and an inhibition of breathing.
Negative pressure applied to the tracheostomy, on the other hand, led to slowing
of respiration, an audible expiratory grunt and often apnoea in the unanaesthetised or lightly anaesthetised lamb (Fig. 5). Under surgical anaesthesia the response to
negative airway pressure was usually one of increased respiratory frequency. It
should be noted that laryngeal adductor activity was often completely abolished
by deeper anaesthesia.

In non-REM sleep it has already been shown that breathing frequency and pattern
as well as the laryngeal activity was influenced by altering airway pressure.
This did not occur in REM sleep. Before concluding that the newborn differs from
the adult in response to increased airway pressure one would wish to see
comparable testing of the unanaesthetised adult. Indeed - because of the
classically described inhibition of breathing with lung inflation, investigators

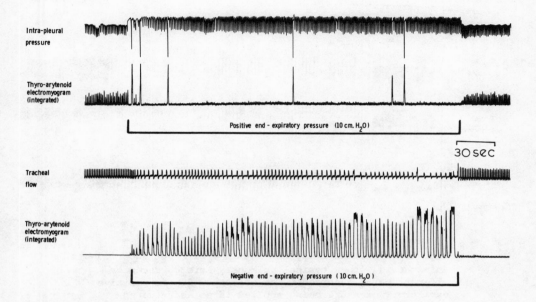

Fig. 3. In the top panel the effect of a sudden increase
of end-expired pressure is seen in an unanaesthetised
lamb. There is an inflation apnoea and thyro-arytenoid
(TA) activity abruptly drops out. However respiratory
frequency gradually increases to be above central values
after 3 minutes of +10 cm H_2O pressure. Removal of
positive pressure sees the instantaneous return of
expiratory TA activity and an initial deflation tachypnoea.
In the lower panel negative pressure is applied to the
tracheostomy in another lamb with no resting TA activity.
A fall in breathing frequency and a large increase in TA
occurs. The high sustained levels represent glottic
closure. After the removal of negative pressure there is
an abrupt return to regular breathing.

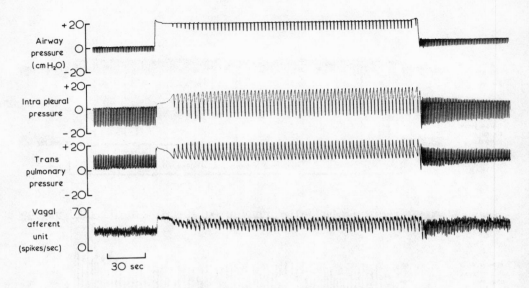

Fig. 4. A similar study to that in Fig. 3 but under deeper
anaesthesia with a typical pulmonary stretch receptor
afferent being recorded. The effect of 20 cms positive
expiratory pressure being applied is an accentuated
inflation apnoea which corresponds well with the trans-
pulmonary pressure change and the integrated vagal afferent
fibre discharge. However breathing frequency remains
below control levels under anaesthesia.

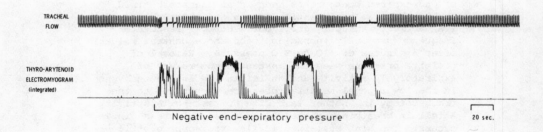

Fig. 5. In this unanaesthetised lamb 10 cm H_2O negative
pressure applied to the tracheostomy caused recurrent
apnoea with glottic closure.

have considered that the beneficial effects of positive airway pressure in treating recurrent apnoea in the premature human must be by improving oxygenation and thus respiratory drive (Ref. 22). In fact adequate lung distention is necessary for the generation of phasic vagal impulses from the lung to provide rhythmic breathing. Conscious man has recently been shown to hyperventilate in response to positive pressure breathing also with a fall in PACO$_2$ (Ref. 23).

It has been suggested that the fall in lung volume that occurs during rapid-eye-movement sleep may explain the altered (delayed) response to airway inflation or deflation. Our experiments would suggest that the difference observed during rapid-eye-movement sleep is greater than would be anticipated from any spontaneously occurring reduction in volume. The changes in respiratory rate occur within a breath or two of a change in sleep state; well before a significant change in FRC would have occurred (see Fig. 2b).

Respiratory stimuli in sleep state. The responses to airway occlusion, respiratory loading, and laryngeal stimuli, hypoxia and hypercapnia differ between rapid-eye-movement and quiet sleep states. A consistent difference is the delayed arousal occurring in rapid-eye-movement sleep. However, this raised threshold to arousal in REM probably does not normally pose a threat to life, since it occurs well within safe limits.

In unanaesthetised newborn lambs restrained on their backs the continued presence of water, but not saline in the larynx caused sustained often fatal apnoea (Ref. 27). This seldom occurred in the unrestrained lamb. None the less environmental temperature (especially when moderately elevated), hypoglycaemia and anaesthetics can interact to turn a transient apneic response to airway stimulation into prolonged often fatal respiratory arrest. These observations serve to underline the importance of 'non-respiratory' stimuli in respiratory control in the newborn. A number of other recent studies have demonstrated the vulnerability of the anaesthetised or sedated newborn to inhibition of breathing by a variety of airway stimuli (Ref. 25,26). These observations have been taken to indicate the likely mechanism of respiratory arrest occurring in neonatal apnoea and sudden infant death. Although these studies follow a traditional approach to testing respiratory control, the conclusions drawn from them are clearly inappropriate and misleading for the reasons just discussed.

Hypoxaemia. Hypoxaemia warrants more detailed consideration. In the adult dog it was shown that while arousal was delayed in REM sleep both to hypercapnia and hypoxaemia, the ventilatory response to hypoxaemia, both increased tidal volume and frequency, was maintained while that to hypercapnia was not. The interaction between hypoxaemia and hypercapnia was also lost in REM sleep. The ventilatory responses to hypoxaemia in the puppy were similar to those reported in the dog, the puppy possibly tolerating a lower PO$_2$ before arousal (Ref. 27). The lamb, on the other hand, differed in that an increase in respiratory frequency was negated by a fall in tidal volume; possibly caused by ineffective diaphragm activity associated with rib-cage collapse.

While acute rapidly occurring hypoxaemia represents one way of testing the chemical drive to breathing, observations on chronic hypoxaemia are of equal interest. Baker (28) has shown that one-third of a group of kittens, submitted to an environmental oxygen of 10% for 10-hour periods, hypoventilated with a reduction in respiratory frequency during quiet sleep but reverted to a normal pattern during REM sleep. Further episodes of quiet sleep saw a return of respiratory failure. Continued hypoxaemia led to a reduction in time spent in REM sleep and thus decreased the opportunity to revert to effective breathing. Apnoea and death occurred in these kittens whereas those that had hyperventilated in response to hypoxaemia in quiet sleep (two-thirds) survived. This would

suggest a defect in quiet sleep rather than in REM sleep. These findings are in
fact consistent with the results observed during acute hypoxia in that a tolerance
to a lower PaO_2 in REM sleep appears to be suggested in both studies. It is
worth noting that in adult man, with obstructive lung disease, that a loss of
high-voltage quiet sleep has been reported (Ref. 29). It should be recalled that
the fetal response to hypoxaemia is one of apnoea.

Hypercapnia. The validity of adding CO_2 to the inspired air as a physiological
test of respiratory drive will be considered here. A great deal has been inferred
from studies employing this technique. It was shown that CO_2 added to the
inspired gas abbreviated the post-inspiratory activity of slowly adapting
pulmonary stretch receptors (Ref. 30). It was further shown that CO_2 from 1 - 5%
was effective in stimulating breathing even when there was no pulmonary
circulation (Ref. 31). Nevertheless it was considered that this was not of
functional significance in adult man breathing in the eupnic range. However, if
breathing were initially stimulated by other pathways, then carbon dioxide may
become a stimulus to breathing via the lung even in adult man. In the unanaesthetised newborn lamb and in two premature human infants it was shown (Ref. 32)
that low levels of inspired CO_2 (1.5%) were a stimulus to breathing and that
minute volume increased while arterial CO_2 decreased significantly. Thus,
hyperventilation with hypocapnia occurred in 9 of 14 lambs. Furthermore the
ventilatory response to hypoxaemia which had been minimal or absent in these
lambs without the addition of CO_2 was now enhanced. At very least minute
ventilation is a poor measure of the arterial chemical drive to breathing. It is
evident that in the newborn CO_2 can be a stimulus to breathing via the lower
airway. The upper airway has chemo-receptors which selectively sense a variaty
of chemical stimuli including carbon dioxide (Ref. 33), reflexly inhibiting
breathing by way of the superior laryngeal nerves. It seems teliologically
appropriate that the organism should sense and attempt to respond to its gaseous
environment before changes are perceived in the circulatory system. Of interest
are the lambs which required an elevation of arterial PCO_2 before an increase in
respiratory frequency or depth occurred. In these studies the increases in
minute ventilation were achieved both by increased tidal volume and respiratory
frequency. The use of anaesthesia in such studies usually modified or abolished
this response. A further important observation was that the unanaesthetised
lambs became apneic at a PaO_2 in the range of 25 - 30 mm Hg when no CO_2 was
added. However they were responsive to other stimuli, for example they would
suck on a teat and often had their eyes open. This apnoea was reminiscent of the
apneic response observed in the fetus.

Discussion

The continuous non-restricted recording of physiological variables during
development has shown that some of the changes in respiratory events e.g.
respiratory frequency do not progress to adult values in a simple fashion as
previously thought. After birth there are high and low points in the levels of
spontaneous activity of the respiratory system. Some of these coincide, e.g.
expiratory laryngeal 'braking' and respiratory frequency, perhaps suggesting a
direct relationship. These changes have been observed in detail in the lamb, a
species comparatively mature at birth. There are reports now of similar
changes in the respiratory frequency of the human with a peak frequency
occurring at three months of age (Ref. 34). One author, Sterman, maintains that
the normal human infant does not establish quiet sleep until 1 - 3 months of
post-natal age. Notwithstanding this wide range of maturation of the central
nervous system at birth, viability is ensured in most species. Only continuous
recording of a selection of species in fetal and post-natal life will clearly
differentiate those changes which are adaptations to extra-uterine life from

HYPOXIC RESPONSE WITH AND WITHOUT pA CO$_2$ "CONTROLLED"

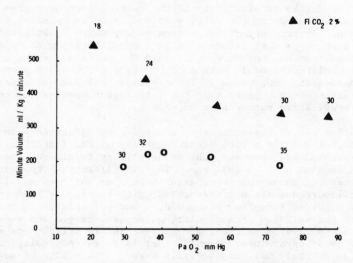

Fig. 6. This is a plot of the minute volume recorded at
the end of 10 minutes of sequential decrements in inspired
oxygen concentrations, without added CO_2 (open circles)
and with 2% CO_2 added (closed triangles) in a newborn
lamb. The $PaCO_2$ is shown at some of the PaO_2 levels.
The minute ventilation is increased over control when 2%
CO_2 is added with a fall in $PaCO_2$. The ventilatory
response to hypoxaemia was converted from a negative one
to a substantial one with 2% CO_2 but with a large fall in
$PaCO_2$ (18 against 30 mm Hg). Also the lamb did not become
apneic as it had without the addition of CO_2 even although
a lower PaO_2 was achieved. Nine out of fourteen lambs
showed this response.

those already established in utero. For instance the comparisons presently being
made between fetal breathing activity observed in the human fetus and that recorded
in the fetal lamb may well prove to be misleading. The influence of behavioural
state, especially the apnoea associated with high voltage electrocortical state, is
evident prenatally in the lamb whereas this stage is not reached until post-term in
the human. It is possible that comparability may exist between the fetal lamb
prior to 110 days of fetal life and the human fetus up to term. It may be
important when interpreting breathing patterns, respiratory responses and the
physiology of the jeopardised pregnancy. The current interest in the relationship
between pre- and post-natal breathing patterns must take account of the maturity
of the particular species at the time of birth.

An active involvement of the respiratory system, both upper airway and diaphragm
in expiration occurs during quiet sleep in an age-dependent fashion. A recent
proposition that the inspiratory phase of the respiratory cycle can be likened to
the "duty cycle" of an electrical pump system, derives from anaesthetised studies
and is probably misconceived when applied to the intact animal (Ref. 35). There is

no paradox in the slowing of breathing that occurs with the removal of end-
expired pressure.

Whether the level of maturation of a species or individual at the time of birth
relates to the degree of plasticity of the central nervous system and could thus
be a critical influence on the ability of the organism to adapt is worth
consideration. In particular the preterm human, which is of great moment to us
all and from which so much information is now collected, must be questionable as
providing normal data. One view would hold the premature to be an anomaly by
defination. Unlike the adult with a rigid rib-cage, the premature has to 'work' to
maintain an adequate lung volume. The rib-cage collapse and apnoea that
frequently occur would suggest that the intercostal muscles may be essential
muscles of respiration rather than accessory.

Labels of defective, depressed or even altered respiratory responses with age or
sleep state should await a better understanding of the functional organisation of
regulatory mechanisms. However, the vulnerability to altered chemical drives to
respiration remains a vexed question. The significance of the activation of
carotid or central chemo-receptors after birth has not been considered here.
While their importance are not discounted, direct evidence from the intact
chronically recorded fetus and newborn does not yet exist. In the meantime,
concern over the validity of manipulating inspired oxygen and especially carbon
dioxide tensions as appropriate tests of ventilatory drive needs resolution.
Paintal's view of paranatural stimuli, that is to say physiological stimuli
applied in an unlikely way, may be valid here.   Their site of action and interaction in the intact neonate has not been clearly established. In any event, the
sensory priorities including non-respiratory input differ in the newborn. Thus
adaptive mechanisms and especially arousal are probably of critical importance.
Indeed arousal is an important respiratory reflex; obliviated by anaesthesia.

Nonetheless the respiratory response to hypoxia is an important factor for
consideration. Evidence from intact studies suggest that the response to
hypoxaemia of the fetus is one of apnoea, an entirely appropriate response; and
that after birth this response takes a variable amount of time to change to one
where an increased respiratory effort will occur.   Other sensory and adaptive
mechanisms usually ensure survival during this period. However, an intriguing
possibility is that an inhibition of breathing, perhaps similar to that
observed in the fetus, may occur at a higher PaO_2 level in quiet sleep than in
REM sleep. Thus an acceptable level of hypoxaemia occurring in REM sleep may be
below the safety limit for quiet sleep. A change in sleep state from REM to quiet
sleep could then lead to apnoea. The commonly held view of hypoxaemic depression
of the central nervous system is almost certainly too simplistic.

The apparent changes in respiratory drive with changing behavioural state which
are suggested by the alterations in respiratory rhythmicity and frequency are of
interest. The possibility that the 'tone ' of the stretch receptors determines
the threshold for chemo-sensitivity could explain the apparent variability in
response to inhaled CO_2 on a peripheral basis. The rapidity of the change in
respiratory frequency that occurs with the change in sleep state suggests that
a 'dynamic' FRC rather than a passive FRC might be the important determinant of
both stretch and chemical thresholds. These considerations do not deny the
contribution of volitionally and behaviourally determined changes in central
thresholds. The view that the Hering Breuer reflex is basically inhibitory has
prevented the real importance of distending airway pressure as a stimulus to
breathing in infantswith recurrent apnoea being recognized (ref. 36). While
acute distension of the lung is inhibitory, continuous distension provides a drive
to breathing which is mediated by vagal afferents from the lung. Thus distending

pressure in the newborn has both a mechanical and a neurogenic effect in preventing alveolar collapse.

Finally acute studies under anaesthesia or even under restraint in the newborn are of limited value and may even produce artefactual results. The search for techniques for chronic recording from the afferent and efferent pathways involved in respiratory mechanisms are now a priority.

Much of this work was supported by NICHD Contract No. 1-HD-3-2772 and the Foundation for Study of Infant Deaths (London).

1.   A.J. Berger, R.A. Mitchell, J.W. Sevringhaus, Regulation of Respiration, NEW England J.Med. 297, 92 (1977).

2.   P.G.F. Swift, J.L. Emery, Clinical observations in response to nasal occulusion in infancy, Arch Dis Childl 48, 997 (1973).

3.   D.J. Henderson-Smart, D.J.C. Read, Depression of intercostal muscle and abdominal muscle activity and vulnerability to asphyxia during active sleep in the newborn. Sleep Apnoea Syndromes. Krog Foundation Vol. III 93 (1978).

4.   H. Rigatto, R. de la T. Verduzio, D.B. Cates, Effects of O_2 on the Ventilatory response to CO_2 in preterm infants. J. Appl. Physiol. 39 (6), 896 (1975).

5.   E.A. Phillipson, Regulation of breathing during sleep. A.M. Rev. Respir. Dis. 115 (Suppl) 217 (1977).

6.   G.H. Schweiler, Respiratory regulation during postnatal development in cats and rabbits and some of its morphological substrates. Acta. Physiol Scand (Suppl) 304, 1 (1968).

7.   W.A. Karczewski, Some effects of anaesthetics on the functional organization of the bulbo-pontine respiratory complex. Bull Path. Physiol. Resp. 9 (3), 731 (1973).

8.   J.E. Molony, Development of Breathing patterns in the fetal lamb, Fifth conference on fetal breathing. University of Nijmegen 1,(1978).

9.   G.S. Dawes, Breathing and rapid-eye-movement sleep before birth. Fetal & Neonatal physiology. Sir Joseph Bancroft Symposium Cambridge University Press. 49, (1972).

10.   K. Boddy, G.S. Dawes, R. Fisher, S. Pinter and J.S. Robinson, Fetal Respiratory movements, electro-corticol and cardiovascular responses to hypoxemia and hypercapnia in sheep. J. Physiol 243, 599 (1974).

11.   R. Harding, P. Johnson, M.E. McClelland, C.N. McCleod, P.L. Whyte, Laryngeal Function during breathing and swallowing in fetal and newborn lambs. J. Physiol. 272 14 P (1977).

12.   Y. Ruckebusch, M.Galejoux, B. Eghboli, Sleep cycles and kinesis in
           the foetal lamb. Electro-encephalog. Clin. meusphysiol. 42 226 (1977)

13.   R. Harding, P. Johnson, M.E. McClelland. Ingestive activity and its
           relation to breathing in fetol and neonatal lambs.
           Fifth Conference on Fetal Breathing. University of Nijmegen.23 (1978).

14.   R. Harding, P. Johnson, M.E. McClelland. The expiratory role of the
           larynx during development and the influence of behavioural state,
           This conference.

15.   P. Karlberg, R.B. Cherry, F.E. Escordo, Respiratory studies in
           newborn infants, II Development of mechanics of breathing during the
           first week of life. Acta. Paediatr. Suppl. 135. 121. (1962).

16.   R.E. Olver, E.O.R. Reynolds, L.B. Strang. Fetal lung liquid in
           Fetal & neonatal physiology. Proceedings of Sir Joseph Barcroft
           Centenary Symposium. Cambridge University Press. 186 (1973).

17.   A.D. Milner & R.A. Saunders. Pressure and volume changes during the
           first breath of human neonates. Arch. Dis. Child. 52 918 (1977).

18.   V.C. Harrison, H. de Heese, M. Klein. The significance of grunting
           in hyaline membrane disease. Pediatrics 41 (3) 549 (1968).

19.   M. Glagowska, A. Stransky, J.G. Widdicombe, Reflex control of
           discharge in motor fibres to the larynx. J. Physiol. 239. 365 (1974).

20.   K.W. Cross, M. Klaus, W.H. Tooley. The response of the newborn baby
           to inflation of the lungs. J. Physiol. 151, 551 (1960).

21.   D. Trenchard. Role of pulmonary stretch receptors during breathing in
           rabbits, cats & dogs. Resp. Physiol. 29. 115. (1977).

22.   G.A. Gregory, J.A. Kitterman, R.H. Phibbs, W.H. Tooley, W.K. Hamilton,
           Treatment of the ideopathic respiratory distress syndrome with
           continuous positive airway pressure. NEW England J. Med.284, 1333(1974)

23.   B. Bishop, J. Hirsh, M. Thursby. Volume, flow and timing of each
           breath during positive-pressure breathing in man.
           J.Appl. Physiol. Respirat.Environ. Exercise Physiol. 45 (4),495 (1978).

24.   P. Johnson, J.S. Robinson, D.S. Salisbury. The onset and control of
           breathing after birth. Sir Joseph Bancroft Symposium on Fetal and
           Neonotal Physiology, Cambridge University Press 217 (1973).

25.   D. Sutton, E.M. Taylor, R.C. Linderman. Prolonged apnoea in infant
           monkeys resulting from stimulation of superior laryngeal nerve.
           Pediatrics. 61. 4. 519 (1978).

26.   S.E. Downing, D.C. Lee, Laryngeal chemo sensitivity. A possible
           mechanism for sudden infant death. Pediatrics. 55. 640 . (1975).

27.   D.S. Henderson-Smart, D.J.C. Read, Depressed ventilatory responses to
           hypoxemia associated with rib-cage paradox during active sleep in the
           newborn. Aust. Paed. Journal. abstract (1978).

28.   T.L. Baker, D.J. McGinty. Reversal of cardiopulmonary failure during
          active sleep in hypoxic kittens. Implications for sudden infant
          death. Science. 198, 419 (1977).

29.   J.W. Wynne, A.J. Black, J. Heringway, L.A. Hunt, D. Shaw, M. Flick.
          Disordered breathing and oxygen desaturation during sleep in patients
          with chronic obstructive pulmonary disease. Chest. 73.2 Suppl.301
          (1978).

30.   G.W. Bradley, M.I.M. Noble, D. Trenchard. The direct effect on
          pulmonary stretch receptor discharge produced by changing the lung
          carbon dioxide concentration in dogs on cardiopulmonary bypass and
          its action on breathing. J. Physiol. 261. 2. 359.(1976).

31.   A. Bartoli, B.Cross, A. Guz et al. The effect of carbon dioxide in
          airways and alveoli on ventilation, a vagal reflex studied in the
          dog. J. Physiol. 240 91 (1974).

32.   P. Johnson. Evidence for lower airway chemo receptors in newborn
          lambs. Pediatric Research. 10. (4) 462 (1976).

33.   R. Harding, P. Johnson, M.E. McClelland. Liquid sensitive laryngeal
          receptors in the developing sheep, cat and monkey.
          J. Physiol. 277 409 (1978).

34.   J. Hoffenbrowers, R.M. Harper, J.E. Hodgeman, M.B. Sterman,
          D.J. McGinty. Polygraphic studies of normal infants during the first
          six months of life. Respiratory rate and variability as a function of
          state. Pediat. Res. 12 120 (1978).

35.   I. Wyszogrodski, B.T. Thach, J. Milic-Emili. Maturation of respirat-
          ory control in unanaesthetized newborn rabbits.
          J. Appl. Physiol. Respirat.   Environ Exercise Physiol. 44(2) 304(1978)

36.   L. Strang in Neonatal Respiration.Physiological and Clinical Studies.
          Blackwells Scientific publications. 60 (1977).

DISCUSSION

Remmers asked if there were changes in respiratory rate mediated by
an increase in T_I and T_E or both when the tracheal window was opened.
Johnson replied that there was a small increase in T_I with a large
increase in T_E. He was then asked to explain the apparently paradoxical effect on respiratory rate i.e. the fall in rate with the open
trachea. Johnson said that the newborn is organized to defend its
lung volume by expiratory laryngeal 'braking' in quiet sleep and diaphragmatic 'braking' in REM sleep. In quiet sleep this produces positive subglottic pressure and therefore a considerable transmural gradient from airway to pleura. This was a stimulus to breathing as we
have shown in the studies in the unanaesthetized lamb. Opening the

tracheal window, thus preventing the positive pressure in expiration,
means a removal of the pressure stimulus and a fall in frequency. At
the same time the laryngeal adductors reciprocate reflexly and
increase adduction in a maximal attempt to impede airflow and thus
prevent lung collapse. However, section of afferent and efferent pathways from the larynx had no effect on effects of positive and negative
breathing via a tracheotomy. This effect was impressively age dependant in this species and mediated by pulmonary vagal afferent pre-
sumptively the stretch receptors. There is no paradox - except with
studies conducted under anaesthesia where negative pressure breathing
causes an increase in respiratory rate, which in Johnson's view is an
experimental artefact.

THE EXPIRATORY ROLE OF THE LARYNX DURING DEVELOPMENT AND THE INFLUENCE OF BEHAVIOURAL STATE

R. HARDING, P. JOHNSON and M. E. McCLELLAND

Nuffield Institute for Medical Research, University of Oxford, U.K.

As a variable and controllable resistance in the upper airway, the larynx can, potentially, be an important influence in the regulation of breathing. Most of the present knowledge of laryngeal function during respiration has been derived from experiments using anaesthetized mature animals which have emphasized the role of abductor muscles in influencing upper airway resistance. The involvement of muscles of adduction is less clear, since anaesthesia is known to diminish their activity (1,2) and there may be differences related to species and maturity. We have examined the behaviour of both adductor and abductor muscles in relation to behavioural state at different stages of development in sheep.

The experiments were performed in foetal lambs between 110 and 140 days of gestation, in lambs from birth to 6 weeks of age and in adult sheep. EMG recording electrodes were introduced, under anaesthesia, into the thyroarytenoid muscle (TA), the largest and most accessible adductor muscle, into posterior cricoarytenoid (PCA), the principal abductor muscle, and into the diaphragm (costal margin). Behavioural state was determined from the frontal electrocorticogram (ECoG), the electro-oculogram (EOG) and, after birth, from video monitoring.

In the post-natal lamb (2 - 6 weeks) expiratory activity of the larynx was most consistent during quiet wakefulness or quiet (non-REM) sleep. TA activity began 20 - 30 ms after cessation of activity in inspiratory muscles (PCA and diaphragm), and continued for a variable proportion of expiratory time. Adductor activity, maximal in early expiration, was coincident with elevated laryngeal resistance and with supra-atmospheric pressure (5 - 10 cm H_2O) in the sub-glottic airway. These events were accompanied by reduced or absent expiratory airflow measured at the nose (Fig. 1). Hence T_E was increased and respiratory frequency lowered in relation to the degree of adductor activity. PCA discharge was essentially in phase with the diaphragm and was absent when TA was active.

The phasic expiratory activity of TA was profoundly reduced and usually absent during REM sleep (Fig. 2). The muscle was active only during periods of apnoea and during swallows. Positive expiratory airway pressure was absent except during apnoea. In

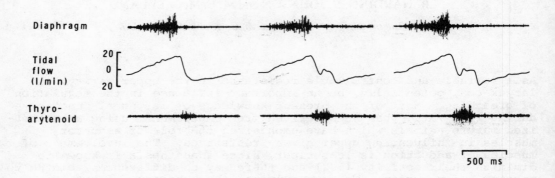

Fig. 1 The effect of laryngeal adductor activity on tidal airflow
        detected at the nose during quiet sleep. Expiratory flow
        (below the mid-point) is interrupted by activity of TA and
        other adductor muscles.

contrast to TA, PCA continued to discharge phasically and often
became active throughout expiration in parallel with the loss of
TA activity.

The relationship between behavioural state and laryngeal function
is well developed in late foetal life (3). During the state
resembling REM sleep (desynchronized ECoG and rapid eye movements)
when breathing movements occur (4), PCA discharged in phase with
the diaphragm but TA activity was negligible. In foetal apnoea,
when the ECoG contained slow waves and rapid eye movements were
absent, the diaphragm and PCA were essentially quiescent but TA
was tonically active. After birth the degree of expiratory TA
activity in quiet sleep was unimpressive, but it gradually
increased in intensity during the first 1 - 2 post-natal weeks.

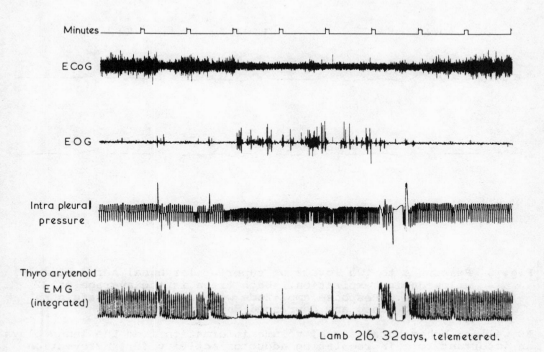

Lamb 216, 32 days, telemetered.

Fig. 2   The influence of sleep state on thyroarytenoid activity.
         The recording shows a short period of REM sleep preceded and
         followed by quiet sleep. TA activity and simultaneous
         positive over-shoot of intra-pleural pressure were absent in
         REM sleep.

The excitability of TA motoneurones was systematically tested in
lambs by measurement of the responses evoked by single stimuli
delivered to the superior laryngeal nerve (internal branch). The
response was always larger during expiration than during inspiration
regardless of whether TA was phasically active; the latency was
constant (13 - 15 ms). During inspiration, the diaphragm and PCA
were inhibited for 25 ms, also after a latency of 13 - 15 ms. In
REM sleep, the amplitudes of sub-maximal responses were reduced,
particularly during expiration (Fig. 3). The excitability of TA
motoneurones was always less during REM sleep than during quiet
sleep, regardless of the degree of TA activity in the latter state.

The reduction of TA activity and excitability during REM sleep was
reflected in the diaphragm electromyogram. The decay of diaphram-
atic activity was more gradual, particularly during the tonic phase
of REM sleep, than during quiet sleep or wakefulness (Fig. 4).
This finding may be interpreted as a disinhibition of inspiratory
neurones by expiratory neurones during REM sleep.

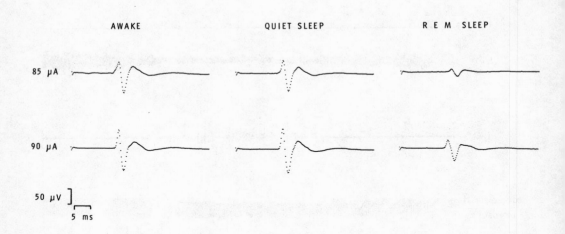

Fig. 3   Responses to two levels of superior laryngeal nerve stimul-
         ation during expiration. Each trace is the average of 32
         responses. Response amplitude was similar in wakefulness
         and quiet sleep and depressed during REM sleep.

As well as behavioural state, volume information from the lungs plays
an important role in regulating adductor activity (5). Prevention
of the development of supra-atmospheric pressure in the trachea by
opening a tracheostomy leads to augmented and prolonged TA activity
during expiration, increased T_E and slower breathing. This response
is further increased, often to the point of apnoea accompanied by
sustained laryngeal adduction, by application of negative end-
expiratory pressures (5 - 10 cm H_2O). The converse response,
reduced TA activity and laryngeal resistance, often with increased
respiratory frequency after an initial apnoea, followed the application of positive end-expiratory pressures. The threshold was as low
as 2 cm H_2O and the response lasted for as long as the pressures
were maintained. Bilateral intra-thoracic vagotomy provoked
prolonged and augmented expiratory adductor activity and abolished
the effects of applied end-expiratory pressures. These results were
obtained in unanaesthetized or lightly anaesthetized animals;
surgical levels of anaesthesia eliminated activity in adductor
muscles.

In adult sheep laryngeal adduction during expiration occurred only in-
frequently. It was often initiated for a short period when the
sheep lay down, possibly due to an increase in intra-pleural pressure
and hence a reduction in trans-pulmonary pressure. In lambs,
adductor activity could be accentuated by sustained compression of
the chest, probably by the same mechanism.

The results show that during development in sheep, laryngeal
adduction is an important means of regulating expiratory airflow and
hence respiratory frequency and perhaps FRC. This important function

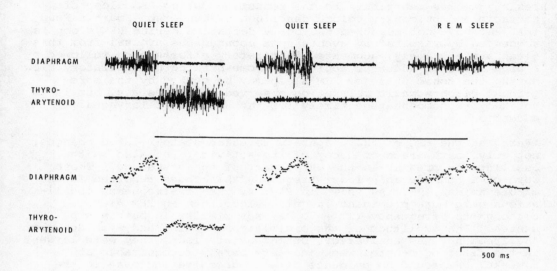

Fig. 4   The influence of sleep state on the diaphragm EMG. In quiet
         sleep, whether TA is active (LHS) or not (centre), activity
         of the diaphragm is terminated abruptly. During REM sleep
         (tonic phase) diaphragmatic relaxation is more gradual. EMG
         activity during single breaths is shown in the upper half.
         Averages of full-wave rectified EMGs during 64 consecutive
         breaths are shown in the lower half.

of the larynx in normal respiration may have been overlooked in the
past because adductor muscles, unlike abductor muscles, are rendered
inactive by surgical levels of anaesthesia. During quiet sleep and
wakefulness in lambs, adduction of the larynx seems to be the
principal means of retarding expiratory airflow. There is little
post-inspiratory activity in the diaphragm, even when the adductors
are inactive. Other species may differ: adult cats, for instance,
appear to depend on post-inspiratory diaphragmatic activity and
reduced PCA activity to retard expiration (6). Sleep related
changes in upper airway resistance in adult cats studied by Orem (7)
were attributed largely to differences in PCA activity. It would be
of interest to establish whether kittens make greater use of
adductor muscles than do adult cats.

During quiet sleep and light anaesthesia, adductor motoneurones and
hence expiratory laryngeal resistance appear to be controlled
principally by afferent traffic arising in vagal slowly-adapting
pulmonary receptors. This mechanism seems well adapted to the
maintainance of pulmonary distension during expiration. The
underlying causes of occasional inactivity in TA during quiet sleep
in lambs, and more so in the adult, requires further investigation.

Laryngeal retardation of expiratory airflow is absent in REM sleep

when adductor motoneurones are less excitable. Laryngeal resistance
during expiration may be further lowered by tonic, or expiratory,
activity in PCA. The absence of an effective expiratory
resistance may contribute to the reduction during REM sleep of
thoracic and pulmonary volume described by Henderson-Smart & Read
(8). We have not measured FRC but a deflation during REM sleep is
suggested by respiratory events upon spontaneous arousal from this
sleep state; namely, augmented inspiratory efforts each followed by
a high level of adductor activity. Some braking of expiratory flow
during the tonic phase of REM sleep may be caused by the more
gradual diaphragmatic relaxation observed in this state, but it is
unlikely to compensate entirely for the absence of laryngeal
adduction.

Averaging the EMG of the diaphragm revealed state-related changes,
not only in the rate of decay of its activity, but also in the
oscillations present in the early part of the discharge. These
were of a considerably lower frequency than those reported in the
mature animal (9). As shown in Fig. 4, the low-frequency oscillations were more prominent in quiet sleep than in REM sleep,
although the frequency (17 - 20 Hz) was similar in both sleep
states. The amplitude of the oscillations diminished with age, but
the frequency was unaltered. During quiet sleep, they were largest
in the first post-natal week and were barely recognizable at
5 weeks. We found no evidence of a progressive increase in the
frequency of the oscillations with age, as has been suggested by
Suthers et al (10). When the oscillations were augmented in the
more mature lamb, for instance by hypercapnia, their frequency was
unchanged from that observed in the same animal when newly born.
We have also detected oscillations with a similar frequency in the
EMG of the fetal diaphragm. The presence of the low-frequency
oscillations in the EMG of the PCA muscle, phase linked to those of
the diaphragm, suggests that they originate in the central
respiratory rhythm generator.

References

(1)   C. Eyzaguirre, & J. R. Taylor. Respiratory discharge of some
      vagal motoneurons. J. Neurophysiol. 26, 61 - 78 (1963).

(2)   J. H. Sherrey & D. Megirian. Spontaneous and reflexly evoked
      laryngeal abductor and adductor muscle activity of cat.
      Exp. Neurobiol. 43, 487 - 498 (1974).

(3)   R. Harding, P. Johnson, M. E. McClelland, C. N. McLeod &
      P. L. Whyte. Laryngeal function during breathing and
      swallowing in foetal and newborn lambs. J. Physiol. 272,
      14 - 15P (1977).

(4)   G. S. Dawes, H. E. Fox, B. M. Leduc, G. C. Liggins &
      R. T. Richards. Respiratory movements and rapid eye move-
      ment sleep in the foetal lamb. J. Physiol. 220, 119 - 143
      (1972).

(5)   R. Harding, P. Johnson & M. E. McClelland. The influence of
      end-expiratory pressure on laryngeal adduction in lambs.
      Proc. Int. Union Physiol. Soc. 13, 305 (1977).

(6)   J. E. Remmers & D. Bartlett.   Reflex control of expiratory
       airflow and duration.   J. Appl. Physiol. 42, 80 - 87 (1977).

(7)   J. Orem, P. Norris, R. Lydic.   Laryngeal abductor activity
       during sleep.   Chest. 73, 300 - 301 (1978).

(8)   D. J. Henderson-Smart & D. J. C. Read.   Depression of
       intercostal and abdominal activity and vulnerability to
       asphyxia during active sleep in the newborn.   In
       Guilleminault, C. & Dement, W. C. (eds): Sleep Apnea
       Syndromes.   A. R. Liss Inc. New York, 93 - 117 (1978).

(9)   M. I. Cohen.   Synchronization of discharge, spontaneous and
       evoked, between inspiratory neurons.   Acta Neurobiol. Exp.
       33, 189 - 218 (1973).

(10) G. K. Suthers, D. J. Henderson-Smart & D. J. C. Read.   Post-
       natal changes in the rate of high frequency bursts of
       inspiratory activity in cats and dogs.   Brain Research,
       132, 537 - 540 (1977).

DISCUSSION

In response to a question by Remmers, Harding made the statement
that the temporal relationship between the diaphragm and thyroarythe-
noid activity remained the same whether the tracheostomy was closed
or open and that opening of the tracheostomy caused no change in the
amount of post-inspiration activity in the diaphragm.

GENERATION AND REGULATION OF PATTERN OF BREATHING

C: Human Physiological and Clinical Aspects

ANALYSIS OF THE DEPTH AND TIMING OF INFANT BREATHING

M. K. S. HATHORN

*Department of Physiology, The London Hospital Medical College,
London E1 2AD, U.K.*

INTRODUCTION

It has been shown that in sleeping, full-term newborn infants, tidal volume (V_T) and instantaneous respiratory rate ($f = 60/T$) show periodic changes, varying from 6.7 to 12.5 sec in duration, super-imposed on more stable background levels (Hathorn, 1978). The amplitude of these oscillations is higher during rapid eye-movement (REM) sleep than during quiet sleep (NREM). The oscillations in V_T tend to be *out of phase* with those for f, particularly during NREM sleep; this contrasts with *in phase* oscillations in V_T and f found in premature infants during episodes of periodic breathing.

The type of frequency analysis used in the above study (Hathorn, 1978) provided information about the *average* amplitude, frequency and phase relationships in the data, and not how these might vary with time. In addition, other variables of the respiratory cycle such as the duration of inspiration (T_I) were not examined. It was therefore decided to examine possible changes, with time, in the oscillations and phase relationships between V_T and f in term newborn infants during both REM and NREM sleep, and to compare these with periodic breathing in premature babies.

METHODS

Thirty healthy term infants were studied with their mothers' informed consent and often with the mother present, during the first week after delivery. Ventilation was recorded using the trunk plethys-mograph (Cross, 1949) as previously described (Hathorn, 1974). REM and NREM sleep states were determined using the criteria of Prechtl & Beintema (1964). Steady-state periods of NREM and REM sleep each lasting from 2 to 6 min were selected, and the amplitude (V_T), and the durations of inspiration (T_I) and expiration (T_E) of each respiratory cycle were measured (Hathorn, 1974). From these were calculated T (= $T_I + T_E$) and f (= 60/T). Five healthy premature infants with long records of periodic breathing were also studied, in order to compare their breathing patterns with those of the term infants.

363

For the analysis of slow periodic changes in ventilation, longer than the individual respiratory cycle, continuous histograms of V_T and f were sampled at equi-spaced intervals of 0.5 sec and the resulting data points were passed through a digital band-pass filter (0.05 - 0.19 Hz) to remove long-term trends in the data incapable of resolution, and high frequency noise introduced by the sampling process (Blackman & Tukey, 1959). Frequency analysis was performed by calculating auto- and cross-covariance functions for V_T and f; these show the time intervals over which periodic components in the data start repeating themselves. The fourier transform of these functions results in the power spectrum, which shows the distribution of variation in the data according to frequency (Bendat & Piersol, 1966). These methods have been described in full elsewhere (Hathorn, 1978).

RESULTS

Table 1 shows the overall mean values for V_T, T_I, T_E and f, calculated for individual respiratory cycles in each infant in both sleep states. This table also shows the mean rate of inspiratory

TABLE 1   Overall mean values in 30 term infants

	NREM	REM	$\dfrac{REM}{NREM}$	No. of* infants
V_T (cm^3)	15.6	13.2	0.85	25/30
T_I (sec)	0.67	0.49	0.73	30/30
T_E (sec)	1.02	0.74	0.73	29/30
V_T/T_I (cm^{3}sec^{-1})	23.9	28.7	1.20	29/30
f (min^{-1})	37.3	54.5	1.46	30/30

* Number (out of total) showing indicated change

airflow, calculated as V_T/T_I. It will be seen that 25 of the 30 infants showed a reduction in mean V_T during REM sleep. Almost all of the babies showed similar proportionate reductions in both T_I and T_E in this sleep state, with a consequent increase in respiration rate (f) in all infants. The mean rate of inspiratory inflow was higher during REM than NREM sleep in 29 of the 30 infants.

Correlation coefficients (r) were calculated between individual values of V_T and T_I, and V_T and T, in all the infants. These are shown in Fig. 1. It will be seen that the correlations, although statistically significant in most infants, showed considerable variation. Since the value of r^2 indicates the proportion of the variation ascribable to the correlated variables, it is evident that in almost all the infants, most of the variation in V_T, T_I and T should be sought elsewhere.

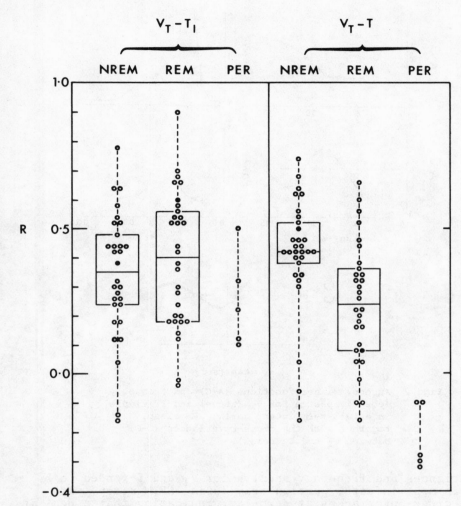

Fig. 1 Correlation coefficients (r) between V_T and
T_I, and V_T and T, in 30 full-term infants
in REM and NREM sleep, and 5 premature
infants during periodic breathing. The
boxed areas cover 50% of the data, the
central bar indicating the median value.

Frequency analysis of V_T and f

The filtered data showed the presence of periodic changes in V_T and f
in both sleep states (e.g. Figs. 5 and 6). These oscillations were
not regular, but showed variation in both amplitude and in the peak-
to-peak intervals between successive oscillations.

M. K. S. Hathorn

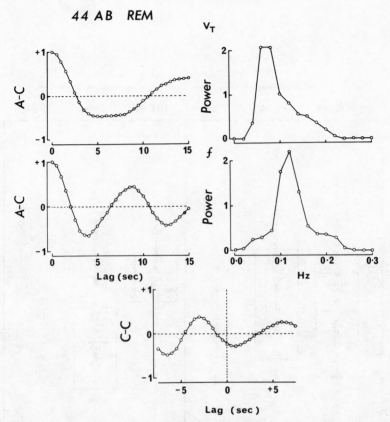

Fig. 2   Autocovariance functions (A-C) and frequency
(power) spectra for V_T (above) and f (middle)
in a full-term infant during REM sleep,
together with the cross-covariances (C-C)
between V_T and f (below).

Autocovariances and frequency spectra for V_T and f tended to be
similar in most infants, particularly during NREM sleep, with
negative cross-covariances at zero-lag, indicating that a peak in V_T
coincides, on average, with a trough in f.   Figure 2 shows an infant
in REM sleep where the main oscillations in V_T and f were somewhat
different.   It will be seen that the periodicity in V_T was about
15 sec (O.08 - O.10 Hz) compared with about 9 sec for f (O.12 Hz).
The cross-covariance in this infant shows a less marked relation
between V_T and f, with some displacement in their average out of
phase relation.

It will be seen from Table 2 that the amplitudes of the oscillations in both V_T and f (expressed as root-mean-square values) were
increased in all infants during REM sleep: about 3-fold for V_T and
more than 4-fold for f.   It should also be noted that the average
frequency of these oscillations was slightly lower during REM sleep
than in NREM sleep in most of the 30 full-term infants.

TABLE 2   Amplitudes and frequencies of oscillations

	NREM	REM	$\dfrac{\text{REM}}{\text{NREM}}$	No. of infants
RMS values of oscillations				
V_T (cm^3)	1.0	2.9	2.90	30/30
f (min^{-1})	1.9	8.4	4.42	30/30
Mean frequency of oscillations (Hz)				
V_T	0.115	0.10	0.87	23/30
f	0.12	0.10	0.83	18/30

The most striking features in the frequency analysis of V_T and f
described above were (a) the increased amplitude of the oscillations
during REM sleep, and (b) changes in the cross-covariances with
alteration in sleep state and in periodic breathing. During NREM sleep
nearly all full-term infants showed negative cross-covariances; in
REM sleep, the results were more variable, while in the premature
infants with periodic breathing, the cross-covariances were positive.

This type of analysis shows the average properties of the data over
the whole duration of the record, and not how they might vary with
time. Two methods are now described to indicate changes occurring
with time: (a) running cross-covariances, and (b) plots of running
phase difference.

Running cross-covariances

Cross-covariances between V_T and f were calculated on the first
100 data points, covering the first 50 seconds of the trace; the
results were then plotted as the first line of a 3-dimensional graph
opposite the midpoint in time, namely 25 sec. The process was then
repeated 1 or 2 sec further on in the trace (depending on the length
of trace available), and the new cross-covariances plotted at the
26 (or 27) sec point. This process was continued until the last
100 data points were reached. In this way, between 100 and
131 running estimates were plotted. The results of this procedure in
a full-term infant, during both REM and NREM sleep, are shown in
Fig. 3. The negative and positive time lags are shown in the horizontal axis, the amplitude of the cross-covariances in the vertical
axis, while in the time axis, the first results are shown at the back
of the plot, and the results from the last part of the trace at the
front of the plot.

During NREM sleep, it will be seen from Fig. 3 (right) that although
there is some change with time in the amplitude and periodicity in
the cross-covariances, they all show a consistently negative
deflection at zero-lag, i.e. throughout the trace, the oscillations
in V_T and f are fairly consistently *out-of-phase* with each other, a
peak in a V_T oscillation coinciding with a trough in the f oscillation. During REM sleep, however, there are several differences: the
amplitude of the cross-covariances is more variable, the periodicity

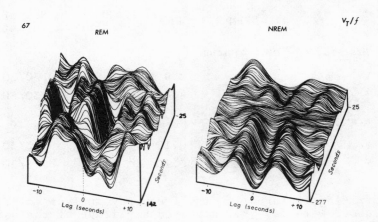

Fig. 3   Three-dimensional plots showing changes in
         cross-covariances between V_T and f with
         time, during both REM and NREM sleep.
         Each line on the REM plot represents an
         increment of 1 sec, while in the NREM plot,
         the increments were 2 sec because of the
         increased length of trace available (see
         text for explanation).

varies more, and although there is a tendency for the cross-
covariances to be negative at zero-lag, this is far more variable
than during NREM sleep. It would appear that during REM sleep, there
is less tendency for the oscillations in V_T and f to cancel each
other out than is the case during NREM sleep.

Figure 4 shows running cross-covariances between V_T and f in a
premature baby during periodic breathing.   It will be seen that the
plots are remarkably stable, and that at zero lag, the cross-
covariances are all positive, i.e. the oscillations in V_T and f are
in-phase with each other.

Plots of running phase differences

The other method developed for examining the relationship between
oscillations in V_T and f is illustrated in Figs. 5, 6 and 7.   In
each of these graphs, a facsimile of the original trace of
ventilation is shown at the bottom. The top two lines are the output
of the band-pass filter, showing the oscillations in V_T and f.   At
each 0.5 sec interval, the phase (or fraction of a complete
oscillation) for each of these two traces is calculated; these are
then subtracted from each other and plotted as the phase difference.
If the two oscillations are completely *in-phase*, the difference would
be zero and a phase difference point would be plotted on each of the
3 dashed lines. *Differences* in phase would result in points lying
between the dashed lines; if the oscillations are completely *out-of-
phase*, the points would be plotted half-way between the dashed lines.

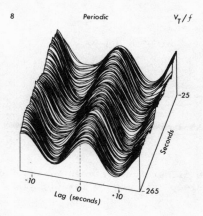

Fig. 4   Running cross-covariances between V_T and f
          in a premature baby during periodic breathing.
          Each increment is 2 seconds (see legend to
          Fig. 3 and text for explanation).

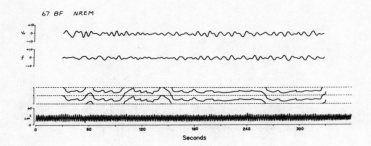

Fig. 5   Phase differences between V_T and f during
          NREM sleep. Top two traces: filtered data
          showing oscillations in V_T and f respect-
          ively; middle traces: running phase differ-
          ences, with dashed lines showing zero phase
          difference; bottom trace: facsimile of
          ventilation. See text for explanation.
          (This is the same infant as shown in Fig. 3.)

During NREM sleep (Fig. 5), the plots of phase difference tend to lie
between the dashed lines, with occasional crossings, indicating that
the oscillations in V_T and f are predominantly out-of-phase in this
sleep state. This is the same infant shown in Fig. 3 (right).
During REM sleep (Fig. 6), the phase differences are far more
unstable - see also Fig. 3 (left).

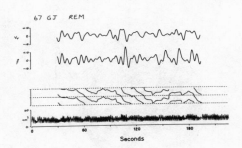

Fig. 6   Phase differences between V_T and f during
         REM sleep (see legend for Fig. 5).

Figure 7 shows a plot of running phase differences in another infant
during REM sleep, who after a time moved into a short interval of
periodic breathing. The phase plot shows the unstable phase
differences typical of REM sleep; with the onset of periodic
breathing, however, the phase lines move towards the dotted lines,
indicating *in-phase* oscillations in V_T and f in this pattern of
breathing.

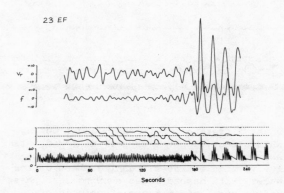

Fig. 7   Phase differences between V_T and f in
         another infant in REM sleep, showing
         transition to periodic breathing. (See
         legend for Fig. 5.)

Figure 8 shows running phase differences between the oscillations in
V_T and f during periodic breathing in the same infant previously
illustrated in Fig. 4. Figure 8 shows that both V_T and f remain
closely *in phase* with each other over the entire period of the
trace.

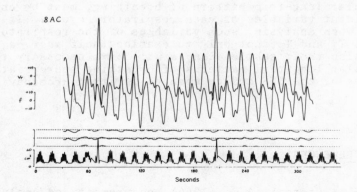

Fig. 8   Phase differences between V_T and f during
         periodic breathing in a premature infant
         (see legend for Fig. 5).

DISCUSSION

The present study shows that in sleeping full-term newborn infants,
both the rate and depth of breathing undergo cyclic variations.
These oscillations, with a mean period of about 8 to 10 seconds, are
compatible with the behaviour of a respiratory feed-back control
system with a time-lag representing the lung-chemoreceptor circulation time. In such a system, the amplitude of these oscillations
would depend both on the degree of damping, and the overall sensitivity of the respiratory controller to fluctuations in blood gases.
The differing amplitudes of these oscillations during REM and NREM
sleep would imply a change in supramedullary influences on the
characteristics of the respiratory centre with change in sleep state.

Another finding of interest is the temporal relation between the
oscillations of V_T and f. In premature infants, in whom periodic
breathing is commonly found, the oscillations of V_T and f are *in
phase* with each other, resulting in marked instability in alveolar
ventilation. In the full-term infant, these oscillations are
maintained relatively *out-of-phase*, leading to more stable ventilation. In addition, the ability to maintain this out-of-phase
relationship appears to be more efficient during NREM than REM sleep.

This change in the phase relationship between V_T and f with increasing maturity of the newborn infant, and the influence of sleep state
on this relationship, raises the question of whether there may be
somewhat differing controls for the rate and depth of breathing:
during periodic breathing, the two controllers operate in phase with
each other, while in the more mature baby, they become more closely
'locked' out of phase with each other, leading to more efficient
ventilation.

All the output of the respiratory controller required to establish any particular long-term pattern of breathing, must be encoded in the significant variables of each respiratory cycle. It is therefore necessary, when analysing such variables of the respiratory cycle such as V_T, T_I and T_E, not only to examine their *average* relationships, but also their subtle *changes with time* necessary to produce the particular long-term patterns of breathing appropriate to both the maturity of the CNS and to changes in its neurobehavioural state.

REFERENCES

Bendat, J.S. & Piersol, A.G. (1966) Measurement and Analysis of Random Data, Wiley, New York.

Blackman, R.B. & Tukey, J.W. (1959) The Measurement of Power Spectra, Dover, New York.

Cross, K.W., The Respiratory Rate and Ventilation in the Newborn Baby, Journal of Physiology, 109, 459 (1949).

Hathorn, M.K.S., The Rate and Depth of Breathing in New-born Infants in Different Sleep States, Journal of Physiology, 243, 101 (1974).

Hathorn, M.K.S., Analysis of Periodic Changes in Ventilation in New-born Infants, Journal of Physiology, 285, 85 (1978).

Prechtl, H.F.R. & Beintema, D. (1964) The Neurological Examination of the Fullterm Newborn Infant, Little Club Clinics in Developmental Medicine, No. 12, Heinemann, London.

DISCUSSION

The need for similar studies of the 'out-of-phase' periodicity in adult humans was expressed, although some scanty data are available from the work of Pribam (J.Physiol. 166, 425, 1963; cf. also Benchetrit & Bertrand, Resp.Physiol. 23, 147, 1975).

Hathorn was asked whether the type of 'out-of-phase' oscillations was influenced by letting the babies breath a gas mixture high in oxygen. He replied that he had observed this type of oscillations also when subjecting the babies to high oxygen. He had found it difficult to get sufficient number of 'runs' in high oxygen and controls in the same baby and in the same sleep state to be able to ascertain whether there is a change in one direction or the other. However, he thought that there might have been a tendency for this type of oscillations to increase in high oxygen. The 'in-phase' type of oscillations, i.e. the Cheyne-Stokes type, has generally been found to decrease or vanish in high oxygen.

Euler pointed out that Cheyne-Stokes type of periodic breathing appears to be due to instability in the chemical feedback controller for ventilation with large swings in chemical stimuli and in ventilation as will be reported later (p. 417). In this type of periodicity the rate of increase of CIA, the inspiratory 'off-switch' thresholds, and the T_E controlling factors are all changing in a manner similar to the responses to changes in chemical stimuli. In contrast, the variations of the parameters in the 'out-of-phase' type of periodicity with its fairly constant ventilation do not resemble the variations seen in response to changes in chemical stimuli. It would therefore seem unlikely that this latter type of periodicity could be due to oscillations in the chemical feedback regulation of ventilation, but rather to periodic variations in the pattern generator, possibly caused by cyclic changes in the thresholds of the inspiratory 'off-switch' mechanisms as has been suggested earlier (Euler & Trippenbach, Acta physiol.scand. 97, 175, 1976).

SPATIAL AND TEMPORAL CHARACTERISTICS
OF FETAL BREATHING MOVEMENTS IN MAN

G. GENNSER

Department of Obstetrics and Gynecology, University Hospital, S-214 01 Malmö,
Sweden

INTRODUCTION

The 'rediscovery' in the present decade of fetal breathing movements (FBM) took
place in two steps. The first was taken when showing, in chronically catheterized
fetal lambs, episodic rhythmic alterations of the intratracheal pressure (1, 2).
The second step was the confirmation by modern technique of the fetal chest wall
movements in man (3, 4) observed and described already by Ahlfeld in 1888 (5).
Ultrasound has been quickly established as the presently best available method to
study in detail the FBM in man without registered side-effects. It is, however,
mainly limited to identify and measure the movements of the fetal trunk interfaces
and does not reveal pressures and flows in the respiratory tract. Our means to investigate the breathing activity and its physiological regulation in the human fetus are therefore severely restricted. It is the object of this paper to summarize
present knowledge on the character and pattern of FBM in man, to compare these
data with corresponding data of newborn infants and to, by analogy, suggest possible mechanisms in this system operating in utero. For a correct appreciation of
available data on FBM, it was estimated necessary to outline the ultrasonic methodology and its limitations.

TECHNIQUE

For non-invasive, harmless registration of FBM only a few methods are avialable.
External pressure gauges, measuring fetal movements transmitted to the maternal
abdominal wall, were used already by Ahlfeld (5) and recently by Timor-Tritch (6).
To its disadvantage, this procedure does not visualize the fetal body and cannot
discriminate between FBM and other fetal or maternal movements.

The first reported study on diagnostic sonar (3) employed a one-dimensional A-mode
method. A single ultrasound beam from a transducer applied to the maternal abdominal wall is directed towards the fetal heart. The echoes, originating from one of
the fetal chest walls, are identified and the movements are detected and measured
by an electronic gate. The A-mode method has, however, inherent short-comings (7),
the major ones being difficulties in identifying the echo-giving structures and
in discriminating signals of FBM from various artefacts caused by non-specific
movements.

The Doppler-principle has been utilized in detecting frequency shifts in fetal echoes of continuous ultrasound (8). Such frequency shifts, synchronous with independently monitored FBM, are found to originate not from movements of the fetal trunk walls but from changes of flow velocity in the inferior caval vein (9), which is accelerated during inspiration. The data obtained by this method seem to contain more information of accompanying circulatory changes than of the breathing movements per se. Pulsed Doppler systems have recently been tried combined with other ultrasound modes, yielding information of FBM velocity within a range gate (10).

Real-time B-mode ultrasonography was first applied for visualizing FBM in 1975 (4) and has since become the most widely applied technique for this purpose. In this mode, repeated B-scanning of the object is performed so rapidly that all echoes from the structures in the section can be displayed simultaneously and reveal movements of the echo origins. The B-scanning is achieved by various transducer arrangements: one or a few crystals moved mechanically (rotating or sector type) or a line of fixed crystals activated sequentially (linear array transducer, phased array transducer). These arrangements are convenient for creating a two-dimensional transsectional image of the fetus. By the full visualization of the fetal trunk it is possible to identify the FBM and to select the optimal part for insonation, i.e. the structure having movements of the largest amplitude. For registering the FBM displayed on the scanner screen, two different methods have been employed.

One method is observing the movements on the scanner screen and manual marking each FBM by pressing an event-marker. This can be performed either on-line or when reviewing event sequences stored on video-tape. The event-marker produces a punched tape, which is subsequently subjected to computer analysis. This method is time-consuming and its time-resolution is limited.

The second method makes it possible to perform objective quantification of the fetal movements by a combination of the real-time B-mode scanner with an A-mode principle. One way is to manually analyse the movements of echoes in a TM-mode display of signals from one of the transducers in a linear array scanner (11). An automatic method was used in the present study. A time-distance (TD-) recorder (12), when attached to a real-time scanner, enables the operator to choose anyone of the lines constituting the image on the scanner oscilloscope screen (Fig. 1).

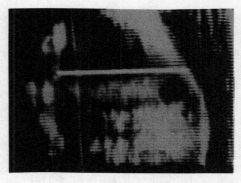 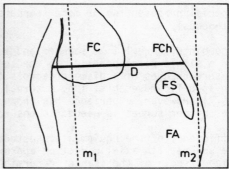

Fig. 1. Real-time B-mode display of a longitudinal section of the fetal trunk. Fine vertical marker lines (m_1,
m_2) are used when chosing echoes to be followed, bright
horizontal line (D) indicates the diameter measured by
the TD-recorder along the selected image line. FC = fetal
heart; FCh = fetal chest; FA = fetal abdomen; FS = fetal
stomach.

This line is displayed intensified and two echo-following devices can be moved in
front of any echo complex along this line. Thus. two echoes can be selected whose
movements are to be recorded, e.g. the proximal and the distal fetal chest wall.
The time for the ultrasound beam to create the two chest wall echoes is measured
digitally and a digital-to-analog converter generates an on-line signal representative for the instant fetal trunk diameter. The signal is produced on a paper
record with the fetal pulse and maternal breathing (Fig. 2) and stored on magnetic
tape.

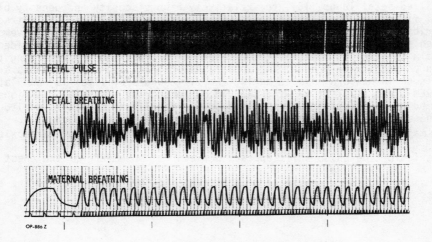

Fig. 2. FBM signal (middle trace) recorded with fetal pulse
(upper trace) and maternal breathing (lower trace). Time is
given in seconds. Missed fetal heart beats are artefacts.

For special purposes two or more scanners with attached TD-recorders can be used simultaneously.

When combined, a real-time scanner and a TD-recorder produce quantification of the FBM in a single plane parallel to the sonar beam. The ability of this equipment to measure changes of a diameter across the fetal trunk minimizes the influence of non-specific movements, i.e. maternal breathing movements transferred to the fetus (7). However, experience has shown that constant supervision of the fetus on the scanner screen is needed to ensure a recording free from artefacts.

The efficiency of the equipment to detect FBM is limited by the range resolution of the scanner (in axial direction approximately 1 mm). The frame frequency (40 images/sec.) of the scanner determines the time resolution. The output signal from the TD-recorder is, when necessary, passed through a slew-rate filter + a bandpass filter: the slew-rate filter permits the FBM, which do not activate the filter, to pass without distortion. The combination of slew-rate and bandpass filter reduces the amplitude of a 1.5 Hz input signal in vitro by 21.3 % (13).

CONFIGURATIVE CHANGES DURING FBM

The physical characteristics of the breathing movements in the human fetus have to some details been evaluated by real-time ultrasound scanning (11, 14). The current concept of the human FBM includes the contraction of the diaphragm as a central event in the breathing cycle, accompanied by a simultaneous retraction of the chest wall and an expansion of the abdominal wall. This phase, which also comprises an increase of the kyphosis of the thoracic spine, is regarded equivalent to an inspiration. During expiration, the diaphragm, the chest wall and the abdominal wall return to their original position.

A prominent feature of the human FBM is their variability in rhythm, rate and amplitude also during periods of continuous, seemingly regular breathing. This variation applies also to the pattern of inverse or paradoxical breathing, which is the predominant one during the last trimester of gestation. The low compliance of the fluid-filled fetal lungs (15), the relatively high viscosity and density of the tracheal fluid, and the pliable chest walls sufficiently explain the retraction of the ribs, when the diaphragm contracts. The paradoxical breathing movements have been evaluated by studying slowmotion replay or frozen frames of video-records using either a single real-time B-scanner or two scanners recording the fetal trunk in perpendicular planes. The appearance of fetal see-saw movements are similar to those in newborn infants during the first hours of life (16) and later during REM-sleep (17). By viewing the video-tapes or by analysing Lissajous figures formed by x-y plotting of signals from two fetal body diameters monitored simultaneously (Fig. 3), the following conclusions have been reached:

(1) The majority of all fetal breathing movements observed are of paradoxical pattern.
(2) A periodic time phase shift appears between the movements of the chest wall and of the abdominal wall.
(3) Occasionally, for a couple of breaths, the site of the fulcrum of the see-saw movements is dislocated in caudal or cephalad direction.

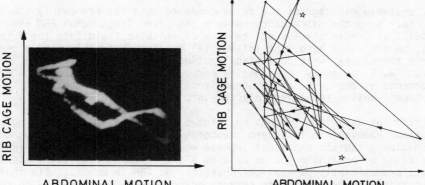

Fig. 3. Relative changes of abdominal diameter (horizontal axis) v chest diameter (vertical axis). Left photo of oscilloscope screen shows basically paradoxical breathing movement but with phase displacement and increased rate of chest cage movement. Right picture shows plot of movements measured manually in single frames of video tape (approximately 0.2 sec. between points of measuring). ☆ denote occasional synchronous undirectional movements.

The observation have two implications for our concept of the breathing movements in the fetus. The first is the picture of instability given by the fetal chest cage in conjunction with the paradoxical breathing. This corresponds with the distortion of the rib cage, which appears in infants during REM-sleep (17) when the intercostal muscles are inhibited (19). The role played by the intercostal muscles during fetal breathing has been elucidated recently by Harding and associates in fetal lambs (20). In sheep, FBM occur almost exclusively in REM-sleep (1), and Harding found in this sleep state absent phasic EMG-activity in the intercostal muscles and positive EMG-activity in the diaphragm. Fetal rib cage instability was directly demonstrated by Poore, who used pairs of ultrasonic transducers implanted on opposite chest walls of fetal lambs and compared the changes of the trunk diameters with the concomitantly registered tracheal pressure (21). The instability of the human fetal chest wall visualized by ultrasound gives indirect support to the idea of the FBM being principally of diaphragmatic pattern.

The second point is the consequence of the rib cage instability for the capacity of FBM to produce flow in the fetal respiratory tract. The phase shift between the movements of the fetal chest walls and those of the diaphragm serves to diminish the changes of the chest volume during the breathing cycle. This movement pattern might explain why, in fetal lambs, the flow in the fetal trachea is very low and seldom exceeds the dead space (22). The amplitude of the human FBM is often large: the maximum distance of movements of the fetal chest wall in the sagittal plane at the level of the heart base in the 32nd week was 2.1 ± 0.5 mm (14). The chest volume changes, exerted by the movements of the external chest wall only (disregarding the movements of the diaphragm), has been estimated in a fetus of 37 weeks showing regular breathing movements. Measurements were performed on two simultaneously displayed on-line B-scan images: one of a mid-line sagittal plane and one of a frontal plane. The chest volume was calculated as the sum of 1 cm high truncated cones with elliptic plane surfaces. In five consecutive cycles the peak-to-peak volume change was 52.02 ± 14.92 (mean $\pm$ SD) cm^3. The pliable, unstable rib cage of the fetus tends to make the FBM mainly isovolumic, thereby clarifying the discrepancy between the often large human FBM and the variable results of tracer studies on the flow of amniotic fluid into the fetal lungs (see 23). On the other hand, the intercostal muscles presumably play a central role for a transitory functional stabilization of the chest wall, when in-phase fetal trunk wall movements occasionally occur (Fig. 3). It is tempting to regard such movements as the cause of the unequivocal entrance into the fetal lungs of radioisotope-labelled red cells injected into the amniotic fluid (24).

Transposition of data from infants to fetuses or between species must be performed with caution. However, in full-term newborns the paradoxical breathing characterizes REM-sleep; thoraco-abdominal inphase movements being exceptions (25). If the phase-relation of breathing can be used as a criterium of activity state in the fetus, the predominantly paradoxical character of FBM in man suggests that these movements mainly occur in a state corresponding to REM-sleep. Such a correlation would agree to that found in fetal lambs (22).

TIME COURSE OF FBM

Single breath cycle characteristics

The human FBM occur episodically (vide infra) and the following data are obtained from periods of <u>continuous</u> breathing.

The average <u>rate</u> of breathing movements varies widely (range 35-70 breaths/min.) with occasional fast rates up to 200 breaths/min., our observations according well with those of Patrick <u>et al</u>. (26). The vast variation, partly due to interspersed periods of apnea, makes the average rate of breathing dependent on the length of observation time and is therefore a less meaningful parameter except for periods of continuous breathing.

The time course of the FBM cycle appears from Table 1.

TABLE 1   Parameters of FBM. Mean $\pm$ SD

Fetus	No. of cycles	Duration of total active cycle, sec	Duration of inspiration, sec	Breath-to-breath interval, sec
EO	56	1.28 $\pm$ 0.21	0.70 $\pm$ 0.16	1.33 $\pm$ 0.19
BO	46	1.00 $\pm$ 0.16	0.44 $\pm$ 0.15	1.05 $\pm$ 0.10
BP	50	1.22 $\pm$ 0.20	0.68 $\pm$ 0.20	1.29 $\pm$ 0.14
ER	20	0.97 $\pm$ 0.14	0.43 $\pm$ 0.16	1.33 $\pm$ 0.20
BS	42	0.87 $\pm$ 0.22	0.49 $\pm$ 0.16	1.02 $\pm$ 0.28

It is obvious that, during spells of continuous breathing, the active movements occupy most of the cycle (73 % - 96 %). For each period of breathing movements, there was a significant correlation between the duration of inspiratory time and the total active breathing time (Fig. 4).

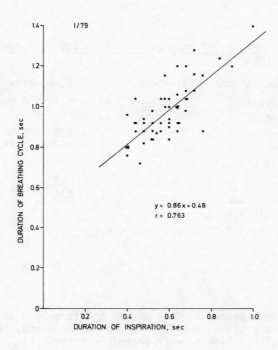

Fig. 4. The duration of the inspiratory phase in relation to the duration of the total breathing cycle in a group of consecutive FBM. Gestational age 39 weeks.

The correlation coefficients in 9 consecutively examined fetuses (gestational age 32 - 40 weeks) were 0.579 - 0.911 (median 0.744). The duration of the expiratory phase was not correlated to the duration of the subsequent cycle (correlation coefficients ranging from -0.260 to 0.693, median 0.180). Thus, like in adults (27), the inspiratory time seems to determine the expiratory time, and the inspiration and the following expiration appear to form an independent entity.

In view of the paradoxical character of the FBM and the consequently reduced possibilities of fetal lung excursions, the 'off-switch' mechanism regulating the inspiratory time in the fetus is less likely to include afferent activity from pulmonary stretch receptors operating at the same setting as after birth. The situation of the fetus might be analogous to that when the lungs are experimentally prevented to expand by tracheal occlusion at the end of an expiration. With feedback signals on volume via the vagus nerve lacking, the centrally generated inspiratory activity is alone responsible for the 'inspiratory off-switch', which in these experiments is attained after a longer inspiratory phase (28). The average duration of the inspiratory time in fetuses is, however, not prolonged in comparison with the inhibited breathing of newborns (Table 2).

TABLE 2 Duration of inspiration in fetuses and newborn infants (mean ± SD)

	Gestational age, weeks	n	Time, sec.
Fetuses	36.4 ± 2.5	11	0.41 ± 0.09[xx]
Preterm infants[x]	29.9 ± 1.5	16	
preocclusion			0.38 ± 0.08
occlusion			0.76 ± 0.28
Term infants[x]	39.8 ± 1.1	14	
preocclusion			0.51 ± 0.11
occlusion			0.70 ± 0.19

[x]From Olinsky et al. 1974 (28).

[xx]In each fetus the mean of 30 consecutive breaths.

It can be assumed from these data that either the threshold of the centrally generated inspiratory activity is lower before than after birth, or signals from other peripheral receptors than lung stretch receptors contribute in utero to the 'inspiratory off-switch'. In infants, rapid distortion of the rib cage observed during REM-sleep is followed by a premature termination of inspiration (29), presumably elicited via the intercostal-phrenic inhibitory reflex reported earlier (30, 31). It is suggested by the present observations that the instability of the fetal chest wall might activate this reflex, thereby contributing to the 'off-switch' of the fetal inspiratory phase.

It was recently pointed out that newborns, because of their very compliant chest walls and their high airway resistance, were breathing at an increased volume level compared to later in life (28). Their high respiratory rate (40-60/min.) does not permit the lungs during passive expiration to return to their functional residual capacity except during apneic periods when the end-expiratory volume is lower than while breathing (Fig. 5).

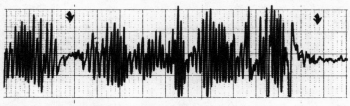

Fetal breathing movements

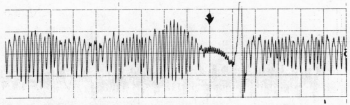

Neonatal breathing movements

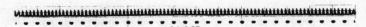

Time, sec

Fig. 5. Trace of FBM recorded by ultrasound and TD-recorder
(upper part) and trace of breathing movements of newborn
infant recorded by measurement of transthoracic impedance.
Arrows indicate different slope of signal during apnea.

In the human fetus, no consistent change in the 'resting respiratory volume' (as
suggested by constant transsectional chest and abdominal diameters) has been observed during fetal apnea (Fig. 5), although the average rate of breathing movements is as high before as after birth. This indirectly evidences that during the
FBM no larger flow occurs in the airways.

Breath-to-breath intervals

Approximately half the number of fetuses observed have demonstrated periods of
seemingly very regular, continuous breathing movements. The breath-to-breath intervals within these periods have varied when measured in fast paper records. In
order to evaluate patterns in the breathing frequency, the output signals from
the TD-recorder were passed through an instrument analysing the instantaneous
breathing rate (Fig. 6) (32).

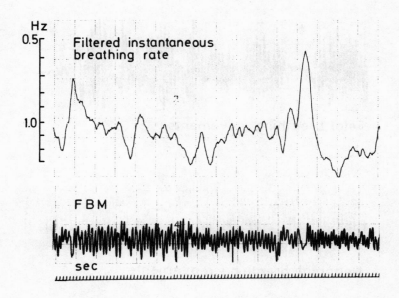

Fig. 6. Trace of continuous FBM obtained from a TD-recorder
(lower curve) and of the instantaneous breathing rate
(upper curve).

This device uses the phase-locked loop principle to avoid the influence of random
noise. Its capture range was set to 1.1 Hz ± 50 %, thereby capturing most of the
observed average rates of human FBM. Processing the fetal breathing signals in
this way revealed a variability of the instantaneous FBM rate, which was higher
during active periods (defined by the appearance of fetal gross movements and by
the increased basal level and variability of the fetal heart rate) than during
resting periods (no gross movements, low basal level and variability of fetal
heart rate) (32). Two types of breath-to-breath interval variations appeared in
the records: one of rapid oscillations with an amplitude of 0.02 - 0.15 Hz, and
one with slow oscillations exceeding 0.2 Hz. In sequences of continuous breathing
movements ranging 1.0 - 9.2 min. in seven fetuses, the mean periods of oscillations of the former type varied between 1.9 and 3.9 sec. (0.26 - 0.53 Hz), and
those of the latter type between 14.3 and 50.0 sec. (0.02 - 0.07 Hz).

Hathorn recently reported oscillations of the respiratory rate in newborn infants
with mean periods ranging 6.7 - 12.5 sec. (33). These figures are compatible
with an oscillatory behaviour of the respiratory feed-back control system, the
transport lag-time in the lung-chemoreceptor circulation in newborn infants being
somewhat longer than 6 sec. The demonstration here, in preliminary form, of rate
oscillations in the FBM is intriguing, as any established fetal feed-back control
system involving chemoreceptor activity and fetal ventilation is highly unlikely.
The cardiovascular undulations associated with breathing in fetal lamb (34) and
also (respiratory arrhythmia) in human fetus (35, 36) might, however, be part
of a mechanism by which the fetus can influence its own distribution of gases
and thereby constitute an active feed-back loop. It cannot be excluded that the
fetal breathing rate oscillations are responses to fluctuations of primarily
maternal origin in P_{A,CO_2} reaching the fetal central chemoreceptors.

Long-term rhythms

The incidence of breathing movements per time unit was (for technical reasons) the quality of FBM to be first evaluated (22) and has hitherto been the most widely studied parameter. An arbitrary definition of fetal apnea as 6 sec. or more without breathing movements is now generally accepted. The marked variability seen in the single FBM is also apparent in the longer time course. It is possible to recognize three patterns of the FBM incidence in the middle of the last trimester of gestation as demonstrated by Patrick (37) in a careful study.

(1) A nyctohemeral rhythm of FBM has peaks of incidence at 0700, 1000 and 1400 hours, and troughs at 1800 and 2400 hours. This pattern is reflected by the circadian profile of maternal plasma glucose concentration - with one notable exception: the steady significant increase in the incidence of FBM between 0100 and 0700 hours is not paralleled by any concomitant increment in blood sugar level (37). An induced hyperglycemic state can clearly augment the activity of FBM (38, 39), hypothetically via an altered wake state of the fetal CNS or an increased central accumulation of CO_2 secondary to an enhanced glucose metabolism. The nocturnal rhythm of the FBM incidence suggests, however, other metabolic or endocrine cycles as influencing the fetal respiratory centers.

(2) Increments of the time spent breathing by the fetus are superimposed on the basal circadian rhythm 2 - 3 hours after each carbohydrate-rich meal. This reactivity can be exploited in clinical practice by administering carbohydrates to the woman before examination in order to ensure optimal FBM activity.

(3) A third rhythm of FBM shows a periodicity of 1.0 to 1.5 hours. Increased activity during 20 - 60 min. is followed by a prolonged period of apnea (37, 40). It is close at hand to conclude that these variations might be expressions of altered rest-activity states of the fetus, in agreement with the relation between sleep-states and breathing patterns in newborn infants (41). Recently was found a persistent individual activity profile in fetuses monitored four periods daily for a week (Gennser and Maršál, to be published). The study of the rhythms of FBM is clearly linked to further analysis of fetal behavioural state.

ACKNOWLEDGEMENTS

Parts of these investigations have been carried out in fruitful collaboration with Karel Maršál, M.D. and Kjell Lindström, D.Sc.. Expert technical assistance was given by Mr. Arbe Bjuvholt, Mrs. Ann Thuring and Mr. Serge Boulanger. The work was supported by the Swedish Medical Research Council (B79-17X-04517-05A), the Medical Faculty, University of Lund, and the Magnus Bergvall Foundation.

REFERENCES

(1) G.S. Dawes, H.E. Fox, B.M. Leduc, G.C. Liggins, and R.T. Richards, Respiratory movements and paradoxical sleep in the foetal lamb, J. Physiol. 210, 47 P (1970).

(2) C. Merlet, J. Hoerter, Ch. Devilleneuve, and C. Tchobroutsky, Mise en évidence de mouvements respiratoires chez le foetus d'agneau in utero au cours du dernier mois de la gestation, C.R. Acad. Sc. Paris 270, 2462 (1970).

(3) K. Boddy and J.S. Robinson, External method for detection of fetal breathing in utero, Lancet ii. 1231 (1971).

(4) G. Gennser and K. Maršál, Fetal breathing movements in man. Film presented
        at the 2nd Conference on Fetal Breathing, Nuffield Institute for
        Medical Research, Oxford, October 3rd, 1975.

(5) F. Ahlfeld, Ueber bisher noch nicht beschriebene intrauterine Bewegungen des
        Kindes, Verh. dtsch. Ges. Gynäk., Zweiter Kongress p. 203, Breitkopf
        und Härtel, Leipzig (1888).

(6) I. Timor-Tritsch, I. Zador, R.H. Hertz, and M.G. Rosen, Human fetal respira-
        tory arrhythmia, Am. J. Obstet. Gynecol. 127, 662 (1977).

(7) K. Maršál, G. Gennser, K. Lindström, and U. Ulmsten, Errors and pitfalls in
        ultrasonic measurements of fetal breathing movements, in Kurjak, A.
        (Ed.) (1978) Recent Advances in Ultrasound Diagnosis, p. 200, Ex-
        cerpta Medica, Amsterdam.

(8) E.S. Boyce, G.S. Dawes, J.D. Gough, and E.R. Poore, Doppler ultrasound
        method for detecting human fetal breathing in utero, Brit. Med. J.
        2, 17 (1976).

(9) J.D. Gough and E.R. Poore, Directional Doppler measurements of foetal
        breathing, J. Physiol. 272, 12 P (1977).

(10) R. McHugh, W.N. McDicken, C.R. Bow, T. Anderson, and K. Boddy, An ultrasonic
        pulsed doppler instrument for monitoring human fetal breathing in
        utero, Ultrasound in Med. and Biol. 3, 381 (1978).

(11) R.S.G. M. Bots, G.H.B. Broeders, and D.J. Farman, The dynamics of human fetal
        breathing movements; a multiscan echofetographic approach, Eur. J.
        Obstet. Gynecol. Reprod. Biol. 6, 339 (1976).

(12) K. Lindström, K. Maršál, G. Gennser, L. Bengtsson, M. Benthin, and P. Dahl,
        Device for measurement of fetal breathing movements. - I. The TD-
        recorder. A new system for recording the distance between two echo-
        generating structures as a function of time, Ultrasound Med.
        Biol. 3, 143 (1977).

(13) K. Maršál, U. Ulmsten, and K. Lindström, Device for measurement of fetal
        breathing movements. II. Accuracy of in vitro measurements, filtering
        of output signals, and clinical application, Ultrasound Med. Biol.
        4, 13 (1978).

(14) Maršál, K. (1977) Ultrasonic measurements of fetal breathing movements in
        man, Thesis, Malmö.

(15) E. Agostoni, A. Taglietti, A. Ferrario Agostoni, and I. Setmikar, Mechanical
        aspects of the first breath, J. Appl. Physiol. 13, 344 (1958).

(16) H.C. Miller and F.C. Behrle, Respiratory patterns in newborn infants as de-
        termined by airflow and pneumographic studies, Pediatrics 10, 272
        (1952).

(17) R. Knill, W. Andrews, A.C. Bryan, and M.H. Bryan, Respiratory load compensa-
        tion in infants, J. Appl. Physiol. 40, 357 (1976).

(19) R. Knill and A.C. Bryan, An intercostal-phrenic inhibitory reflex in human newborn infants, J. Appl. Physiol. 40, 352 (1976).

(20) R. Harding, P. Johnson, M.E. McClelland, C.W. McLeod, and P.L. Whyte, Laryngeal function during breathing and swallowing in foetal and newborn lambs, J. Physiol. 272, 14 P (1977).

(21) E.R. Poore, The relationship between fetal breathing movements as measured by thoracic pressure changes and the movement of the chest measured directly in vivo, Eskes, R. (1978) in Proceedings of the Fifth Conference on Fetal Breathing, Nijmegen.

(22) G.S. Dawes, H.E. Fox, B.M. Leduc, G.C. Liggins, and R.T. Richards, Respiratory movements and rapid eye movement sleep in the foetal lamb, J. Physiol. 220, 119 (1972).

(23) P.L. Wilds, Observations of intrauterine fetal breathing movements - A review, Am. J. Obstet Gynecol. 131, 315 (1978).

(24) J.H. Duenholter and J.A. Pritchard, Fetal respiration, quantitative measurements of amniotic fluid inspired near term by human and rhesus fetuses. Am. J. Obstet. Gynecol. 125, 306 (1976).

(25) L. Curzi-Dascalova and E. Plassart, Respiratory and motor events in sleeping infants: their correlation with thoracico-abdominal respiratory relationships, Early Human Development 2, 39 (1978).

(26) J. Patrick, R. Natale, and B. Richardson, Patterns of human fetal breathing activity at 34 to 35 weeks´ gestational age, Am. J. Obstet. Gynecol. 132, 507 (1978).

(27) F.J. Clark and C. von Euler, On the regulation of depth and rate of breathing, J. Physiol. 222, 267 (1972).

(28) A. Olinsky, M.H. Bryan, and A.C. Bryan, Influence of lung inflation on respiratory control in neonates, J. Appl. Physiol. 36, 426 (1974).

(29) R. Knill and A.C. Bryan, An intercostal-phrenic inhibitory reflex in human newborn infants, J. Appl. Physiol. 40, 352 (1976).

(30) E.E. Decima, C. von Euler, and U. Thoden, Intercostal to phrenic reflexes in the spinal cat, Acta Physiol. Scand. 75, 568 (1969).

(31) J.E. Remmers, Inhibition of respiratory activity by intercostal muscle afferents, Respiration Physiol. 10, 358 (1970).

(32) J. Stagg and G. Gennser, Electronic analysis of foetal breathing movements: A practical application of phase-lock-loop principles, J. Med. Engin. Technol. 2, 246 (1978).

(33) M.K.S. Hathorn, Analysis of periodic changes in ventilation in new-born infants, J. Physiol. 285, 85 (1978).

(34) J.C. Fouron, Y. Korcaz, and B. Leduc, Cardiovascular changes associated with fetal breathing, Am. J. Obstet. Gynecol. 123, 868 (1975).

(35) I. Timor-Tritsch, I. Zador, R.H. Hertz, and M.G. Rosen, Human fetal respira-
     tory arrhythmia, Am. J. Obstet. Gynecol. 127, 662 (1977).

(36) T. Wheeler, G. Gennser, A.J. Murrills, and R. Lindvall, Combined recordings
     of fetal breathing and fetal heart rate in the human, Proc. Fifth
     Conf. Fetal Breathing, p. 37, Nijmegen (1978).

(37) J. Patrick, R. Natale, and B. Richardson, Patterns of human fetal breathing
     activity at 34 to 35 week's gestational age, Am. J. Obstet. Gynecol.
     132, 507 (1978).

(38) P.J. Lewis, B.J. Trudinger, and J. Mangez, Effect of maternal glucose inge-
     stion on fetal breathing and body movements in late pregnancy, Brit.
     J. Obstet. Gynaecol., 85, 86 (1978).

(39) R. Natale, J. Patrick, and B. Richardson, Effects of human maternal venous
     plasma glucose concentrations on fetal breathing movements, Am. J.
     Obstet. Gynecol. 132, 36 (1978).

(40) I.E. Timor-Tritsch, LeR. J. Dierker, R.H. Hertz, N.C. Deagan, and M.G. Rosen,
     Studies on antepartum behavioral state in the human fetus at term,
     Am. J. Obstet. Gynecol. 132, 524 (1978).

(41) H.F.R. Prechtl, The behavioural states of the newborn infant, A review,
     Brain Res. 76, 185 (1974).

NON-CHEMICAL FACTORS IN THE CONTROL OF BREATHING IN PATIENTS WITH PULMONARY DISORDERS

M. D. ALTOSE, N. S. CHERNIACK, B. GOTHE, S. G. KELSEN
and N. WOLKOVE

*Case Western Reserve University, Cleveland, Ohio and University of Pennsylvania,
Philadelphia, Pennsylvania, U.S.A.*

INTRODUCTION

Arterial blood gas tensions can differ considerably in patients with pulmonary disorders of apparently similar severity. Variations among individuals in the sensitivity of the respiratory chemoreceptors may in part account for these differences. This is based on the findings that patients with blunted ventilatory responses are more likely than those with brisk responses to develop alveolar hypoventilation when the mechanical properties of the ventilatory apparatus are deranged (1,2). However, the observations that arterial blood gas tensions may be normal in individuals with only minimal ventilatory responses to hypoxia and hypercapnia suggest that other, presumably non-chemical stimuli arising, for example, from the excitation of thoracic mechanoreceptors may also play a role in maintaining alveolar ventilation at appropriate levels (3,4).

The assessment of non-chemical factors in the control of breathing is complicated by the lack of clear delineation of the specific receptors and of neural pathways. Consequently, indirect methods must be employed. In the present study, this has been accomplished by examining the effects of mechanical ventilatory loading. The effects on respiratory motor output have been evaluated from changes in ventilation and occlusion pressure, i.e., the force generated by the contraction of the inspiratory muscles against a closed airway. The sensations produced by ventilatory loading have been quantitated using the psychophysical techniques of magnitude estimation and just noticeable differences to assess the effects on mechanoreceptor excitability and afferent activity.

METHODS

Studies were performed on normal subjects and in patients with asthma and chronic obstructive lung disease. They ranged in age from 21 to 62 years. The patients with chronic obstructive lung disease all complained of exertional dyspnea, cough and expectoration. The asthmatics had experienced episodes of wheezing and had demonstrated at least a 15 per cent increase in forced expiratory volume in one second after the inhalation of isoproterenol. Some of the asthmatics and all of the patients with chronic obstructive lung disease had reduction in forced expiratory volume in one second and elevations of airway resistance at the time of the study.

Mechanical ventilatory loads of several different types were employed. Airflow resistance was increased by adding fine mesh screen discs to the inspiratory and/or the expiratory lines of the breathing circuit. Elastic loading was

389

achieved by having the subjects breathe from rigid containers. Selective restriction of either rib cage or abdominal movement was produced by securing rigid restraints anteriorly and posteriorly at the mid-thoracic or mid-abdominal levels, respectively.

The effects of ventilatory loading were assessed both during progressive hypercapnia and progressive hypoxia produced by rebreathing techniques so that respiratory responses during mechanical loading could be compared to those under control conditions at the same level of chemical drive (5).

Ventilation was determined by electrical integration of the flow signal from a pneumotachygraph and the occlusion pressure was determined from the moutn pressure 100 ms after the onset of an inspiratory effort against a closed airway. Considerations regarding the use of occlusion pressure to assess respiratory motor activity have been described previously (6,7).

The perception of changes in airflow resistance was assessed by determining just noticeable differences and from magnitude estimation. Just noticeable differences i.e., the threshold change in airflow resistance required for detection was measured with the subjects breathing quietly through a circuit consisting of a mouthpiece and a low-resistance one-way valve. Randomly, small flow-resistances of different magnitudes were added to the inspiratory side of the circuit. Each resistance was applied at least six times. Subjects signalled whenever the added resistance was detected. The smallest added resistance detected during half of the presentations was referred to as the just noticeable difference. Just noticeable differences were also determined after the baseline resistance of the circuit was increased by the application of additional loads to the inspiratory line.

Studies of magnitude estimation involved the quantitation of the sensations produced by breathing against a series of easily detectable flow-resistive loads. A series of flow-resistive loads ranging from 6 to 72 $cmH_2O/L/s$ were employed. Subjects were made to breathe against one of the loads of intermediate severity and to assign arbitrarily a number based on their perception of the severity of the load. This served as a reference. Next, each of the remaining loads was randomly applied to the inspiratory line and the subjects assigned a numerical value to each load according to their estimate of the magnitude of the resistance based on the value given to the reference load.

RESULTS

Effects of Ventilatory Loading on Respiratory Motor Activity in Normal Subjects

Resistive loading of inspiration reduces the ventilatory responses to both hypercapnia and hypoxia in normal subjects. However, the occlusion pressure responses rise, an alteration not explained by changing chemical drive. Since inspiratory flow-resistive loading does not alter functional residual capacity and presumably does not affect resting inspiratory muscle length, the increased occlusion pressure seems to reflect an elevated respiratory motor output. Figure 1 illustrates the effects of inspiratory flow-resistive loading on occlusion pressure response. The occlusion pressure increases proportionally with progressive hypercapnia. The values for occlusion pressure (P_{100}) at any given P_{CO_2} and the slope of the occlusion pressure response are greater with an added inspiratory flow-resistive load (interrupted line) then during free rebreathing (solid line).

The magnitude of the increase in occlusion pressure during both flow-resistive and elastic loading varies considerably among subjects. At any level of chemical

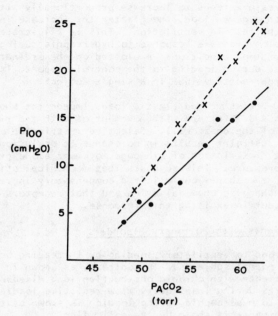

Fig. 1. Effects of inspiratory loading on occlusion pressure.

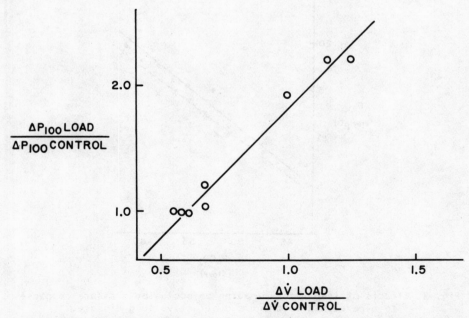

Fig. 2. Relationship between changes in ventilatory and occlusion pressure
responses during inspiratory loading.

drive, the occlusion pressure tends to increase proportionally with the severity
of the load. Also, with a given load, the greater the increase in occlusion
pressure, the smaller the fall in ventilation. This is illustrated in Fig. 2.
The ratio of the occlusion pressure response to hypercapnia during flow-resistive
loading to that under control conditions is plotted on the ordinate. The ratio of
the ventilatory response during loading to the control response is shown on the
abscissa. Each point represents values in a single subject.

Externally applied flow-resistive and elastic loads impede the shortening of all
the respiratory muscles and interfere with movement of both the rib cage and
abdominal compartments of the chest wall. Selective restriction of abdominal
movement by a physical restraint results in no change in occlusion pressure
responses. In contrast, restriction of rib cage movement alone produces an
increase in occlusion pressure. This suggests that mechanical stimuli even when
limited to only part of the thorax can elicit a compensatory increase in respiratory output not due to changing chemical drive and that receptors in the rib cage
may be particularly potent in exciting this response.

Motor Responses in Patients with Pulmonary Disorders

Asthmatic patients respond to ventilatory loading by increasing occlusion pressure
in a manner similar to normal subjects. In contrast, as shown in Fig. 3, in a
typical individual, patients with chronic obstructive lung disease do not increase
their occlusion pressures during inspiratory flow-resistive loading. The occlusion pressure response to hypercapnia during loading is shown by the interrupted
line and the control response is shown by the solid line.

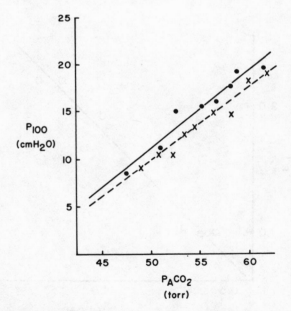

Fig. 3. Effects of inspiratory loading on occlusion pressure responses
to hypercapnia in chronic obstructive lung disease.

Hyperinflation of the thorax in chronic obstructive lung disease and the resulting decrease in resting inspiratory muscle length place the inspiratory muscles at
a mechanical disadvantage and could interfere with the ability of those muscles to

contract forcibly, thus preventing the occlusion pressure from increasing during ventilatory loading. That this is not the case is suggested by the observations that an acute increase in the end-expiratory level in normal subjects produced by an expiratory resistance fails to affect the normal response to mechanical loading.

The differences in the responses of the asthmatic whose airway obstruction is episodic and of the patients with chronic obstructive lung disease whose airway disease is permanent and relatively fixed raises the possibility that chronic persistent elevations in airway resistance blunt the responses to mechanical loading much as chronic elevations in CO_2 tension decrease the respiratory responses to hypercapnia. Impaired respiratory compensation during ventilatory loading could result if chronically disordered lung function were to interfere with mechanoreceptor activation.

The importance of the sensory effects of mechanical loading on the respiratory responses is suggested by the findings that the increase in the occlusion pressure during ventilatory loading in healthy man and in animals is abolished by general anesthesia (9,10). To further evaluate these sensory effects, the conscious perception of mechanical loads was examined.

Perception of Changes in Airflow Resistance

In normal subjects the just noticeable difference in airflow resistance increases proportionally with increases in the baseline resistance. The baseline resistance was determined from the sum of the resistance of the breathing circuit and the subject's own airway resistance. As the resistance of breathing circuit is increased, larger changes in airflow resistance are required for detection. However, the just noticeable difference expressed as a percentage of the baseline resistance (JND%) remains constant in a given subject over a wide range of baseline resistances, in accordance with the Weber-Fechner law (11). The JND% in normal subjects is approximately 20 per cent.

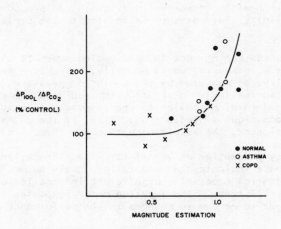

Fig. 4. Relationship between magnitude estimation and responsiveness to flow-resistive loading.

Asthmatic patients demonstrate an increased just noticeable difference. This can
be explained by their elevated airway resistance since the JND% is, in fact, no
different from that in normal individuals. In contrast, patients with chronic
obstructive lung disease exhibit elevations in just noticeable differences which
cannot be accounted for simply on the basis of increased airway resistance. In
the group of patients with chronic obstructive lung disease the just noticeable
differences in airflow resistance expressed as a percentage of the baseline
resistance was 49 ± SE 7%.

Similarly, the exponent for magnitude estimation of airflow resistance is the
same in normal subjects and in asthmatics, but is significantly lower in patients
with chronic obstructive lung disease further indicating an impaired sensory
effect of easily detectable ventilatory loads.

That changes in respiratory output during ventilatory loading are related to the
sensory effects of the load itself is suggested by the findings that normal subjects and asthmatics with the highest exponents for magnitude estimation and the
lowest just noticeable differences in airflow resistance exhibit the greatest
increases in occlusion pressure during inspiratory loading while the patients
with lower exponents for magnitude estimation and higher just noticeable differences demonstrate little change in occlusion pressure response during loading.
The relationship between the exponent for magnitude estimation of airflow resistance and the change in occlusion pressure responses to hypercapnia during inspiratory flow-resistive loading is illustrated in Fig. 4.

DISCUSSION

In anesthetized animals, respiratory mechanoreceptor stimulation affects the
level and pattern of ventilation and the respiratory responses to chemical
stimuli (12,13,14). These findings suggest that the activity of receptors in the
lung and chest wall play a role in ventilatory control and in the maintenance of
normal levels of alveolar ventilation.

The present study, using external ventilatory loads to excite respiratory mechanoreceptor activity indicates that changes in the mechanical characteristics of the
breathing apparatus in healthy conscious individuals can produce an increase in
respiratory motor activity that seems to be related to the sensations produced by
ventilatory loading.

The respiratory responses during ventilatory loading resemble the responses to
hypercapnia and hypoxia in several ways. Normally, there is a progressive increase
in respiratory activity, as measured by the occlusion pressure, with graded ventilatory loads which increasingly interfere with respiratory movements. The
responses to mechanical loading similar to the responses to chemical stimulation
are diminished in unconscious subjects (10). Also, if the mechanical stimulation
is persistent and prolonged, the respiratory responses become blunted.

The studies of sensory perception of ventilatory loads in patients with chronic
obstructive lung disease indicate that adaptation involving mechanoreceptor
activity and/or the central processing of afferent information occurs with chronic
elevations in airway resistance. The impaired motor responses to ventilatory
loading does not appear to be due to changes in the performance of the respiratory muscles alone.

In normal individuals, occlusion pressure increases if rib cage movement is
selectively restricted. If adaptation were to occur, it would be expected that
this increased response would not be seen during chronic rib cage restriction.
In fact in two patients with rheumatoid spondylitis thus far examined who have

chronically restricted rib cage movement, the occlusion pressure responses to hypercapnia were not increased.

There is considerable evidence that depressed chemosensitivity can contribute to respiratory failure in patients with lung disease. For example, CO_2 retention during an acute attack of bronchospasm seems to occur only in those asthmatics with low ventilatory responses to hypercapnia (2). Also, children who develop hypercapnia because of upper airway obstruction produced by hypertrophied adenoids demonstrate blunted CO_2 responses even after the adenoids are removed (1). Depressed mechanoreceptor sensitivity could also conceivably lead to respiratory failure. This, however, is difficult to demonstrate since chemical drive itself is sufficient to maintain ventilation in most individuals.

We have recently studied five patients with normal lung function but with sub-normal ventilatory responses to hypoxia and hypercapnia (4). Three of the patients while at rest had normal arterial oxygen and carbon dioxide tensions while the other two had resting arterial hypercapnia and hypoxemia. Mechanore-ceptor function was evaluated from the ability of the patients to estimate and to produce specified changes in their own tidal volume. In the patients with alveo-lar hypoventilation, breathing was more irregular, with much wider variation in tidal volume. Also, the accuracy of producing tidal volumes of specified sizes and of estimating the volumes of breaths produced by different degrees of volun-tary effort was markedly impaired. In those individuals with depressed chemo-sensitivity, a concommitant impairment in mechanoreceptor function may indeed result in alveolar hypoventilation and respiratory failure.

The methods for assessing mechanoreceptor function are indirect but probably no more indirect than are the methods for evaluating chemosensitivity. Certainly, external ventilatory loads are not strictly comparable to lung disease in affect-ing pulmonary mechanical function. Also, it is difficult to separate the psycho-logical effects of ventilatory loading from the specific effects on mechanore-ceptor activity.

The present study, however, has shown that the mechanical alterations of the ventilatory apparatus can produce substantial respiratory responses and suggests that abnormalities in the non-chemical control of breathing may be important in the development of respiratory failure.

REFERENCES

(1) R. H. Ingram and B. J. Bishop, Ventilatory responses to carbon dioxide after removal of chronic upper airway obstruction. Am. Rev. Resp. Dis. 102, 645 (1970).

(2) A.S. Rebuck and J. Read, Patterns of ventilatory response to carbon dioxide during recovery from severe asthma, Clin. Sci. 41, 13 (1971).

(3) G.B. Irsigler, Carbon dioxide response lines in young adults: the limits of the normal response, Am. Rev. Respir. Dis. 114, 529 (1976).

(4) N. Wolkove, M.D. Altose, S.G. Kelsen and N.S. Cherniack, Chemical and neural mechanisms in alveolar hypoventilation, Clin. Res. 24, 291 A (1976).

(5) A.S. Rebuck, M. Kangalee, L.D. Pengelly and E. J. M. Campbell, Correlation of ventilatory responses to hypoxia and hypercapnia, J. Appl. Physiol. 35, 173 (1973).

(6) W.A. Whitelaw, J-Ph. Derenne and J. Milic-Emili, Occlusion pressure as a
     measure of respiratory center output in conscious man, Respir.
     Physiol. 23, 181 (1975).

(7) M.D. Altose, S.G. Kelsen, N.N. Stanley, R.S. Levinson, N.S. Cherniack and
     A.P. Fishman, Effects of hypercapnia on mouth pressure during airway
     occlusion in conscious man, J. Appl. Physiol. 40, 338 (1976).

(8) S.S. Stevens, On the psychophysical law, Psychol. Rev. 64, 153 (1957).

(9) G.D. Isaza, J.D. Posner, M.D. Altose, S.G. Kelsen and N.S. Cherniack,
     Airway occlusion pressure in awake and anesthetized goats, Respir.
     Physiol. 27, 87 (1976).

(10) W.A. Whitelaw, J-Ph. Derenne, J. Couture and J. Milic-Emili, J. Appl.
     Physiol. 41, 285 (1976).

(11) Schiffman, H.R. (1976) Sensation and Perception: an integrated approach,
     Wiley, New York.

(12) E.J.M. Campbell, C.J. Dickinson and J.B.L. Howell, The immediate effects of
     added loads on the inspiratory musculature of the rabbit, J. Physiol.
     (London) 172:321 (1964).

(13) M.D. Altose, N.N. Stanley, N.S. Cherniack and A.P. Fishman, The effects of
     mechanical loading and hypercapnia on the inspiratory muscle EMG,
     J. Appl. Physiol. 38, 467 (1975).

(14) S.G. Kelsen, M.D. Altose, N.N. Stanley, R.S. Levinson, N.S. Cherniack and
     A.P. Fishman, Electromyographic response of respiratory muscles during
     elastic loading, Am. J. Physiol. 230, 675 (1976).

DISCUSSION

Cherniack was asked about his view on the nature of the afferent information underlying the sensations and respiratory responses of his patients and whether the cerebral cortex might be involved both in terms of awareness of the loads and in terms of providing a cortical drive to the respiratory control system which would embrace also the motor response to added loads. Cherniack replied that a cortical component is certainly present both in normal breathing at rest and in the responses to loads and to CO_2 and that this cortical component is part of the normal response. The receptors which provide the cortex with the necessary information about changes in respiratory mechanics and reflex   drives are probably not only those situated in the ribcage and the respiratory muscles. Also the receptors in the lungs seem to be of importance in this respect. This was suggested by the experiments employing bronchoconstricting agents. The results of these experiments had shown that for the same change in airway resistance a bronchoconstricting agent caused a larger change in occlusion pressure than did a change in external resistance.

THE PATTERNS OF CHANGE OF TIDAL VOLUME AND OF INSPIRATORY AND EXPIRATORY TIME DURING STEP CHANGES OF ALVEOLAR P_{CO_2} AND/OR P_{O_2}

W. N. GARDNER, D. J. C. CUNNINGHAM and E. S. PETERSEN

University Laboratory of Physiology, Oxford, U.K.

When a man or anaesthetized animal rebreathes from a confined space, the ventilation increases as the inspiratory gas composition changes. If hypoxia predominates, and thus stimulation comes mainly from the arterial chemoreceptors, the pattern of response involves more change of respiratory frequency than when most of the stimulation comes from the intracranial chemoreceptors: in the second case the emphasis is on change of tidal volume (e.g. Haldane, Meakins & Priestley (1) and, recently, Rebuck, Rigg & Saunders (2)). There is a corresponding distinction between the primary responses to sudden de-activation of the two groups of chemoreceptors (Hanson, Nye & Torrance (3)), and also to their separate activation in paralyzed animals, i.e., even in the total absence of lung movements (Cherniack, Kelsen & Lahiri (4)). It follows that volume feedback from the lungs and chest wall is not essential for the difference to be manifest, and, furthermore, that the two sets of chemoreceptors are capable of influencing different parts of the central neural apparatus along more or less separate afferent pathways within the central nervous system.

On the other hand, when a steady hyperpnoea has become established, any one level of ventilation comprises the same combination of mean tidal volume (V_T) and mean breath duration (T_T) and its constituent inspiratory and expiratory components T_I and T_E whether the drives are from one or the other set of chemoreceptors or from both, or, for that matter, from exercise. This phenomenon first became apparent in the 1950's, and is now well established. Figure 1, from data of Cunningham & Gardner (5), shows V_T plotted against T_I and T_E (the latter extends leftward from the origin) during steady states of hyperpnoea driven by hypercapnia in high oxygen (open symbols) and by hypercapnia in hypoxia (filled symbols): the two sets

of points are intermingled. The same is true of the points representing the
steady states in the experiments on three new subjects to be described below.

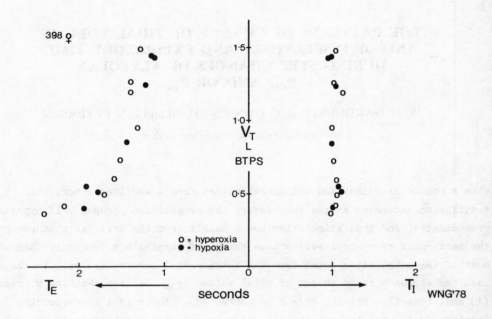

Fig. 1. Steady-state relations between mean tidal volume V_T
and mean inspiratory and expiratory durations T_I, T_E.

It appears that something occurs between the onset of the change in the drive and
the subsequent steady state, and it is this transition that has now been studied.
Step changes of drive, involving mainly intra-cranial and/or mainly arterial
chemoreceptors, have been imposed repeatedly on each subject and the average time
courses of the approaches to the steady states have been determined. The findings
have already appeared in abstracts (6, 7).

In nearly all earlier work of this kind the step changes have been of <u>inspiratory</u>
gas composition, and much of the analysis of the results has been concerned with
the slow washing in of the fresh gas mixtures to the alveoli, the rate of which
itself depends upon the simultaneously developing hyperpnoea. The present work
has been concerned with step changes of <u>alveolar</u> gas composition. These are
technically difficult to execute and success depends upon well practised

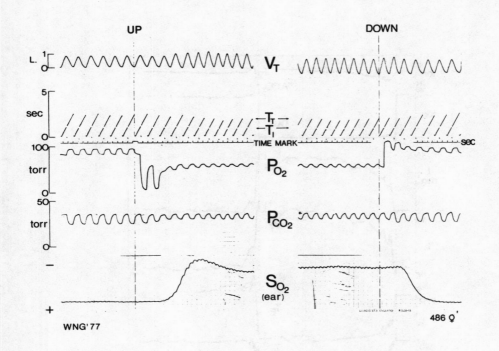

Fig. 2. Specimen experimental record of isocapnic hypoxic
steps of drive up and down. From above downwards,
(1) inspiratory-expiratory volumes (pneumotachograph);
(2) voltage-time ramp, re-set at onset, and interrupted at
end of, inspiration; (3) time, sec.; (4 and 5), P_{O_2} and
P_{CO_2} at mouth (mass spectrometer, transit delay ~ 1 sec)
(6) uncalibrated high-gain ear oximeter record, desaturation
upwards.

manipulation of inspiratory gases. The analysis of the results is, however, much
more straightforward. Figure 2 illustrates single steps of drive up and down
(P_{A,O_2} down and up), P_{A,CO_2} in this case being held constant. On the step up of
drive the initial fall of P_{A,O_2} was induced quickly by two inspirates of O_2-free
gas followed by a gradual approach from below to what would become the steady
inspiratory P_{O_2}. Meanwhile, inspiratory P_{CO_2} was gradually and slightly
increased in anticipation of the hypocapnia that would otherwise have accompanied

the respiratory response to hypoxia. The "steady state" at 7 – 8 min served as the starting point of the next down-step of drive.

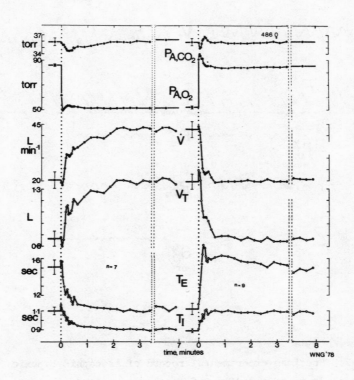

Fig. 3. Mean results on one subject of isocapnic hypoxic steps. Bars on control points indicate ± 2 S.E.M.

Between 7 and 13 such steps in each direction, in which the time profiles of the alveolar gas were satisfactory, were analysed and averaged for each subject. A typical time plot, averaged for all the isocapnic hypoxic steps on one subject, is shown in Fig. 3: from above downward are shown the alveolar P_{CO_2} and P_{O_2}, inspiratory ventilation $\dot{V}$, V_T, T_E and T_I. All 1st, 2nd, ... $\underline{i}$th breaths were averaged up to 30 sec and then the averages ran over longer periods. V_T, after a latent period of one respiratory cycle, moved smoothly towards its final value with a half time of about 10 sec. T_I followed a slower time course but the change in it was small. Changes in T_E were considerable, and on the step down of drive there was a large overshoot which lasted for 3 – 4 min, the final value being

approached from above. This unexpected pattern of T_E was seen in all 3 subjects.
Undershoot was not apparent in the up step.

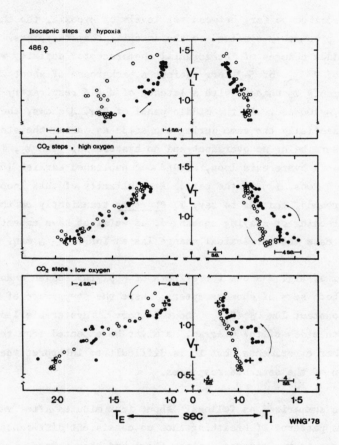

Fig. 4. Relations between V_T, T_I and T_E during the three
types of transition between steady states. Bars denote
4 x average S.E.M. for the nearest set of points. This
subject also shows clear breaks between ranges 1 and 2.

Such changes are easily appreciated on the V_T, T_I, T_E plot. Figure 4 shows
averaged figures for one subject with T_E again plotted leftwards from the origin.
The crosses (some of them obscured by points) are the steady states, the filled
circles are the averaged single breaths of the up steps and the open circles are
the averaged single breaths of the down steps. The data of Fig. 3 appear in the

top panel. Note that the V_T, T_I relation in these hypoxic steps is the same in both directions; the marked overshoot shown by T_E in Fig. 3 appears here as a substantial hysteresis loop.

In the steps described so far, between two levels of hypoxia, the change of stimulation was presumably confined to the arterial chemoreceptors. The responses to sudden changes of intracranial chemoreceptor activity were studied by imposing steps of P_{A,CO_2} of 5-7 torr against a background of about 200 torr O_2. In these experiments V_T changed with a latency of 4 - 5 respiratory cycles and a half time of 40 - 100 sec. As the middle panel of Fig. 4 shows, the V_T, T_E relation was essentially the same during the steps as during the steady state (cf. Fig. 1), there being no overshoot and no hysteresis. The V_T, T_I plot, on the other hand, shows a hysteresis loop, as did one published earlier (6; cf. Bradley, Euler, Marttila & Roos, (8) in the cat). A peculiarity of this loop is that it is the "wrong way round", that is to say, T_I shortens transiently on the downstep instead of lengthening or staying unchanged, as we might have expected, and vice versa. In this case the paradoxical change lasted for 1.5 - 3 min.

The bottom panel of Fig. 4 shows the effects of applying sudden change of stimulation to both sets of chemoreceptors; here the steps were of CO_2 against a background of constant low O_2 (P_{A,O_2} about 50 torr). Hysteresis loops can be discerned on both sides of the diagram, as might be expected from the results shown in the other experiments, but it is difficult to interpret the results as a simple summation of the separate responses.

This work may be summarised as follows. About four minutes after various kinds of step change, the patterns of breathing show no consistent differences; in the same subjects, one to two minutes earlier there had been substantial differences in pattern that were highly dependent on the nature of the change of stimulus.

It seems that something similar may occur in exercise, though results in the literature are rather scattered. Changes of frequency are often more prominent than changes of tidal volume at the onset of exercise and of recovery from it (9; 10; 11; 12). In the steady state, however, the V_T, T_I, T_E relations in exercise are essentially the same as in hyperpnoea at rest (13; 14).

DISCUSSION

There thus appear to be separate afferent pathways for different kinds of
stimulation, each producing its characteristic pattern of immediate response.
However, it looks as if some co-ordinating mechanism soon comes into operation;
over a period of some 3 - 4 min it imposes a straitjacket on the mean pattern such
that the early differences disappear.

The mean steady-state pattern selected is highly characteristic of the individual,
and its parameters are well correlated with CO_2 and hypoxia sensitivities (13; 15;
16;   17) and with other anthropometric quantities (15).

The criteria on which the mean pattern is selected have received sporadic
attention for many years from, for example, Röhrer, Otis, Fenn, Rahn, Mead and
Priban, to mention only a few. As Professor Grodins has told us here and elsewhere, it is still not clear what these criteria are, but they seem to be related
to the optimization of the energy cost of breathing and possibly also of gas
exchange.

Our results raise the possibility that the generation of individual breaths is
separate from a second, longer-term controller that monitors the performance of
the system within a wider frame of reference. In a system that has to tolerate
the gross short-term interruptions of rhythm imposed by the vagaries of everyday
life, a separate element of control working on a longer time scale and involving
averaging might be advantageous. There has been little experimental evidence
besides our own bearing on this possibility, but the methods used at present for
studying cat brainstem neurophysiology are not of the kind that would provide such
evidence. However, Hämäläinen & Viljanen (18) have published a model that seems
to echo some features of our own results; it embodies a two-tier hierarchical
control of patterning, the lower concerned with air-flow patterns (expiration
being independent), and the higher concerned with driving pressures, volumes and
times. It remains to be seen whether this model, or another like it, can form the
basis for making experimentally testable predictions.

This work was supported by the Medical Research Council.

REFERENCES

(1) J. S. Haldane, J. C. Meakins & J. G. Priestley,   The respiratory response to anoxaemia, J. Physiol. 52, 420 (1919).

(2) A. S. Rebuck, J. R. A. Rigg & N. A. Saunders, Respiratory frequency response to progressive isocapnic hypoxia, J. Physiol. 258, 19 (1976).

(3) M. Hanson, P. C. G. Nye & R. W. Torrance, Convergence of hypoxia and hypercapnia (this symposium).

(4) N. S. Cherniack, S. G. Kelsen & S. Lahiri, The effects of hypoxia and hypercapnia on central nervous system output. In Respiratory Adaptations, Capillary Exchange and Reflex Mechanisms, pp.312-324. Ed. Paintal, A. S. & Gill-Kumar, P.   V. Patel Chest Inst., Delhi (1977)

(5) D. J. C. Cunningham & W. N. Gardner, The relation between tidal volume and inspiratory and expiratory times during steady-state CO_2 inhalation in man, J. Physiol. 227, 50 (1972).

(6) W. N. Gardner, The pattern of breathing following step changes of alveolar P_{CO_2} in man, J. Physiol. 242, 75P (1974).

(7) W. N. Gardner, The pattern of human respiratory response to step change of P_{A,O_2}, J. Physiol. 275, 33P (1978).

(8) G. W. Bradley, C. von Euler, I. Marttila & B. Roos, Transient and steady-state effects of CO_2 on mechanisms determining rate and depth of breathing, Acta physiol. scand. 92, 341 (1974).

(9) P. Dejours, Control of respiration in muscular exercise, In Handbook of Physiology - Respiration I, pp.631-648. Ed. Fenn, W. O. & Rahn, H. Amer. Physiol. Soc., Washington, D.C.

(10) D. J. C. Cunningham, B. B. Lloyd & D. Spurr, The relationship between the increase in breathing during the first respiratory cycle in exercise and the prevailing background of chemical stimulation, J. Physiol. 185, 73P (1966).

(11) W. L. Beaver & K. Wasserman, Tidal volume and respiratory rate changes at start and end of exercise, J. appl. Physiol. 29, 872 (1970).

(12) J. I. Jensen, H. Vejby-Christensen & E. S. Petersen, Ventilation in man at onset of work employing different standardized starting orders, Respir. Physiol. 13, 209 (1971).

(13) E. N. Hey, B. B. Lloyd, D. J. C. Cunningham, M. G. M. Jukes & D. P. G. Bolton, Effects of various respiratory stimuli on the depth and frequency of breathing in man, Respir. Physiol. 1, 193 (1966).

(14) J. D. S. Kay, E. Strange Petersen & H. Vejby-Christensen, Mean and breath-by-breath pattern of breathing in man during steady-state exercise, J. Physiol. 251, 657 (1975).

(15) J. M. Patrick & A. Howard, The influence of age, sex, body size and lung size on the control and pattern of breathing during CO_2 inhalation in Caucasians. Respir. Physiol. 16, 337 (1972).

(16) D. J. C. Cunningham & W. N. Gardner, A quantitative description of the
       pattern of breathing during steady-state CO_2 inhalation in man, with
       special emphasis on expiration, J. Physiol. 272, 613 (1977).

(17) E. Strange Petersen & H. Vejby-Christensen, Effects of body temperature on
       ventilatory response to hypoxia and breathing pattern in man, J. appl.
       Physiol. 42, 492 (1977).

(18) R. P. Hämäläinen & A. A. Viljanen, A hierarchical goal-seeking model of the
       control of breathing, Biol. Cybernetics 29, 151 & 159 (1978).

DISCUSSION

Eldridge suggested that the after-discharge phenomena might be of
significance for the results on timing now presented by Cunningham.
Although he had not made any specific studies of the on- and off-
time constants of the stimulus and post-stimulus effects on T_I, T_E
and breath duration, he stated that not only the peak phrenic amplitudes but also the rate of rise of phrenic activity and breath duration were involved in these kinds of stimulus and post-stimulus
effects.

Cunningham replied that afterdischarge might play a significant
role. He based this view on the considerable difference in off-
transients between the afferent neural activity from the arterial
chemoreceptors, as judged from published records and the effects on
$\dot{V}$ and V_T obtained in their own experiments involving hypoxic stimuli.

RESPIRATORY PATTERN OF HUMAN SUBJECTS DURING HYPOXIA, HYPERCAPNIA OR CHANGES IN THE LEVEL OF WAKEFULNESS

H. GAUTIER

Laboratoire de Physiologie, Faculté de Médecine Saint-Antoine,
75012 Paris, France

This paper reviews some data which have been obtained by us several years ago in a study concerning the analysis of variables which characterize the human spirogram during specific (hypoxia or hypercapnia) and non-specific respiratory stimulations inducing arousal (attention tests) (1). The purpose of the above experiments was to investigate whether the model proposed for the control of respiration based on results obtained in animals during both hypercapnia and stimulation of the supra-pontine reticular formation (2) could also be applied to humans. Although the results obtained in men were slightly different from those observed in cats, it was nevertheless confirmed that in the both species breathing pattern was differently affected depending on the nature of the stimulus. These results are further analyzed in the present paper, taking into account the model for the genesis and control of respiratory activity recently proposed by von Euler (3).

METHODS

Three groups of young, healthy subjects (most of them medical students) participated in the experiments. The first group of nine subjects was subjected to both hypoxia (FI_{O2} = 0.12) and hypercapnia (FI_{CO2} = 0.03), the ventilation ($\dot{V}_E$) being increased by about 30 % with both stimuli. The second group of six subjects was subjected to hypercapnia (FI_{CO2} = 0.12) or to attention tests. The latter consisted in counting mentally, as fast as possible, a given letter or a sequence of letters (*e.g.* "e" following a consonant and preceding a vowel) in a text written in a foreign language. During the attention tests, ventilation increased approximatively 20 % and the level of hypercapnia was chosen to match for the increase in ventilation. The third group of five subjects was subjected to two different attention tests. The first was identical to that described above. The other consisted in drawing circles on a X-Y recorder by operating a pair of knobs. In humans, these tests elicit changes in the electro-encephalogram, spinal reflexes, heart rate and galvanic skin response identical to those observed in animals during reticular stimulation (4). Since Winkler (5), it is also known that attention results in consistent changes in the breathing pattern.

All specific and non-specific stimulations lasted three minutes, during which period a steady-state in the ventilatory response was always observed. The tests were repeated 6 to 10 times, separated by control periods. The 10 respiratory cycles preceding the test and the last 10 cycles of the test were measured and averaged. The changes in ventilation elicited by all the above tests were barely sensed by the subjects.

RESULTS AND DISCUSSION

The breathing pattern is differently modified by specific respiratory stimuli (increase in tidal volume with relatively small changes in respiratory phase durations) as compared to non-specific respiratory stimuli (decrease in tidal volume with large decreases in phase durations) (Fig. 1). The breathing pattern is also differently modified by hypoxia (decrease in T_I and T_E) as compared to hypercapnia (decrease in T_E only).

The different response patterns of the spirogram result obviously from different inputs to the respiratory center :

With hypercapnia, respiratory stimulation originates in the peripheral and central chemoreceptors. An increase in the mean inspiratory flow ($\bar{V}_I = V_T/T_I$) and therefore in V_T is observed, since T_I does not change significantly, at least in the range of stimulations used in the present study. The relative contributions from peripheral and central chemoreceptors to the observed hypercapnic response is unknown.

With hypoxia, a peripheral component due to stimulation of the arterial chemoreceptors is associated with a central component which causes a depression of respiratory activity (6). From animal studies, it seems that this depression affects mainly the mean inspiratory flow (7). The net effect of these opposing actions results in an increase in mean inspiratory flow causing an increased V_T in spite of a shortening of T_I. In addition, there is a decrease in T_E which is more marked than with hypercapnia. The differing effects of hypoxia, as compared to hypercapnia, have already been reported in awake men (8, 9). Others workers, however, have described identical changes in V_T and breath duration, irrespective of the nature of the humoral stimulus (10).

With attention tests, a marked decrease in respiratory phase durations is observed. In spite of a consistent increase in the mean inspiratory flow, the decrease in T_I is associated with a marked reduction in V_T. Using these attention tests, considerable inter-individual variability in response is noted. Of course, the stimulation is less easily quantifiable and the response is less predictable than with hypercapnia or hypoxia, because in attention tests the response depends, among other factors, on the motivation of the subject to comply with the instructions given by the experimenter. During specific respiratory stimulation, a change in ventilation (especially in alveolar ventilation) is made necessary in order to limit the possible modifications of the *milieu intérieur* by the various inhaled gas mixtures. During changes in the level of consciousness, on the other hand, the modifications in ventilation are not essential for the homeostasis of the body. In fact, because of the peculiar breathing pattern observed during attention tests (decrease in V_T and large increase in breathing frequency), the alveolar ventilation is barely modified in spite of an increase in the overall ventilation. It is of interest to note that the breathing pattern observed in humans during attention tests (decrease in respiratory phase durations without corresponding increase in tidal volume) is quite similar to that observed during hyperthermia in lightly anesthetized cats (11) or during passive limb movements in anesthetized dogs and rabbits (12). These experiments have in common an increase in ventilation caused by non-humoral respiratory stimuli.

Although there are considerable inter-individual differences in the response of
the breathing pattern to attention tests, in any given individual the response
is rather reproducible. It is of interest to note that during attention tests,
the magnitude of the response of any given variable appears to be closely related
to its absolute control value ; the greater the control value, the larger the

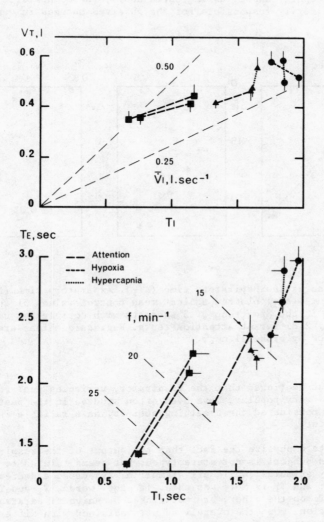

Fig. 1. Tidal volume (V_T) plotted against inspiratory time (T_I), (upper
         panel) and expiratory time (T_E) plotted against T_I, (lower panel).
         Thin dashed lines represent the mean inspiratory flow ($\dot{V}_I$) in upper
         panel, and breathing frequency (f) in lower panel. Mean values
         (with standard error) are shown for 1st group of subjects (circles),
         2nd group (triangles) and 3rd group (squares).

modifications brought about by the stimulus (Fig. 2). This is especially true for T_I and T_E. These results are in agreement with the *law of initial value* (13) which applies to many biological variables. This law has already been verified in another study dealing with the changes in ventilation associated with short-lasting increases in the level of vigilance (14). Although an extensive analysis has as yet not been made, it appears that this law does not apply to the modifications of respiratory variables obtained during specific stimulations (hypoxia or hypercapnia) where, as indicated above, the homeostatic function of the body is primarily responsible for the observed changes in ventilation.

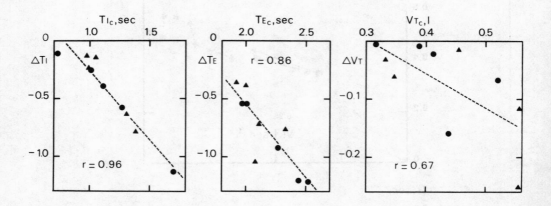

Fig. 2.   Mean changes in inspiratory time (ΔT_I), expiratory time (ΔT_E) and
          tidal volume (ΔV_T) plotted against mean control values of these
          variables in the 3rd group of 5 subjects with correlation coefficient
          (r) during 2 different attention tests. Regression lines are
          represented by broken lines.

Finally, it must be mentioned that the respiratory variables analyzed above, which are nowadays very popular, have been often studied in the past by psychologists who considered the breathing activity as a reliable index of changes in behaviour.

The present results emphasize the fact that the output of the respiratory center of the awake human subject is not stereotyped, but seems related to the nature of the respiratory stimulus. While all stimuli always cause a decrease in T_E, the response of V_T and T_I is more variable. In other words, V_T and T_I on the one hand, and T_I and T_E on the other, are not linked by univocal relationships (Fig. 1). In addition, when the overall results obtained with different stimuli are considered, it appears that two variables, namely *mean inspiratory flow* and *expiratory duration* are consistently affected in a similar manner, irrespective of the nature of the stimulus (Fig. 3). These two variables show an inverse relationship in most of the subjects, as confirmed also by a previous study during rebreathing with different gas mixtures (Fig. 4). In the latter study,

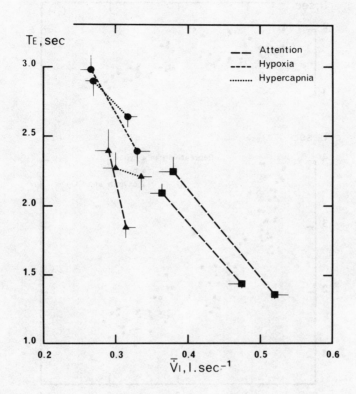

Fig. 3. Mean expiratory time (T_E) plotted against mean inspiratory flow
($\bar{V}_I = V_T/T_I$) in the 3 groups of subjects. Same symbols as in Fig. 1.

it was also observed that T_I does not consistently change, except at high
inspiratory flows, whereas T_E decreases steadily when inspiratory flow increases.
The fact that, in general, the V_T/T_I *vs* T_E relationship is not linear, does not
preclude the possibility of a causal relationship between these two variables.

The mean inspiratory flow represents an index of the recruitment of neurons
during inspiration or of the rate of rise of the *Central Inspiratory Activity
(CIA)*. It depends on the drives originating in the chemoreceptors or in the
reticular activating system. Expiratory duration, which represents an easily
monitored index of expiratory activity, is a variable which, probably is not
directly controlled *per se* by the respiratory center. It results from the
interaction of several as yet not too well quantified factors such as (a) the
braking effect of residual contraction of inspiratory muscles during the early

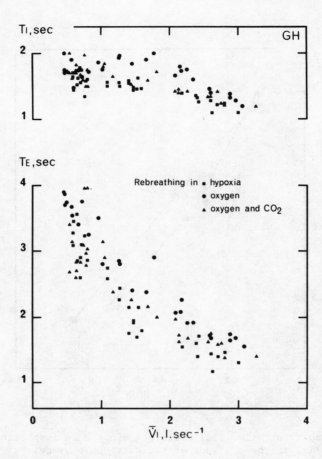

Fig. 4.   Inspiratory time (T_I) and expiratory time (T_E) of individual breaths
          plotted against mean inspiratory flow ($\bar{V}_I$) in a typical subject during
          rebreathing from a bag containing initially hypoxic mixture (F_{O2} = 0.14),
          oxygen or CO_2 (F_{CO2} = 0.07) in oxygen.

part of expiration, (b) the control of laryngeal resistances and (c) the
accelerating effect of expiratory muscle contraction (15, 16). Consequently,
the precise nature of the link between the mean inspiratory flow and the
expiratory duration remains highly speculative, and further work in both humans
and animals is clearly needed to elucidate this point.

Acknowledgement. The author is grateful Monique Bonora for her assistance in
carrying out experiments and preparation of the manuscript.

REFERENCES

(1) H. Gautier, Effets comparés de stimulations respiratoires spécifiques et de l'activité mentale sur la forme du spirogramme de l'homme, J. Physiol. 61, 31 (1969).

(2) M.I. Cohen and A. Hugelin, Supra-pontine reticular control of intrinsic respiratory mechanisms, Arch. Ital. Biol. 103, 317 (1965).

(3) C. von Euler, The functional organization of the respiratory phase-switching mechanisms, Fed. Proc. 36, 2375 (1977).

(4) A. Hugelin, Bodily changes during arousal, attention and emotion in Hockman, C.H. (1972) Limbic system mechanisms and autonomic function, Thomas, Springfield, p. 202.

(5) C. Winkler, Attention and respiration, Konink. Akad. Wetenschap. Amsterdam Proc. Section Sci. 1, 121 (1899).

(6) M.J. Miller and S.M. Tenney, Hyperoxic hyperventilation in carotid-deafferented cats, Respir. Physiol. 23, 23 (1975).

(7) H. Gautier and M. Bonora, Effects of carotid body denervation on respiratory pattern of awake cats, In preparation.

(8) J.S. Haldane, J.C. Meakins and J.G. Priestley, The respiratory response to anoxaemia, J. Physiol. 52, 420 (1919).

(9) A.S. Rebuck, J.R.A. Rigg and N.A. Saunders, Respiratory frequency response to progressive isocapnic hypoxia, J. Physiol. 258, 19 (1976).

(10) W.N. Gardner, D.J.C. Cunningham and E.S. Petersen, The patterns of change of tidal volume, and of inspiratory and expiratory time during step changes in alveolar P_{CO_2} and/or P_{O_2}, This Symposium.

(11) G.W. Bradley, C. von Euler, I. Marttila and B. Roos, Steady state effects of CO_2 and temperature on the relationship between lung volume and inspiratory duration (Hering-Breuer Threshold curve), Acta Physiol. Scand. 92, 351 (1974).

(12) E. Agostoni and E. D'Angelo, The effect of limb movements on the regulation of depth and rate of breathing, Respir. Physiol. 27, 33 (1976).

(13) J. Wilder (1967) Stimulus and response. The law of initial value, Wright, Bristol.

(14) H. Gautier, Respiratory and heart rate responses to auditory stimulations, Physiol. and Behav. 8, 327 (1972).

(15) H. Gautier, J.E. Remmers and D. Bartlett Jr, Control of the duration of expiration, Respir. Physiol. 18, 205 (1973).

(16) J.E. Remmers and D. Bartlett Jr, Reflex control of expiratory airflow and duration, J. Appl. Physiol. 42, 80 (1977).

CAUSES OF INSTABILITY IN THE CONTROL OF BREATHING IN THE ADULT AND NEONATAL STATES

ANIMAL MODELS OF CHEYNE-STOKES BREATHING

N. S. CHERNIACK, C. VON EULER, I. HOMMA and F. KAO

Nobel Institute for Neurophysiology, Karolinska Institutet, Stockholm, Sweden

INTRODUCTION

The striking crescendo and decrescendo swings of ventilation seen in Cheyne-Stokes breathing have provoked considerable speculation but no agreement concerning its origins (1-5). One reasonable hypothesis is that Cheyne-Stokes breathing is a manifestation of instability in the feedback control of breathing similar to the cyclic fluctuations in output that occur in man-made control systems when they become unstable (6-8). The complex and often precarious clinical state of patients exhibiting Cheyne-Stokes breathing has precluded rigorous testing of this or any other theory in man. However, experiments in animals in which Cheyne-Stokes breathing has been deliberately produced are informative and tend in general to support the idea that periodic breathing of the Cheyne-Stokes variety can occur in circumstances that favor unstable ventilatory control (9-11). In order to understand these experiments better, the circumstances in which instability arises in man-made systems need to be reviewed.

THEORETICAL CONSIDERATIONS

A control system consists of a controller which directs the operation of a controlled system via a communication channel (6,8,12,13). Because of the occurrence of random disturbances which prevent the controlled system from precisely executing the instructions of the controller, an additional communications channel is often included. This channel allows information on the output to be fed back to the controller so that it can take corrective action. The controller is subdivided into the controlling element itself, a sensor which tests the output and a comparator which compares the information obtained from the sensor to some desired or "reference value". In the ventilatory control system, the controllers are the central respiratory neurons and the central and peripheral chemoreceptors which act as sensors and comparators. The controlled system consists of the respiratory muscles, the lungs, and the gas stores of O_2 and CO_2 (the CO_2 and O_2 in physical solution and in chemical combination in the body). The controller and the controlled system are interconnected by nerve fibers and the blood.

Feedback control reduces the steady state error of the system, but also introduces the possibility that the corrective action taken by the controller may be inappropriate, reinforcing rather than reducing the error and producing a perpetually oscillating output (8). Inappropriate corrective actions may occur if the controller action is delayed as a result of the time required to receive and process the data relayed from the sensors and to transmit controller commands (9). This sort of delay occurs in physiological systems whenever information is carried over nervous or circulatory pathways.

If these delays are sufficiently great, controller action to correct the effects of a disturbance may result in the output overshooting the desired level (9). When the controller is ultimately informed of this overshoot, it takes excessive

417

action, now in the opposite direction, causing the output to undershoot the level desired. When the undershoots and overshoots are the same in amplitude, the output will continue to swing about endlessly never reaching a steady state in which the output is stable.

It is possible for the output of physiological or physical systems to oscillate even in the absence of delays. Components of physiological systems have properties of inertia, friction, and elasticity like the elements of physical systems and cannot instantaneously attain a steady state after a disturbance (11,12). The terms compliance (a measure of elasticity), resistance (a measure of friction), and the inertance (a measure of mass) are commonly used, for example, to describe the behavior of the lungs and chest wall. Neurons and sensory receptors have similar characteristics. These properties make oscillations in output possible in the immediate postdisturbance period before a steady state is reached. Whether or not such oscillations occur during transient states and how rapidly they will decay will depend on the damping ratio of the system. The damping ratio is greater when the frictional resistance and compliance of the system is increased and is reduced when inertia is increased. The use of feedback control decreases the damping of a system. Increasing the sensitivity of a feedback controller further diminishes damping even though it enhances the accuracy of control system performance (6,8).

Further insights into the causes of instability in the ventilatory control system can be obtained by considering O_2 and CO_2 control of breathing separately. Below about 30 mm Hg change in CO_2 tension seem to have little or no effect on ventilation so that controller gain is zero (14). Over a wide range of CO_2 tensions (above 30 mm Hg Pco_2 at constant oxygen tension), ventilation increases linearly with Pco_2 indicating a constant CO_2 controller gain. On the other hand, arterial chemoreceptor discharge and ventilation increase hyperbolically with decreasing PaO_2 levels, resulting in an increasing O_2 controller gain with hypoxia (14).

The dissimilar characteristics of the O_2 and the CO_2 stores also contribute to the difference in the stability of the two systems (15). The ratio between the volume of CO_2 or O_2 stored in the body for a given change in gas tension is a measure of the compliance of the stores. The larger the change in gas stored for a given change in gas tension, the greater the compliance and the greater the damping. The compliance of the CO_2 stores exceed that of the O_2 stores because large amounts of CO_2, but only minute amounts of O_2, are stored in the tissues. Since the damping ratio is reduced by increases in compliance, the damping effect of the CO_2 stores is far greater than that of the O_2 stores. Because of the large damping influence of the CO_2 stores and the nearly linear response of the CO_2 receptors, the CO_2 control system is by itself very stable. CO_2 control is further stabilized by the increase and decrease in cerebral blood flow that occurs with changes in arterial Pco_2 which slow the rate of change of Pco_2 in the surroundings of the central chemoreceptors (16). On the other hand, the O_2 control system tends to be much more unstable than that for CO_2 because of low damping characteristics of the O_2 stores and the alinear characteristics of the O_2 controller. While the usual stability of ventilatory responses to hypoxia is explained by the multiple physiological connections between the O_2 and CO_2 system, through ventilation, the Bohr and Haldane effects on the affinity of hemoglobin for CO_2 and O_2, metabolism, and the circulation; these same interconnections decrease the stability of CO_2 control.

Despite the stability of CO_2 control, large increase in CO_2 gain produced, for example, by removal of inhibiting cortical influences, could result in Cheyne-Stokes breathing. Great increases in respiratory controller gain have been measured in some patients with cerebrovascular disease who have bilateral hemispheric lesions. Since both O_2 and CO_2 chemoreceptors receive data directly or indirectly through the blood, it is apparent that reductions in the speed of the circulation will

increase the transportation lag in both control systems and will promote instability
The time required for the blood to traverse the blood vessels between the lung and
the chemoreceptors seem to explalin the peculiar relationship between alveolar and
arterial gas tensions observed during Cheyne-Stokes breathing. During Cheyne-
Stokes breathing, the arterial CO_2 tends to be highest and O_2 lowest during hyperpnea while the reverse is true of alveolar gas levels (2,14). It is apparent that
during the instability, the arterial gas tensions reflect the input to the receptors
i.e. the respiratory drive; while the alveolar gas tensions reflect the changing
ventilatory output. In addition, the duration of the cycle of hyperpnea and apnea
tends to vary directly with the circulation time and cycles are generally shorter
when Cheyne-Stokes breathing occurs at altitude in normal individuals than in
patients with cardiac disease and slowed blood circulation (2).

ANIMAL STUDIES

Prolongation of circulation has been shown to cause Cheyne-Stokes breathing in
anesthetized animals. Guyton produced periodic breathing in dogs by inserting
loops in the carotid artery which artificially lengthened the circulation time
between lungs and brain to as much as five minutes (9). Prolonged cycles of
hyperventilation and apnea were observed. Cycle length was proportional to the
length of the artificial loop.

In a different study, periodic breathing occurred in anesthetized dogs with normal
circulation times following a period of artificial hyperventilation (10).

Arterial Pco_2 was 15 to 20 mm Hg in the dogs after several minutes of artificial
hyperventilation with air. When artificial ventilation was stopped, the animals
became apneic for varying lengths of time. Arterial Pco_2 and arterial O_2 saturation
were less than control values when spontaneous breathing resumed. In one-half the
trials, spontaneous breathing, when it resumed, was periodic for a time. The
lower the arterial O_2 saturation at the start of spontaneous breathing, the more
likely was periodic breathing to occur. Enforced asphyxia which produced equivalent
decreases in arterial O_2 saturation but raised arterial Pco_2 was not followed by
periodic breathing when the asphyxia was relieved. Periodic breathing could follow
post-hyperventilation apnea whether or not the vagi were intact. Cerebral ischemia
failed to produce periodic breathing unless it caused cyclic changes in blood
pressure (Mayer Waves) (17).

These findings were compatible with the idea that Cheyne-Stokes breathing occurs
whenever hypoxic rather than hypercapnic drive dominates breathing. The period
of apnea that followed artificial ventilation allowed breathing to begin in hypocapnic and hypoxemic circumstances. With the return of spontaneous breathing,
arterial O_2 saturation and Pco_2 gradually rose and Cheyne-Stokes breathing disappeared as blood gas conditions reverted to normal. The transient nature of the
periodic breathing prevented detailed study of the periodic breathing, but the
findings were compatible with the idea that Cheyne-Stokes breathing resulted from
unstable ventilatory control.

Persistent periodic breathing was produced in cats anesthetized with pentobarbitol
by Cherniack, von Euler, Homma, and Kao (11). In these studies, the cats were
ventilated with a respirator governed by changes in phrenic nerve output so that
feedback loops remained intact. Periodic breathing was elicited in 15 anesthetized
or decerebrate cats by increasing "servorespirator" gain alone or in addition by
lung deflation and/or respiring the cats with hypoxic gas mixtures.

In five cats breathing air, regular waxing and wanning of tidal volume and tidal
phrenic nerve activity, as shown in Fig. 1, could be produced just by increasing

"servorespiratory" gain to magnify the usual effect of phrenic nerve activity on
respiratory tidal volume.

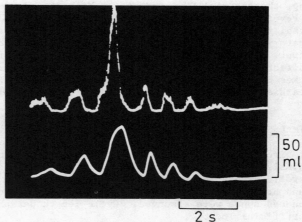

Fig. 1   Periodic breathing in a cat
Phrenic nerve activity is shown above; tidal volume below.

In another 7 cats, lung deflation with negative end-expiratory pressures of 5 to
15 cm H_2O produced periodic breathing after controller gain had been approximately
doubled with the respirator.   In the other 3 cats, ventilation with 6, 9, or 12%
O_2 was necessary to produce cyclic swings in instantaneous levels of ventilation.

These procedures all reduced alveolar Pco_2 to 30 mm Hg or less when periodic
breathing appeared.   Arterial Po_2 was 5 to 15 mm Hg less during the phases of
hyperventilation than during the apneic phases similar to findings obtained in man
during Cheyne-Stokes breathing (2,3).   Prevention of fluctuations in gas tensions
by placing the cat on a fixed level of artificial ventilation eliminated periodic
breathing as shown in Fig. 2.

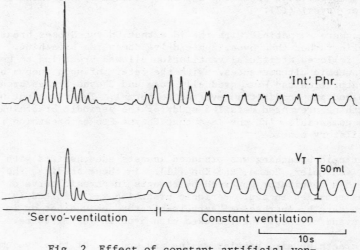

Fig. 2   Effect of constant artificial ventilation on periodic breathing

Lung deflation tended to reduce mean PaO_2 (on the average 6 torr) and it was as
low as 34 torr in animals which developed periodic breathing while inspiring
hypoxic gas mixtures. More severe hypoxia tended to depress breathing and to
eliminate periodicity.

The length of a cycle of hyper- and hypoventilation averaged 18 seconds with a
range of 6 to 30 seconds. The number of breaths per cycle was variable ranging
between 5 to 40 with a mean of 12. The higher breathing rates occurred with lung
deflation. With more rapid breathing, some phrenic nerve activity often continued
at a low level even during the apneic phase as shown in Fig. 3.

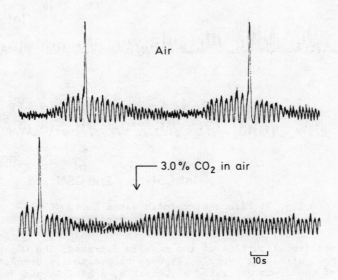

Fig. 3 Effect of CO_2 on phrenic nerve activity during
periodic breathing induced by lung deflation

Once periodic breathing appeared, it was sustained and showed no sign of disappearing if conditions were not changed. Further increases in controller gain
had little effect on the total length of a cycle of hyper- and hypoventilation.
However, the increase in tidal volume during the hyperventilation period at
elevated controller gain was usually associated with an increase in the duration
of apnea at the expense of the length of the phase of hyperventilation.

Decreasing respirator gain eliminated breathing periodicity as did lung deflation
if deflation was needed to produce periodic breathing.

Raising the gain of the servorespirator increased both the absolute level of ventilation at a given $PaCO_2$ and increased the change in ventilation which occurred
for a given change in CO_2. Similar changes in the relationship of ventilation to
hypoxia were observed when servorespirator gain was made greater.

Deflation increased the slope of the ventilatory response as well as the relationship of phrenic activity to Pco_2. Ventilatory response was greater when the lungs

were deflated despite the mechanical interference caused by continuous negative
pressure to inspiratory air movement.

In 3 of the 15 cats, periodic breathing could be produced only when hypoxic gases
(6-12% O_2) were inspired to lower PaO_2 to 45, 40, and 34 torr. Administrations
of 100% O_2 on the other hand caused a gradual disappearance of periodic breathing.
Blockade or surgical interruption of the carotid sinus nerves after vagotomy to
eliminate both carotid and aortic body input also eliminated periodic breathing
as shown in Fig. 4.

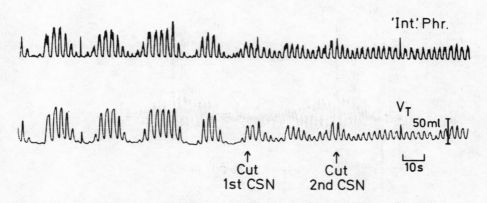

Fig. 4 Effect of carotid sinus nerve (CNS)
section on periodic breathing

Cooling the ventolateral surface of the medulla depressed the CO_2 response relationship without affecting hypoxic response as previously demonstrated (18-20).
Focal cooling of the areas described by Loeschke, Schlafke, and Mitchell on the
ventrolateral medullary surface produced periodic breathing in animals respired
at large servorespirator gains or with hypoxic gas mixtures (18-20). In contrast,
inspiring gas mixtures enriched with CO_2 regularly converted periodic to steady
breathing (see Fig. 3).

Periodic breathing could be produced also after bilateral vagotomy by increasing
respiratory gain and by hypoxia. The total length of the periods of hyper- and
hypoventilation was unaffected by vagotomy but the number of breaths per cycle
decreased and the amplitude of the breaths increased similar to the effect of
vagotomy on respiratory pattern during regular breathing.

Increased controller gain in this study by manipulation of the servorespirator or
reflexly through lung deflation caused sustained periodic breathing in most of
the cats tested during ambient air breathing. By magnifying the effects of
chemical changes on ventilation, increased controller gain caused hyperventilation
in the cats, moving the resting Pco_2 closer to the point of the CO_2 response
curve where alinear changes in gain can occur, i.e. close to the apnea point.

Hypoxemia increased tendencies toward instability. Lung deflation, probably by
causing atelectasis, also reduced arterial Po_2. This may have contributed to
the destabilizing effects provoked by this experimental intervention. Deflation
of the lung would also decrease CO_2 and O_2 reserves in the alveolar air, thereby
reducing damping (15). On the other hand, oxygen breathing, which increased lung

stores and minimized the role of O_2 drive on ventilation, stabilized breathing. Peripheral chemoreceptor denervation also eliminated periodic breathing. Focal cooling areas ventrolateral medullary surface described has been shown to shift CO_2 response to the right decreasing the level of ventilation at a given pCO_2 (21). The resulting decrease in the influence of CO_2 on respiration, in accordance with theory, led to periodic breathing. Increasing the influence of CO_2 by inspiring the CO_2 enriched air made periodic breathing disappear.

DISCUSSION

Theoretically, instability in control with resulting periodic breathing can occur in at least three kinds of situations.

1. Predominant control of breathing by hypoxia. This may account for the periodic breathing seen at altitudes and in sleep where CO_2 response is depressed (2,22).

2. Overall increase in controller gain which may explain the periodic breathing seen in certain types of cerebrovascular disease which affect both cerebral hemispheres (3).

3. Prolonged circulation time which seems to be responsible for the periodic breathing seen in patients with congestive heart failure (4).

All three types of disturbances have been shown in animal experiments to produce periodic breathing.

While it seems to be conclusively established that instabilities in control are a cause of periodic breathing, all periodic breathing in animals and Cheyne-Stokes breathing in man need not arise from this mechanism.

In hemorrhaged animals, instability in circulatory control can lead to cyclic changes in blood pressure, ventilation, and phrenic nerve activity (17). Fig. 5 shows regularly recurring apneas in an animal with Mayer Waves.

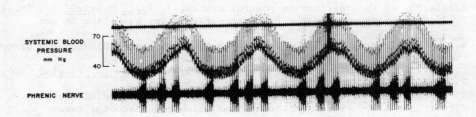

Fig. 5 Periodic breathing associated with
systemic blood pressure oscillations

This kind of periodicity in breathing usually vanishes when sympathetic system antagonists eliminate the vasomotor oscillation. Preiss, Iscoe, and Polosa found that cycles of phrenic nerve activity lasting 24 seconds persisted even after artificial ventilation was begun and blood pressure stabilized (23). They suggested that the residual oscillations were due to an intrinsic rhythmicity in central nervous system drive.

Since clinically Cheyne-Stokes breathing can usually be eliminated by measures which tend to stabilize ventilatory control, i.e. O_2 or CO_2 inhalation or by intravenous aminophylline which shift the response curve to the left, it seems likely that most if not all instances of Cheyne-Stokes breathing in man are caused by unstable ventilatory control (4).

REFERENCES

1. C. G. Douglas and J. S. Haldane, The causes of periodic or Cheyne-Stokes breathing, J. Physiol. 38, 401 (1909).
2. R. L. Lange and H. Hecht, The mechanism of. Cheyne-Stokes respiration, J. Clin. Invest. 41, 42 (1962).
3. F. H. Plum and H. W. Brown, The neurologic bases of Cheyne-Stokes respiration, Am. J. Med. 30, 849 (1961).
4. A. R. Dowell, E. Buckley III, R. Cohen, R. E. Whalen, and H. O. Sieker, Cheyne-Stokes respiration, Arch. Intern. Med. 127, 713 (1971).
5. D. J. C. Cunningham, A model illustrating the importance of timing in the regulation of breathing, Nature 253, 440 (1975).
6. H. T. Milhorn and A. C. Guyton, An analog computer analysis of Cheyne-Stokes breathing, J. Appl. Physiol. 20, 328 (1965).
7. G. S. Longobardo, N. S. Cherniack, and A. P. Fishman, Cheyne-Stokes breathing produced by a model of the human respiratory system, J. Appl. Physiol. 21, 1839 (1966).
8. J. P. Horgan and R. L. Lange, Digital computer simulation of the human respiratory system, IEEE Intern, Conv. Record II, Part 9, 149 (1963).
9. A. C. Guyton, J. W. Crowell, and J. W. Moore, Basic oscillating mechanism of Cheyne-Stokes breathing, Am. J. Physiol. 187, 395 (1956).
10. N. S. Cherniack, G. S. Longobardo, O. R. Levine, R. Mellins, and A. P. Fishman, Periodic breathing in dogs, J. Appl. Physiol. 21, 1847 (1966).
11. N. S. Cherniack, C. von Euler, I. Homma, and F. F. Kao, The role of hypoxia and hypercapnia in inducing periodic breathing in cats, (in press).
12. F. S. Grodins, J. S. Gray, R. R. Schroeder, A. L. Norins, and R. W. Jones, Respiratory responses to CO_2 inhalation. A theoretical study of a non-linear biological regulator, J. Appl. Physiol. 7, 238 (1954).
13. F. A. Grodins, J. Buell, and A. J. Bart, Mathematical analysis and digital simulation of the respiratory control system, J. Appl. Physiol. 22, 260 (1967).
14. D. J. C. Cunningham, The control system regulating breathing in man, Q. Rev. Biophys. 6, 433 (1974).
15. N. S. Cherniack and G. S. Longobardo, Oxygen and carbon dioxide gas stores of the body, Physiol. Rev. 50, 171 (1970).
16. M. Reivich, Arterial pCO_2 and cerebral hemodynamics, Am. J. Physiol. 206, 25 (1964).
17. R. Ferretti, N. S. Cherniack, G. Longobardo, O. R. Levine, E. Morkin, D. H. Singer, and A. P. Fishman, Systemic and pulmonary vasomotor waves, Am. J. Physiol. 209, 37 (1965).
18. H. H. Loeschcke, J. de Lattre, M. E. Schlafke, and C. O. Trouth, Effects of respiration and circulation of electrically stimulating the ventral surface of the medulla oblongata, Respirat. Physiol. 10, 184 (1970).
19. M. E. Schlafke, W. R. Sec, and H. H. Loeschcke, Ventilatory response to altered H^+ ion concentration in small areas of the ventral medullary surface, Respirat. Physiol. 10, 198 (1970).
20. R. R. Mitchell, H. H. Loeschcke, J. W. Severinghaus, B. W. Richardson, and H. H. Massion, Regions of respiratory chemosensitivity on the surface of the medulla, Am. N.Y. Acad. Sci. 109, 661 (1963).
21. N. S. Cherniack, C. von Euler, I. Homma, and F. F. Kao, Graded changes in

central chemoreceptor input by local temperature changes on the ventral
surface of the medulla, J. Physiol. (in press) (1978).

22. E. A. Phillipson, Respiratory adaptations in sleep, Ann. Rev. Physiol.
     40, 133 (1978).

23. G. Preiss, S. Iscoe, and C. Polosa, Analysis of periodic breathing pattern
     associated with Mayer waves, Am. J. Physiol. 228, 768 (1975).

DISCUSSION

In agreement with the results that periodic breathing was elicited
by focal cooling of the 'intermediate' areas Schlaefke reported that
she had observed periodic breathing in an awake cat following coagulation of the superficial layer of the 'intermediate' areas.

Eldridge speculated that a defect in the 'T-pool' mechanism which
causes after-discharges in the respiratory control mechanisms (see
Eldridge and Gill-Kumar, p 101, this volume) might have the effect of the
removal of a stabilizing mechanism and thereby increasing the pro-
pensity for periodic breathing. Similarly it was suggested that a
delay in the maturation of this mechanism might be a causal factor
for periodic breathing in infants.

B.Jonsson pointed out that in the preterm infants the pattern of
periodic breathing often has features different from the crescendo-
decrescendo pattern which might make it necessary to postulate that
periodic breathing of preterm babies is influenced also by other
factors involving profound hysteresis.

With reference also to Jonsson's comment Thach spoke about the
relationship between periodic breathing in sleep and obstructive
apnoea by atonia in the genioglossal muscle. He mentioned that in
the rabbit the hypocapnic threshold for diaphragmatic 'silence' is
higher than that for genioglossal 'silence', the consequence being
that when the activity of the diaphragm returned, it did so prior to
the return of genioglossal respiratory activity. This would be a
model of 'mixed' apnoea in which 'obstructed' breaths occur at the
beginning and at the end of diaphragmatic apnoea during periodic
breathing in infants.

Koepchen drew attention to earlier studies of cardiovascular rhythms
(H.P.Koepchen, Die Blutdruckrhythmik, Steinkopf, Darmstadt, 1962)
where periodic respiration sometimes had appeared as a secondary
effect of a pre-existing third order blood pressure rhythmicity
whereas, at other occasions, blood pressure waves had arisen secondary to a primary periodic type of respiration. Furthermore records
from respiratory neurons during hypoxia occasionally showed periodic
variations in activity appearing synchronously both in inspiratory
and expiratory neurons. This could occur also during constant artificial ventilation and at constant levels of chemical stimuli. Thus,
in addition to feedback oscillations in chemoreceptor or baroreceptor
control circuits one should consider the possibility also of intrinsic brain stem rhythms which may be manifested differently in the
different systems.

LESSONS FROM REINITIATION OF BREATHING
AFTER APNEA

S. LAHIRI and T. NISHINO

Department of Physiology and Institute for Environmental Medicine,
University of Pennsylvania School of Medicine, Philadelphia, PA 19104, U.S.A.

ABSTRACT

Apnea that follows active or passive hyperventilation and the subsequent reinitiation of breathing apparently represent the transition from a nonrhythmic to a rhythmic central state and may provide clues to the role of central and peripheral chemoreceptor inputs and to the central mechanisms of rhythmic respiration. We titrated termination of apnea with peripheral and central chemoreceptor drives in anesthetized cats and found that the greater the peripheral chemoreceptor drive, the lower the central chemoreceptor drive necessary to terminate apnea, even at as low an arterial P_{CO_2} as 12 torr. This reciprocal relationship indicates the complementary contributions of the two sensory inputs toward attaining the inspiratory threshold. If the central chemoreceptors were inactive at these low levels of arterial P_{CO_2}, only a finite peripheral chemoreceptor input would be required to reach the inspiratory threshold. The central chemoreceptor threshold, then, is below 12 torr arterial P_{CO_2}.

Unlike the excitatory input of peripheral and central chemoreceptors, pulmonary stretch receptor input, which normally inhibits inspiration, was found to play little or no role in terminating apnea. The timing effect, a characteristic of rhythmic breathing, was absent during apnea. It is proposed that the Breuer-Hering inhibitory effect depends on the earlier excitation of the inspiratory neurons, which initiates the central activity that generates respiratory rhythm. This central generator in turn activates the reflex-sensitivity of the off-switch mechanism, thus opening a gate by which inhibitory inputs may reach the off-switch. As the generator activity decays during expiration, the off-switch mechanism develops insensitivity in parallel, making the inspiratory neurons free from the inhibitory Breuer-Hering effect.

INTRODUCTION

Respiration, like any other rhythmic reflex activity, requires initiation and termination of central activity. The study of reinitiation of rhythmic breathing
following apnea, an eventful phenomenon in respiratory physiology, provides an
opportunity to further our understanding of the genesis of rhythmicity, as it was
recognized by Lumsden (1). The absence of rhythmic discharge during apnea allows
us to probe the center by manipulating afferent sensory input and to learn about
the role of afferent input in rhythm generation.

EXPERIMENTAL RESULTS AND DISCUSSION

Sensory Inputs and Initiation of Inspiration

Apnea occurs in anesthetized animals following passive (mechanical) hyperventilation; it can also occur after active hyperventilation driven physiologically by
hypoxia. The events leading to the reinitiation of breathing in both these cases
appear similar. An example of apnea following withdrawal of hypoxic stimulation
in the cat is illustrated in Fig. 1 to reiterate the fact that it is a normal
occurrence (2), although a prolonged after-discharge is seen under certain circumstances (3).

The animal, anesthetized with α-chloralose, was prepared so that tracheal air
flow, tidal volume on inspiration, carotid chemoreceptor activity from the peripheral end of one cut sinus nerve, arterial pressure, and end-tidal O_2 and CO_2
partial pressures could be measured, as described previously (4). The animal was
intact otherwise. After the cat had breathed a hypoxic gas mixture (end-tidal
P_{O_2} = 50 torr) for 5 min, inspired O_2 concentration was raised abruptly to 100%.
The first succeeding inspiration was small, and the expiratory phase, 2.5 to 3.0
sec during rhythmic breathing, extended over a period of 38 sec (apnea). The
carotid chemoreceptor activity declined sharply after the first breath of 100% O_2.

During apnea the carotid chemoreceptor activity increased. After the first
breath, the activity again declined. If the carotid chemoreceptor activity had
been withdrawn by infusing oxygenated saline into the contralateral carotid at the
instant of the first breath, the animal would have slipped briefly into apnea
again.

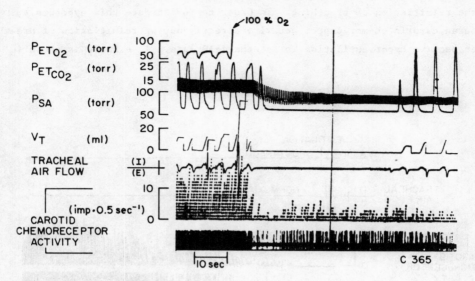

Fig. 1. Reinitiation of breathing following spontaneous
hyperventilation and apnea. Cat, α-chloralose. Effects of
breathing 100% O_2 after hypocapnic hypoxia on carotid chemoreceptor activity and ventilation. Apnea occurred following
the depression of carotid chemoreceptor activity. The apnea
was terminated by a prolonged shallow inspiration and a
short expiration seen in the tracheal air flow trace.

It is well known that the duration of apnea becomes shorter with lowered initial
arterial P_{O_2} at the same initial arterial P_{CO_2} (see 4). The lower the initial
arterial P_{O_2}, the lower the arterial P_{CO_2} at the reinitiation of breathing. This
arterial P_{O_2}-P_{CO_2} relationship implicates peripheral and central chemoreceptors,
but it does not alone define the contribution of each. More often than not it is
believed that the central P_{CO_2}-H^+ drive is zero during apnea because P_{CO_2}-H^+ at
the central chemoreceptors is below a threshold level. However, if the P_{CO_2} is
below the central chemoreceptor threshold, then inspiration should always be reinitiated as soon as peripheral chemoreceptor input reaches the same critical level,
which could occur at any of the observed combinations of arterial P_{O_2} and P_{CO_2}

at the reinitiation of breathing. In order to investigate this hypothesis, we
measured carotid chemoreceptor activity directly during reinitiation of breathing
after passive hyperventilation in anesthetized cats. An example is shown in
Fig. 2.

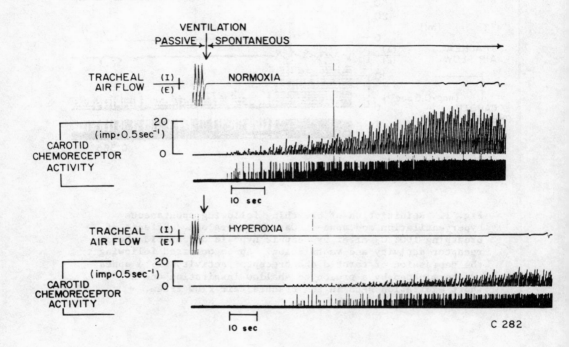

Fig. 2. Effect of P_{O_2} on carotid chemoreceptor activity
during apnea and reinitiation of breathing after passive
hyperventilation. Cat, α-chloralose. During the apneic
period beginning with normoxia, the rate of development and
magnitude of carotid chemoreceptor activity were greater,
and the apneic period was shorter, than after hyperoxia.
[Reproduced from Respiration Physiology with permission (4).]

The animal was hyperventilated for 3 min to hypocapnia of 15 torr, with inspired
P_{O_2} of 150 torr and 660 torr. Both conditions silenced carotid chemoreceptor
activity. During hyperoxia the afferent discharges started and rose slowly,

whereas during normoxia they started earlier, rose sharply, achieved a greater magnitude and terminated apnea in a shorter period. A series of such results is presented in Fig. 3 to show the characteristic rise in carotid chemoreceptor activity after passive hyperventilation and before reinitiation of breathing. We found that the carotid chemoreceptor discharge rate at which the breathing was reinitiated increased with the intensity of hypoxia. The greater the hypoxia, the shorter the apneic period, and consequently, the lower the arterial P_{CO_2} at the termination of apnea.

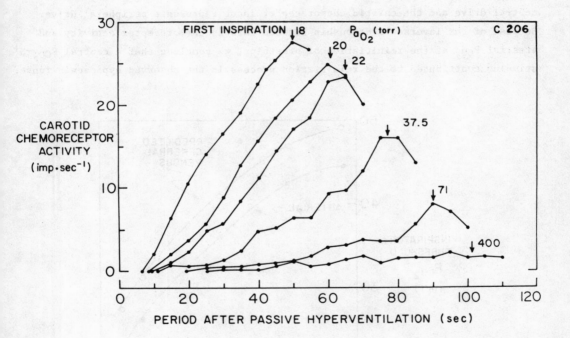

Fig. 3. Carotid chemoreceptor discharge following constant hyperventilation with various levels of inspired P_{O_2}. Cat, α-chloralose. The relationship between carotid chemoreceptor activity and apneic period is inverse.

These titration results can be used to focus on two aspects of respiration: (i) P_{CO_2} threshold for central chemoreceptors, and (ii) rhythm generation and phase-switching after apnea.

Central Chemoreceptor P_{CO_2} Threshold vs. Inspiratory P_{CO_2} Threshold

The relationship between the carotid chemoreceptor input and the inspiratory threshold P_{CO_2} after apnea is shown in Fig. 4. As the carotid chemoreceptor activity increased, the inspiratory threshold arterial P_{CO_2} decreased, and so did cerebral venous P_{CO_2}, as predicted from studies in other cats. This inverse relationship between carotid chemoreceptor input and inspiratory threshold P_{CO_2} at unsteady states holds good for steady states as well, the major difference being that the P_{CO_2} threshold was found to be lower during the steady state at a given peripheral chemoreceptor input. We assume that the arterial P_{CO_2} is an index of central drive and the carotid chemoreceptor input represents peripheral drive. Because of the inverse relationship between carotid chemoreceptor activity and arterial P_{CO_2} at the reinitiation of breathing, we conclude that a central $P_{CO_2}-H^+$ stimulus contributed to the reinitiation process in the observed hypocapnic range.

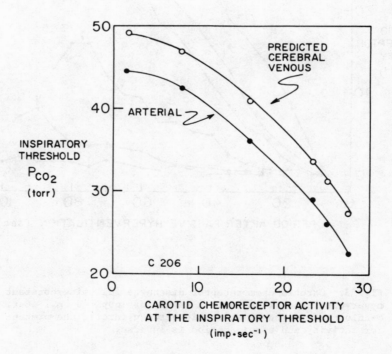

Fig. 4. Relationship between carotid chemoreceptor activity and inspiratory threshold P_{CO_2}. Cat, α-chloralose. The relationship between carotid chemoreceptor activity and inspiratory P_{CO_2} threshold is inverse. [Reproduced from Respiration Physiology with permission (4).]

The source of the central $P_{CO_2}-H^+$ effects is not totally clear. However, in view of the reports that hypercapnia and a local increase of the central $[H^+]$ slightly hyperpolarize some of the bulbospinal respiratory neurons (5, 6) as well as the phrenic motoneurone (7), the excitation by $P_{CO_2}-H^+$ cannot be attributed to direct effects on the respiratory neurons. The evidence has been mounting that there is a separate element on the ventral surface of the medulla which provides the source of excitation (8-10).

The input from the central chemoreceptors gives rise to an output from the bulbospinal respiratory neurons, leading to a linear increase in phrenic discharge and ventilation. On the other hand, partial depolarization by hypocapnia does not by itself trigger the phrenic burst, nor does it make the inspiratory neurons more sensitive to the synaptic input. If it did, the reinitiation of breathing would occur at a lower peripheral chemoreceptor activity as the intensity of hypocapnia was increased. Experimental findings, however, are contrary to the prediction: we found that the greater the hypocapnia, the greater the carotid chemoreceptor input needed to reinitiate breathing.

The relationship between input from central and peripheral chemoreceptor drives and threshold of inspiration is schematically presented in Fig. 5.

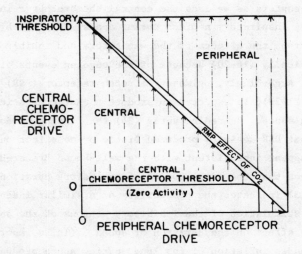

Fig. 5. Schematic representation of peripheral and central chemoreceptor drives to inspiratory threshold at which apnea is terminated. Below the central chemoreceptor $P_{CO_2}-H^+$ threshold (zero activity), peripheral chemoreceptor input alone terminates apnea. A direct depolarizing effect of hypocapnia on the resting membrane potential of inspiratory neurons is included.

A possible direct effect of $P_{CO_2}-H^+$ on the resting membrane potential of the inspiratory neurons and its contribution to reinitiation of breathing is also shown. According to this model, the central chemoreceptor drive is diminished with hypocapnia until its P_{CO_2} threshold is reached, when a single value of peripheral chemoreceptor drive, independent of central $P_{CO_2}-H^+$, is all that is needed to cause inspiratory discharge. In our experiments the central P_{CO_2} threshold was not reached, although arterial P_{CO_2} was as low as 12 torr; i.e., the arterial P_{CO_2} threshold for the central chemoreceptors was below 12 torr arterial P_{CO_2} in the anesthetized cat. The report by Sears and his colleagues (11) that the expiratory muscles continue to discharge during hypocapnia in the absence of inspiratory muscle activity can be cited in support. We have also documented (T. Nishino and S. Lahiri, unpublished) that some expiratory intercostal muscles continued to discharge during severe hypocapnia, although the animal was in a state of apnea. Many bulbospinal expiratory neurons have been documented as discharging tonically during hypocapnic apnea (e.g., 12-15).

Rhythm Generation and Phase Switching after Apnea

Central state and Breuer-Hering reflex sensitivity during apnea.

Clearly the peripheral chemoreceptors as well as the central chemoreceptor inputs are effective in stimulating inspiratory neurons during apnea. During rhythmic discharge of respiratory neurons the effects of the excitatory and inhibitory synaptic inputs vary rhythmically (16-20) because of the ongoing events of the respiratory neuronal network. Accordingly, pulmonary stretch receptor (PSR) input, which prolongs expiration (21-23), is expected to produce a characteristic Breuer-Hering effect, prolonging apnea. We rediscovered (24) the finding of Rosenthal, cited by Breuer (21), that PSR activity produced little or no effect on apnea. These observations may appear inconsistent with the well-known Breuer-Hering inhibitory reflex, but the fact that the final 20-30% of expiratory duration is reflex-insensitive (22, 23) indicates the possibility of a similar insensitivity during apnea. Likewise, stimulation of the inhibitory neurons of the pneumotaxic center (PC) would have no effect on the duration of apnea. (It is important to note, however, that a sudden inflation of the lungs during apnea produced a short phrenic burst, confirming the effectiveness of excitatory input under apneic conditions.)

A plausible explanation for this Breuer-Hering reflex-insensitivity can be offered in the form of a hypothesis relating to the excitatory state of central

generator activity (CGA). Following apnea and subsequent inspiration, the CGA
develops after a delay; it decays, after a delay, with the termination of inspiration. This pattern is consistent with numerous observations on rhythmic
breathing (see 20). We propose that the inhibitory effects of PSR and PC not
only add to the CGA (20); they depend on it as well. In the absence of CGA, the
inhibitory reflexes cannot occur. The idea is incorporated in a simplified model
later.

Initiation of inspiration-- the primary event. In all our observations, inspiration was the first breathing event after apnea: a respiratory cycle never
started with expiration, although many bulbospinal expiratory neurons may discharge tonically during apnea (12-15) and respond to carotid chemoreceptor input
(25, 26), like inspiratory neurons (27). It appears that the central generator
was not activated by the expiratory neurons.

The first phrenic burst of activity did not produce any significant inspiratory
air flow except for a very brief period (Fig. 6; see also Fig. 1), and it was
apneustic.

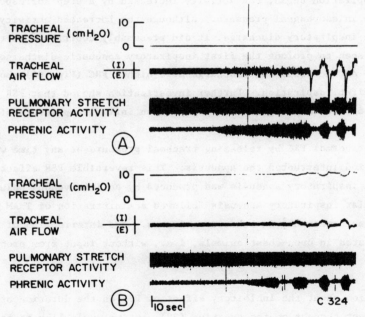

Fig. 6. Effects of lung inflation on inspiratory apneusis
after apnea. Cat, α-chloralose. (A) Under normal conditions, the first air flow signal and phrenic nerve discharge
were apneustic. (B) Lung inflation by an increased end-
expiratory pressure interrupted the apneusis.

The inspiratory burst occurred first both at normal functional residual capacity (FRC) (Fig. 6A) and at increased FRC under positive pressure lung inflation (Fig. 6B). Breuer's claim (21) that inflation of lungs during apnea reverses the respiratory movement (i.e., causes expiration first) was not substantiated. It may be that the available technique obscured his results.

The first breath and the effect of PSR input. Once the first inspiration occurred, PSR input showed a profound effect. The first inspiration was shortened and expiration was prolonged by an increase in tracheal pressure (Fig. 6B)-- demonstrating the classical Breuer-Hering inhibitory reflex. In this context, it is relevant to examine the stretch receptor activity during transition from apnea to the first inspiration. PSR, which oscillates with the respiratory cycles and is practically silent during the expiratory flow, discharged continuously during apnea both at the normal (Fig. 6A) and increased FRC (Fig. 6B). Fig. 7 illustrates further points: (i) a few seconds after hyperventilation, PSR activity increased to a stable value, the change presumably caused by a slow deformation in the receptors (28); (ii) it did not change with the changing blood gases during apnea; (iii) as the first inspiration began, PSR activity increased by a step corresponding to the step decrease in esophageal pressure. Although the increased activity did not terminate the inspiratory discharge, it did presumably contribute to the process: vagotomy was seen to prolong the first inspiratory apneustic discharge in other experiments. An increased PSR discharge at a higher FRC (Fig. 6B) shortened the time of the first inspiration. Further investigation showed that PSR's inhibitory effects did not increase significantly beyond an inflation pressure of 5 cm H_2O.

Restoration of normal FRC by releasing tracheal pressure at any time within the apneustic period interrupted the apneusis. This reversible PSR effect is shown in Fig. 8, where inspiratory apneusis was produced by an intravenous bolus of pentothal. A similar inspiratory apneusis followed administration of THAM [tris (hydroxymethyl)-aminomethane] in other experiments. And interruption of apneusis was also demonstrated in open-chest animals, i.e., without input from proprioceptive receptors.

This information about the inhibitory effect of PSR on the duration of apneusis supports current thought on the question (29), but we would like to point out the boundary condition of the PSR inhibitory effect: the reflex works only after development of CGA has reached a certain level. At this level, CGA opens the gate to the mechanism that terminates inspiration (the off-switch).

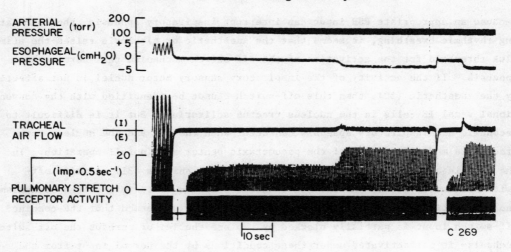

Fig. 7. Pulmonary stretch receptor activity during apnea
and reinitiation of breathing. Cat, α-chloralose. The
relationship of pulmonary stretch receptor activity to
esophageal pressure and tracheal air flow was measured.

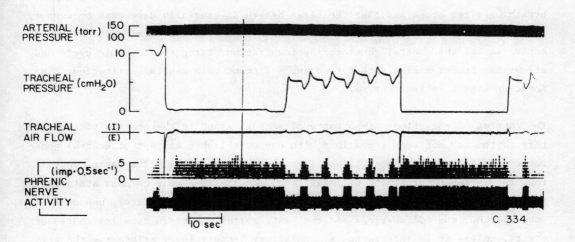

Fig. 8. Reversal of inspiratory apneusis by increasing
tracheal pressure. Cat, α-chloralose. Lung inflation by
increasing tracheal pressure (i.e., increasing pulmonary
stretch receptor and proprioceptive sensory input) caused
reversible interruption of inspiratory apneusis.

Because an appropriate PSR input can interrupt inspiratory apneusis, thus simulating rhythmic breathing, it seems that the anesthetic or alkalosis raises the stimulus threshold for the activation of the off-switch mechanism that terminates
apneusis. If the activity of the inspiratory sensory motor nuclei is not affected
by the anesthetic (30), then this off-switch cannot be identified with the conventional vagal Iβ cells in the nucleus tractus solitarius. But it is difficult to
reconcile how inspiratory apneusis can occur when the PSR and the nucleus parabrachialis medialis (NPBM) of the pneumotaxic center are in full operation. In
the chronic absence of PSR and NPBM input in awake animals (31), a third off-
switch becomes evident, but the simultaneous presence of the off-switch mechanisms
and the continued apneusis is paradoxical unless it is assumed that the combined
off-switch input is partially blocked by the anesthetic; or perhaps the off-switch
mechanism is not activated under these conditions by the normal input from the
PSR, PC and CGA. Clearly the inspiratory neurons themselves and the phrenic
motoneurons are not inhibited during the apneusis.

CONCLUSION

This study demonstrates that inspiration is the primary event in reinitiation of
breathing after apnea and that the first breath is crucially dependent on sensory
input. The act of inspiration itself sets the wheel of its termination in motion.
Activation of the central generator by inspiration starts the rhythmic cycle and
allows the Breuer-Hering effect to occur. Without this central activation, PSR
input by itself is ineffective.

The concept of the primary importance of sensory input in the genesis of respiratory rhythm may not seem compatible with the established concept of central generators for other cyclic activities like locomotion (see 32). The basic central
respiratory generator at the cellular level may lie at a near-dormant state during
apnea. The sensory input provides the spark through the inspiratory neurons.
Once sparked, the CGA develops and the basic rhythmic pattern runs its course of
events, unless it is interrupted by inhibitory sensory input triggering the off-
switch mechanisms. The inhibitory sensory input cannot trigger these by itself
in the absence of CGA during apnea: we therefore postulate a gating mechanism
(to the off-switch) which is opened by the CGA. The inhibitory input then enters
the gate and supplements CGA to trigger the off-switch mechanism. A conceptual
framework based upon the preceding discussion is presented in Fig. 9.

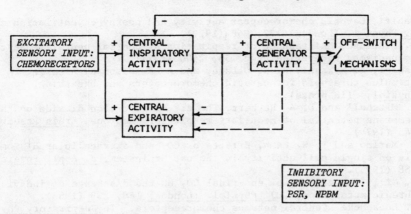

Fig. 9. Simplified model of respiratory rhythm. The
functional relationship between sensory inputs and genesis
of rhythmic breathing is indicated. Two features are emphasized: (i) the excitatory sensory inputs (e.g., chemoreceptors) excite the inspiratory neurons to produce the central
generator activity (CGA); and (ii) until this activity has
developed sufficiently, the off-switch mechanism for termination of inspiration remains insensitive to the inhibitory
PSR and NPBM inputs (the gate is closed). The gating mechanism is opened by the CGA, whereupon the inhibitory activities combine to activate the off-switch mechanisms. The
sensitivity to inhibitory inputs grows with the development
of CGA, which decays following the termination of inspiration. Insensitivity to these inputs occurs after the CGA
decays.

With this discussion, the question of respiratory rhythm generation is certainly
not settled, but it is certain that a study of reinitiation of breathing can guide
us to the source of rhythmicity.

ACKNOWLEDGEMENTS

Supported in part by USPHS-NIH Grants HL-19737-02 and HL-08899-14. We are grateful to Ms. Sandy Dechert and Mr. Anil Mokashi for assistance.

REFERENCES

1. T. Lumsden, Observations on the respiratory centres, _J. Physiol. (London)_ 57,
    354 (1923).

2. S. Lahiri, Carotid chemoreceptor activity and posthyperventilation apnoea, J. Physiol. (London) 272, 84P (1977).
3. F. L. Eldridge, Maintenance of respiration by central neural feedback mechanisms, Federation Proc. 36, 2400 (1977).
4. S. Lahiri, A. Mokashi, R. G. DeLaney and A. P. Fishman, Arterial P_{O_2} and P_{CO_2} stimulus threshold for carotid chemoreceptors and breathing, Respir. Physiol. (in press).
5. R. A. Mitchell and D. A. Herbert, The effect of carbon dioxide on the membrane potential of medullary respiratory neurons, Brain Research 75, 345 (1974).
6. P. L. Marino and T. W. Lamb, Effects of CO_2 and extracellular H^+ iontophoresis on single cell activity in the cat brainstem, J. Appl. Physiol. 38, 688 (1975).
7. P. K. Gill, The effects of end-tidal CO_2 on the discharge of individual phrenic motoneurones, J. Physiol. (London) 168, 239 (1963).
8. H. H. Loeschcke, Central nervous chemoreceptors. In Respiratory Physiology, Physiology Series One, Vol. 2 (1974), ed. J. G. Widdicombe, MTP International Review of Science, University Park Press, Baltimore, p. 167.
9. M. E. Schläfke, Central chemosensitivity: neurophysiology, and contribution to regulation. In Acid Base Homeostasis of the Brain Extracellular Fluid and the Respiratory Control System (1976), ed. H. H. Loeschcke, Georg Frieuse Publishers, Stuttgart, p. 66.
10. Y. Fukuda and H. H. Loeschcke, Effect of H^+ on spontaneous neuronal activity in the surface layer of the rat medulla oblongata in vitro, Pflügers Arch. 371, 125 (1977).
11. T. A. Sears, The respiratory motoneuron and apneusis, Federation Proc. 36, 2412 (1977).
12. H. L. Batsel, Activity of bulbar respiratory neurons during passive hyperventilation, Exp. Neurol. 19, 357 (1967)
13. M. I. Cohen, Discharge patterns of brain-stem respiratory neurons in relation to carbon dioxide tension, J. Neurophysiol. 31, 142 (1968).
14. M. Fallert, G. Böhmer and H. R. O. Dinse, Pattern of bulbar respiratory neurons during and after artificial hyperventilation, Respir. Physiol. 29, 143 (1977).
15. H. Gromysz and W. A. Karczewski, Responses of respiratory neurons of the rabbit to some excitatory and inhibitory stimuli. In Neural Control of Breathing, ed. W. A. Karczewski and J. G. Widdicombe, Acta Neurobiol. Exp. 33, 245 (1973).
16. R. Gesell and F. White, Recruitment of muscular activity and the central neurone after-discharge of hyperpnea, Am. J. Physiol. 122, 48 (1938).
17. M. G. Larrabee and R. Hodes, Cyclic changes in the respiratory centers revealed by the effects of afferent impulses, Am. J. Physiol. 155, 147 (1948).
18. A. M. S. Black and R. W. Torrance, Respiratory oscillations in chemoreceptor discharge in the control of breathing, Respir. Physiol. 13, 221 (1971).
19. F. L. Eldridge, The importance of timing on the respiratory effects of intermittent carotid body chemoreceptor stimulation, J. Physiol. (London) 222, 319 (1972).
20. C. von Euler, The functional organization of the respiratory phase-switching mechanisms, Federation Proc. 36, 2375 (1977).
21. J. Breuer, Die Selbststeuerung der Atmung durch den Nervus Vagus, Sber. Akad. Wiss. Wien 58 (II), 909 (1868).
22. C. K. Knox, Characteristics of inflation and deflation reflexes during expiration in the cat, J. Neurophysiol. 36, 284 (1973).
23. C. K. Knox and G. W. King, Changes in the Breuer-Hering reflexes following rostral pontine lesion, Respir. Physiol. 28, 189 (1976).

24. T. Nishino, A. Mokashi and S. Lahiri, Dependence of inspiratory Pa_{CO_2} threshold on respiratory proprioceptive reflexes, Federation Proc. 37, 532 (1978).

25. H. P. Koepchen, D. Klüssendrof and U. Philipp, Mechanisms of Central transmission of respiratory reflexes. In Neural Control of Breathing, ed. W. A. Karczewski and J. G. Widdicombe, Acta Neurobiol. Exp. 33, 287 (1973).

26. J. Lipski, R. M. McAllen and K. M. Spyer, The carotid chemoreceptor input to the respiratory neurones of the nucleus tractus solitarius, J. Physiol. (London) 269, 797 (1977).

27. R. O. Davies and McI. W. Edwards, Jr., Medullary relay neurons in the carotid body chemoreceptor pathway of cats, Respir. Physiol. 24, 69 (1975).

28. G. Sant'Ambrogio, J. P. Mortola and C. M. Severin, Stretch receptors of the trachea. In The Regulation of Respiration During Sleep and Anesthesia (1978), ed. R. S. Fitzgerald, H. Gautier and S. Lahiri, Plenum Press, New York, p. 307.

29. M. Younes, J. P. Baker, J. Polacheck and J. E. Remmers, Termination of inspiration through graded inhibition of inspiratory activity. In The Regulation of Respiration During Sleep and Anesthesia (1978), ed. R. S. Fitzgerald, H. Gautier and S. Lahiri, Plenum Press, New York, p. 383.

30. A. Hugelin, Regional effects of anesthesia on brainstem respiratory neurons. In The Regulation of Respiration During Sleep and Anesthesia (1978), ed. R. S. Fitzgerald, H. Gautier and S. Lahiri, Plenum Press, New York, p. 5.

31. W. M. St. John, R. L. Glasser and R. A. King, Apneustic breathing after vagotomy in cats with chronic pneumotaxic center lesions, Respir. Physiol. 12, 239 (1971).

32. S. Grillner, Locomotion in vertebrates: central mechanisms and reflex interaction, Physiol. Rev. 55, 247 (1975).

DISCUSSION

The discussion brought out that there was full agreement on the point of central subliminal summation of sensory drive inputs from peripheral and central chemoreceptors even at PCO_2 values so low that no manifest rhythmic respiratory activity is present in the phrenic nerve and that the central chemoreceptive threshold is considerably lower than that indicated by the PCO_2 threshold for inspiratory activity (see Cherniack et al., and Eldridge and Gill-Kumar in Session I in this volume).

NEONATAL BREATHING IN DIFFERENT STATES
OF SLEEP AND WAKEFULNESS

H. F. R. PRECHTL, M. J. O'BRIEN and L. A. VAN EYKERN

Department of Developmental Neurology, University Hospital, Groningen,
The Netherlands

ABSTRACT

When many neurobehavioural and physiological studies in infants are related to state,
a reduction in unexplained variability often emerges. Quantitative intra-state
variability does not invalidate a qualitative state concept, but appropriate modes
of assessment are imperative. Using a hybrid technique to eliminate ECG artefact,
we study the characteristics of the surface EMG of respiratory muscles in human
infants in relation to state and posture. Typical patterns are described and
illustrated, and results of cross-correlating the EMG root mean square signals
are discussed. Tonic activity found in the diaphragm in behavioural states 1 and
3 suggest the presence of functioning muscle spindles in this muscle in the human
infant. Principles developed in neonatal polygraphic research have application in
other fields of research and clinical monitoring.

INTRODUCTION

The Concept of Behavioural States

Classification into behavioural states is a convenient method of categorizing
relatively stable constellations of physiological variables which change
cyclically over time. The application of the state concept has led to a considerable reduction of the variations of outcomes in physiological and neurological
testing of young infants.

Different scales for behavioural states have been introduced depending on the
selection of variables as state criterion. Although in normal infants these
different scales give globally similar results, significant discrepancies may
occur as soon as more distinct analyses of responses are concerned. Another
important point concerns the way in which states are assessed. Traditionally
states have been analysed in consecutive epochs of 10 seconds, 20 seconds,
1 minute or 3 minutes duration. For reasons of stochastic properties of the
signals included in the assessment of states, continuous as opposed to
sequential methods of analysis are preferable. Therefore we have employed a
moving window of 3 minutes duration for state identification. Furthermore only
reliable and easily observable variables should be used as state criteria. These
considerations form the background to our choice of the following state criteria:
open/closed eyes; regular/irregular respiration; gross movements/quiescence;

crying/not crying. Five mutually exclusive states with consistently applied
criteria can be designed as four-dimensional vectors. Because descriptive names
for states are potentially misleading, adjective terms are replaced by numbers.
The criteria of our five states are given in Table 1.
(For a more detailed discussion see Prechtl, 1974, 1977).

TABLE 1   Vectors of Behavioural States

	Eyes open	Respiration regular	Gross movements	Vocalization
state 1	-1	+1	-1	-1
state 2	-1	-1	0	-1
state 3	+1	+1	-1	-1
state 4	+1	-1	+1	-1
state 5	0	-1	+1	+1

signs: +1 = true; -1 = false; 0 = true or false

If a change in the constellation of variables occurs it must last for 3 minutes
or longer to be accepted as a transition to a new state. A detailed analysis of
the "morphology" of sleep state transitions revealed large intra-individual
variations in the manner in which changes in eye-movements and EEG patterns are
related to changes in the regularity of respiration (Shirataki & Prechtl,1977).

From studying the input-output state relation by exploring responses to stimulation of various modalities it became clear that these five different states
represent mutually exclusive and specific modes of nervous activity. Responses to
stimulation of muscle spindles and sacculus-utriculus are exaggerated in state 1,
absent or diminished during state 2 and present during state 3 (and 4 and 5 if
testable). Exteroceptive skin reflexes to tactile and pressure stimuli, auditory
orienting responses and the vestibulo-ocular responses are absent in state 1,
weak but present in state 2, and vigorous during the other states. Responses to
painful stimuli are practically state independent. (For summary see Prechtl,1972).
We are now interested in how these input-output state relations relate to the
regulations of posture and spontaneous respiratory patterns in young infants.
For this purpose we have begun to analyse spontaneous changes in respiratory
muscle EMG in normal and sick infants studied in polygraphic experiments under
standardized conditions and with particular attention to changes associated with
state and posture.

SUBJECTS AND METHODS

Our experience with electromyography of respiratory muscles now includes 48 full-
term and 5 slightly older infants or young children. Most underwent 6 hour polygraphic study with recording of multiple surface EMG, EOG and EEG in addition
to surface EMG of respiratory muscles. In nine instances the EMG of extrinsic
laryngeal and external abdominal muscles were also recorded. Nasal airflow was
monitored by thermistor. Continuous behavioural observations were supplemented
by time-lapse photographic documentation of posture. Infants were either recorded
in prone and supine or in lateral positions. Visual analysis was made of the
polygraphic record and of off-line generated playbacks of the signals recorded
on tape. A PDP-15 computer was used for further analyses such as cross-correlation.

Technical Note

In a previous publication, Prechtl et al., 1977, we described in detail our method of signal measurement and a method of dealing with the large ECG artefact present in the surface EMG of respiratory muscles. Our approach to the problem has been further refined and the processing technique we now follow is illustrated, in Fig. 1.

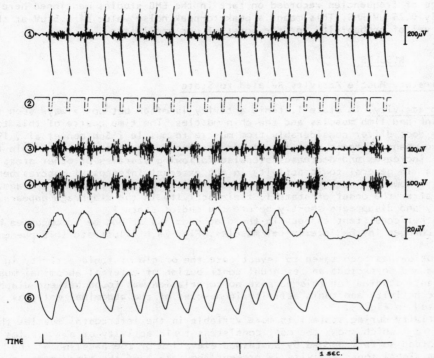

Fig. 1.   Steps in handling respiratory muscle signals
          using a hybrid processing technique. For
          explanation, see text. Signal shown is diaphragm.

The QRS complex in the measured EMG signal, 1, is detected by a level detector and a pulse, slightly longer than the QRS complex is generated, 2. The pulse controls an electronic switch which gates out the QRS complex from the electronically delayed EMG signal, 3. The root mean square value of the gated signal is calculated (rectangular moving time window, T = 300 - 600 msec) and during gating, the QRS complex is replaced by the ongoing RMS value by means of a feedback loop giving signal 4. The final RMS output signal, 5, is only minimally distorted by the ECG complex, although the P wave still causes slight distortion. If necessary the length of the gate can be increased to also include the P wave. As reference the respiration signal as measured by means of a nasal thermistor, 6, is also shown. The RMS signal may be displayed either linearly as in this figure or logarithmically as in many of the other figures. The log output enables comparison of signals independent of amplification factor and emphasizes changes in the lower range of the signal amplitudes.

We have chosen to work with the root mean square value (standard deviation) of the EMG signals for signal technical and statistical reasons. In exploring different methods of signal averaging we found that the ongoing RMS value best represents both the tonic and the phasic components of the EMG signal. This is not surprising since the surface EMG signal has a spiky appearance. The signals of interest are often weak, the intercostal EMG in state 2 for instance, and only slightly above amplifier noise level. In this situation the ongoing RMS value of a surface EMG which has 1/f noise characteristics emerges more clearly from the basic more white noise amplifier signal than does the ongoing average value. The amount of amplifier noise in the frequency band from 30 - 600 Hz, which was the range of frequencies recorded on tape in the EMG studies mentioned here, was maximally 0,25 µV RMS. This means a peak-to-peak noise value of 1.6 µV at the 0.1 % level of probability for the worst of our amplifiers.

RESULTS

A. Respiratory Muscle Activity Related to State

1. Tonic activity. In state 1, tonic activity is often but not always seen in many trunk and limb muscles and the chin muscles. The time course of this tonic activity does differ considerably from muscle to muscle (Schloon et al., 1976) and by no means is tonic activity always present during state 1. As a rule tonic activity increases and decreases stepwise following startles or other gross movements. In general tonic activity in the external intercostal muscles behaves similarly. However, such stepwise changes are less evident in the diaphragm. Shortly after the onset of state 1, tonic activity in the diaphragm appears gradually and disappears shortly before the end of state 1.
These rather consistent changes in the diaphragm may or not be accompanied by similar changes in the intercostal muscles. Fig. 2a,b illustrate this phenomenon.

Great caution has been taken to investigate the origin of tonic activity in the diaphragm and to exclude an eventual contribution of external abdominal muscles. In 9 infants studied for this purpose no correlation was found between diaphragmatic tonic activity and tonic activity in muscles of the abdominal wall, as illustrated in Fig. 3.
Tonic activity during state 1 is more variable in the intercostal muscles than in the diaphragm which shows the most consistent tonic activity of all muscles we have recorded so far. Judged by sustained elevation of the baseline of the diaphragm signal tonic activity is present about 80 % of the time spent in state 1. This is a higher percentage than seen in the chin muscles, tonic activity of which is often taken as one of the state criteria in the assessment of polygraphic sleep recordings. On the other hand tonic activity in the intercostal muscles is present about 60 % of the time of state 1 but varies considerably in its expression, being influenced by factors such as electrode placement and body position, prone, supine or side.

A different picture is seen during state 2. Sustained tonic activity is virtually absent in all muscles including the respiratory muscles, see Fig. 3. However, gross movements may be followed by some tonic activity but a rapid decay within 50 seconds is characteristic. Though sustained tonic activity is thus absent in all muscles during state 2, phasic activity is often present. Thus in state 2 the signal baselines are formed by the noise generated by the amplifier system. The respiratory muscles differ from others in that, though they too demonstrate an absence of sustained tonic activity in state 2, their signal baselines frequently fluctuate widely from breath to breath, inspiratory activities being superimposed on an unpredictably varying baseline which however often returns to the amplifier noise level, see Figs. 2a and b, 3, 6, 8. This feature is more pronounced in diaphragm than in intercostal signals.

In the awake and quiet newborn, thus during state 3, there is a considerable amount of tonic activity in the respiratory muscles, often exceeding the amount

found during state 1 (Fig. 4). During state 4 and 5 high but widely fluctuating
levels of basic activity are present in all muscles including muscles of respiration.

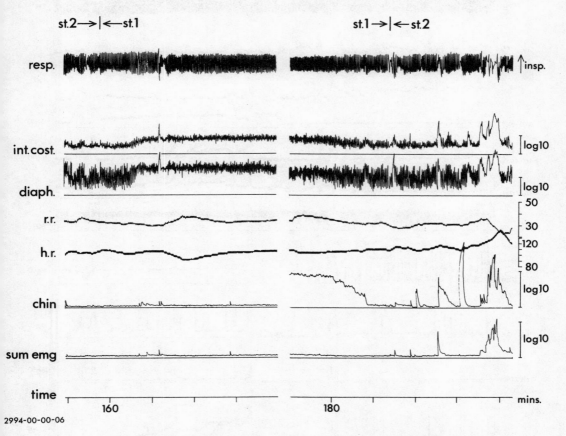

Fig. 2a. The typical pattern of development of tonic activity
in respiratory muscles at beginning of state 1.
In this case its appearance precedes that in other
muscles. Abbreviations: r.r. = respiratory rate;
h.r. = heart rate, both calculated as number of
events in 30 second width, moving window; chin =
chin EMG moving average; sum EMG = moving average
of sum of 4 neck and 1 limb muscle.
b. Decay of tonic activity approaching transition
to state 2. Note reduction also in intercostal
inspiratory amplitude.

A clear relationship appears to exist between periodic breathing and tonic activity
in respiratory muscles in that periodic breathing, if present in quiet sleep, gives
way to a continuous breathing pattern when tonic activity in respiratory muscles
reaches its highest level though a clear amplitude modulation with the same periodicity may persist, Fig. 5.

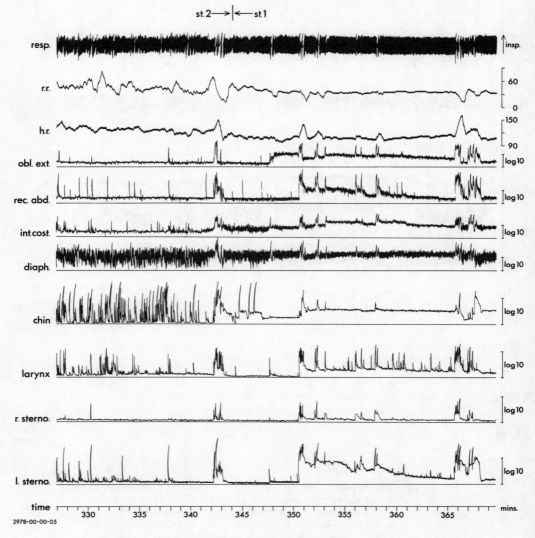

Fig. 3.   45 minutes of a 6 hour polygraphic record showing
          changes in tonic activity in many muscles, including
          abdominal and laryngeal and illustrating the
          independent behaviour of the various signals.

2. Respiratory muscle activity related to type of respiration. Sustained regular
respiration is by definition characteristic for state 1. The EMG signal is spindle
shaped but amplitude modulation is seen in the EMG of diaphragmatic and intercostal
muscles as it is in the thermistor signal. The amplitude of the intercostal activity varies more than that of the diaphragm. These variations are minor in comparison
to the waxing and waning of intercostal inspiratory activity during the irregular
breathing of state 2. Not only does the shape of each inspiratory EMG activity in
both muscles vary but they also vary greatly in burst-burst interval and amplitude.
There are many episodes when intercostal activity is hardly discernible but it is

often clearly present after gross movements. Since the intercostal muscles are
involved in gross movements this augmentation may be based on post-tetanic potention
of the motoneurons from proprioceptive feedback. This augmented activity usually
fades out again after 30 - 60 seconds.

The strong participation of intercostal muscles in the breathing during state 3
is obvious from Fig. 4.

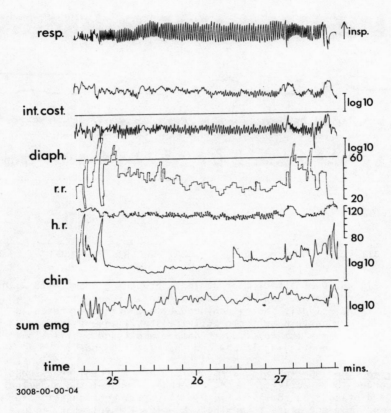

3008-00-00-04

Fig. 4. 2 minutes of state 3 showing high levels of tonic
        activity in respiratory muscles with superimposed
        inspiratory activity. r.r. and h.r. = respiro-
        tachogram and cardiotachogram signals respectively

Inspiratory activity is highly irregular in state 4 and 5, though somewhat more
organized in appearance in state 5 when the large inspirations preceding each cry
are clear to see in both respiratory muscles. During the actual cry the diaphragmatic activity falls while abdominal muscle EMG activity rises. This observation
constitutes another proof of the reliability of our diaphragm.signal.
An interesting aspect is the complex relationship between tonic activity and the
rate and amplitude of inspiratory muscle activity. At the transition from state 2
to state 1 respiration rate generally falls gradually as tonic activity begins to
build up, see Fig. 2a. Within state 1, however, upward resets in tonic activity,
particularly of the intercostal, are often accompanied also by slight upward resets
in respiratory frequency and a downward reset in heart rate. As a tonic (and phasic)

intercostal activity decays, frequency also declines and heart rate rises, see
Fig. 2b. Diaphragmatic activity at times can be seen to rise as intercostal
activity declines, see Fig. 7. At the end of state 1 as tonic activity finally decays, respiration rate may be declining only to become very variable again
with the onset of state 2.

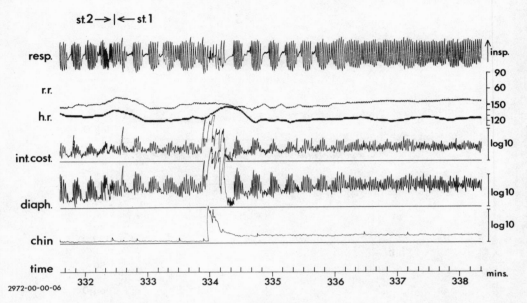

Fig. 5. Demonstration of periodic breathing associated with
marked amplitude oscillation in respiratory EMG
signals, being replaced by a continuous breathing
pattern as tonic activity stabilizes at its
maximum level, with damped amplitude oscillations
continuing in EMG and thermistor signals.

3. Activity in other muscles with a potential role in respiratory regulation.
We have recorded tonic activity in the external laryngeal and abdominal muscles
in state 1 and state 3 as shown in Fig. 3. It varies considerably from one infant
to another and from one state to another. Low level inspiratory modulation of
larynx, neck and abdominal muscles appears to be present at times, but needs
further investigation. More obvious brief increments of extrinsic laryngeal activity
coinciding with chin or neck muscle activity or as isolated phenomena are also seen,
quite prominent at times in state 2. As shown in Fig. 6, they are often but not
exclusively associated with minor disruptions of the ongoing respiratory pattern.
An expiratory modulation of rectus abdominis and obliquus externus EMG activities
was clearly visible in one exceptionally "tonic" newborn in state 1. This infant
studied in supine showed such activity superimposed on a high level of tonic
activity. This phenomenon was most easily seen following startles when, in association with increments in tonic activity, the infant adopted sustained antigravity
postures with legs extended and slightly elevated. Tonic stretch reflexes triggered
by the descent of the diaphragm stretching the tonically active abdominal muscles
may account for this phenomenon.

4. Application of cross-correlation technique. A cross correlation technique has
been employed to investigate the manner in which the respiratory muscles are

dynamically related to each other and to air-flow as monitored by nasal thermistor. This technique allows the estimation of the maximum correlation between two signals in a given frequency band and of the time shift at which the maximum value is found. We cross-correlate, within the expected respiration frequency band, the EMG RMS signals with each other and each separately with the nasal air-flow signal over epochs of chosen length (we have investigated epochs of 10 to 40 seconds). Interesting and reproducible results have been obtained in detailed studies of a group of 5 infants.

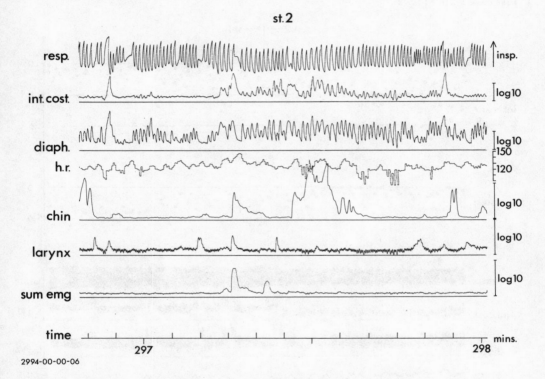

2994-00-00-06

Fig. 6. Typical state 2 showing fluctuating intercostal and
diaphragmatic activity with brief augmentation of
intercostal activity following the gross movements
at 297'30''. The "larynx" signal is derived from a
pair of electrodes, one over each cricothyroid
muscle. Ungated ECG artefact causes the oscillations
in baseline of the moving average signal. Note
intermittent phasic activity in this signal often
associated with respiration rhythm disturbances.

The pattern of change in correlation of delay time illustrated in Fig. 7 has been found with some variation in all 5 infants.

The correlation between the RMS value of intercostal (2nd or 3rd intercostal space, parasternal electrodes) and diaphragm (electrodes on costal margin just outside nipple line, right and left) EMG signals is extremely high for most of state 1, values generally being above 0.85 reaching on occasion 1.0. Some short term fluctuation in level of correlation occurs. Thus the coupling between the two muscles is highly controlled in this state and this holds true even when epochs of as long as 40 seconds are analysed.

Maximum correlation values in state 2 are much more variable, both inter- and intra-
individually, mean values always being significantly lower than in state 1 but the
range of values is such that some values overlap those found in state 1. These
higher values are found when the intercostal signal is visibly larger such as
following a general movement or during a relatively quiet state 2 epoch such as
occasionally occurs, particularly leading up to a transition to state 1 as is
illustrated in Fig. 7.

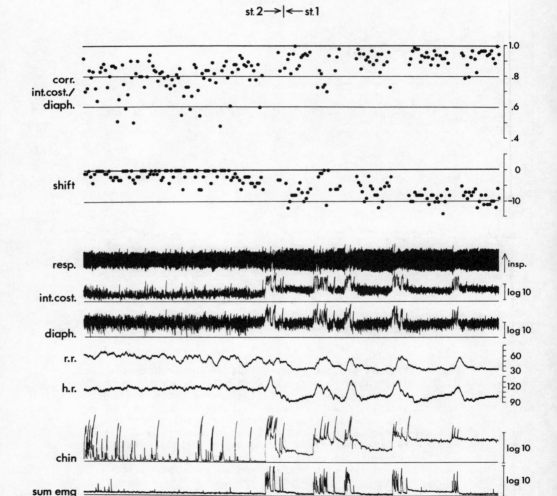

Fig. 7. Results of 50 % overlapping 20 second cross-corre-
lations of intercostal and diaphragm RMS signals

displayed with polygraphic record for comparison. 5
day old healthy infant studied in supine. Note that
all values for shift are 0 or -ve indicating that
intercostal is in phase or slightly leads diaphragm
in state 2, but leads markedly in state 1. A value
of 1 = a shift of 20 milliseconds.

The delay time between intercostal and diaphragm is much greater in state 1, being
of the order of 150 - 200 milliseconds, than in state 2 where there is often no
delay or the intercostal leads only slightly. This state difference is not
explicable on the basis of respiration frequency differences but is related
temporally at least to the presence of tonic activity in the intercostal muscles.
As can be seen from the figure, high correlations are not necessarily linked to
long delay time. These differences in delay time point to a fundamental difference
in the temporal organization of respiratory motor output in the two sleep states
and taken together with the findings for values of maximum correlation suggest
weaker more variable linking of the different respiratory motor outputs in state 2
than in state 1.
The fact that the linking of intercostal and diaphragm differs in the two sleep
states and is not simply a function of signal amplitude is further illustrated
by findings in the infant with upper-airway obstruction illustrated in Fig. 8 ,
who generated high amplitude intercostal activity in state 2. Despite this higher
than normal amplitude, levels of peak correlation in state 2, though higher than
usual, were still not as high as when the infant was in state 1 even though the
intercostal signal in state 1 was smaller than in state 2. In addition the usual
state variations in delay time were seen.

As mentioned we have also performed independent cross-correlation between intercostal and air-flow signal and diaphragm and air-flow. These analyses show not
only that the correlation between intercostal and air-flow is considerably higher
in state 1 than in state 2, i.e. respiration is more costal in state 1 than state
2, but that the correlation between diaphragm and air-flow is also slightly higher
in state 1 than 2, implying more effective diaphragmatic work also in this state.
Analyses of the changes in delay time show that the major shift in timing affects
the intercostal but there is also a slight shift in the diaphragm with respect to
air-flow in state 1 as compared to state 2, air-flow occurring slightly later
following diaphragmatic activity in state 1 than state 2.

DISCUSSION

In the full-term infant Finkel (1975) showed tonic activity in the raw EMG of
intercostal muscles (not clear which) and the diaphragm (intraoesophageal
electrodes), during "orthodoxical" sleep and quiet wakefulness and its absence
during "paradoxical" sleep. In long recordings with surface electrodes we were
able to confirm this observation but also found marked intra-state fluctuations.
This factor of variability is of crucial importance if shortlasting respiratory
experiments are carried out. Even if state is controlled for,quantitative changes
within state of many physiological variables can influence the results of
stimulus-response experiments. The presence of this variability within states does
not invalidate the qualitative state concept but makes careful monitoring of relevant physiological variables necessary. Our studies in normal infants suggest
that changes in body posture and position in space may alter the respiratory
motor output in both sleep states and thus posture is another crucial variable in
experiments related to respiratory regulation in intact infants.

Our findings are relevant to published illustrations of chest and abdominal
movement patterns in sleeping infants. In Fig. 2 of the paper by Curzi-Dascalova

1978, the chest wall expansion in quiet sleep clearly precedes that of the abdomen whereas in active sleep they appear to move simultaneously (though 180° out of phase).This fact can be explained by our findings on the state related shift in lead of the intercostal muscles over the diaphragm. The variability in costo-abdominal movement relationships these authors report relates nicely to the variability in tonic and phasic activity in the respiratory muscles that we find.

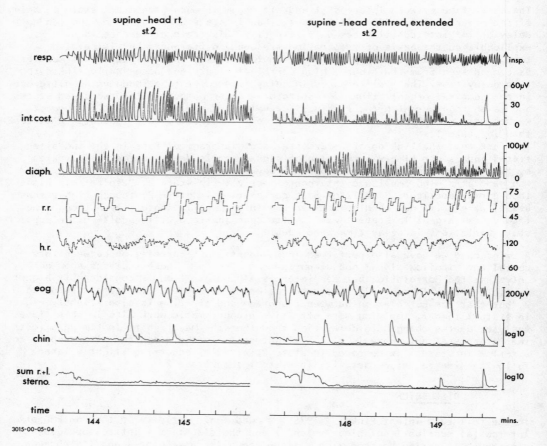

Fig. 8.   This infant had macroglossia and had a mild inter-
          mittent stridor. Respiratory muscles EMG showed
          markedly elevated inspiratory activity particularly
          in intercostal in state 2 when the infant was in
          supine with head to the right, at minutes 144' and
          145'. The dramatic effects of alleviating the partial
          obstruction by centering and extending the head
          are evident at minutes 148' and 149'. Respiratory
          rate was slower when the upper airway obstruction
          was present.

With our sensitive technique complete absence of intercostal inspiratory EMG activity in state 2 for more than a few breaths at a time is rare though the activity measured is often extremely low. This low level of inspiratory activity plus the absence of any sustained tonic activity is obviously not enough to counter-

act the increased negative intrathoracic pressure generated by the contracting
diaphragm. Since the intercostals do not ordinarily lag behind the diaphragm it is
highly unlikely that this intercostal activity could result from peripheral reflexes.

Our speculations in an earlier publication (Prechtl et al., 1977) that the marked
tonic activity we found in the diaphragm might mean the significant presence of
muscle spindles in the human infant has been confirmed by the histological findings
of Bryan reported in this volume of abundant muscle spindles in the tendon area
of the diaphragm in infants.

The signal technical and analysis principles which have evolved in the development
of the polygraphic approach to the study of newborn behaviour and physiology have
wide application in both clinical and research fields. The technique of surface
electromyography described here has many potential applications in clinical
respiratory monitoring and in many lines of respiratory regulation research.

REFERENCES

L. Curzi-Dascalova, Thoracico-abdominal respiratory correlations in infants:
     constancy and variability in different sleep states, Early Hum. Develop.
     2, 25 (1978).

M.L. Finkel, Activity of respiratory muscles in newborn infants during wakening
     and sleep, Zhurnal Evolyutsionnoi Biokhimii i Fiziologii, 11, 92 (1975).

H.F.R. Prechtl, Patterns of reflex behavior related to sleep in the human infant,
     In: C.D. Clemente, D.P. Purpura, F.E. Mayer (Eds.) Sleep and the Maturing
     Nervous System, Academic Press, New York, 1972, 287.

H.F.R. Prechtl, The behavioural states of the newborn infant (a review),
     Brain Res., 76, 185   (1974).

H.F.R. Prechtl, L.A. van Eykern, M.J. O'Brien, Respiratory muscle EMG in newborns:
     a non-intrusive method, Early Hum.Develop. 1, 265 (1977).

H. Schloon, M.J. O'Brien, C.A. Scholten, H.F.R. Prechtl, Muscle activity and
     postural behaviour in newborn infants, Neuropädiat., 7, 384 (1976).

S. Shirataki, H.F.R. Prechtl, Sleep state transitions in newborn infants:
     preliminary study, Dev.Med.Child Neurol., 19, 316 (1977).

Discussion after the next paper

RESPIRATION DURING SLEEP IN INFANTS

M. H. BRYAN and A. C. BRYAN

Research Institute, Hospital for Sick Children, Toronto, Canada

To obtain a "normal" ventilatory response Severinghaus warned that the sound of high heels must be avoided (1). Purves, in this Symposium, recommends reading tomes on political economy. Such a joyless world. The objective is clear, although unattainable: to study the ventilatory response of decerebrate man. The same objective is sought studying the ventilatory response in anaesthetised animals. Again the aim may not be achievable because as Milic-Emili in this Symposium has shown, anaesthetic agents have a profound and variable effect on respiratory control. The other alternative - studying decerebrate animals - is hardly more physiological.

Recently there has been increasing use of trained animals that can be studied awake and during sleep, with results that sometimes conflict sharply with previous data. However, there is still a species problem and extrapolation of, for example, vagal control, to humans is perilous. Another alternative is to study sleeping humans and as it is very tedious studying sleeping adults, it is more convenient to study infants. They sleep a lot, their arousal threshold is high and, as there is continuing post natal development, some insight can be gained into how the system is put together. Breathing starts in utero as an apparently useless act, in terms of gas exchange, although the pattern does appear to respond to conventional chemical and neural stimuli. The premature infant is born with a very uncertain grasp of respiratory rhythmicity and there are substantial changes in both chemical and neural control in the post natal period.

SLEEP STATES

Studies during sleep introduce some problems, but considerable advantages, as there are different sleep states. The taxonomy of sleep states in infants is unsatisfactory and even the nomenclature is not standardised. A state can be identified very specifically, as Rapid Eye Movement or Active Sleep or non-specifically, as State 2 or Paradoxical sleep. It is preferable to avoid a phenomenological definition as one can be in this state without rapid eye movements or activity. We prefer the term Paradoxical sleep as it retains our puzzlement about this state. In infants the states are not well organized or homogeneous. Quiet sleep cannot with certainty be identified below 36 weeks gestational age. Within Paradoxical sleep there can be phasic periods with a lot of small muscle activity and tonic periods with little or no activity. It is important to distinguish these two periods as they have important physiological

differences. In phasic periods there is almost complete suppression of the
intercostal EMG, the ventilatory response to CO_2 is very depressed and the
Hering-Breuer reflex is extinguished. In the tonic phase all these are fairly
well preserved. However, when the definition depends on a phrase like 'a lot of'
it does not encourage comparative work and some of the current controversies
probably hinge on this definition.

Control of breathing in the two sleep states appears to be quite different.
In Quiet sleep the drive is metabolic whereas in Paradoxical sleep the drive is
supra-pontine. The best evidence for this is that, in Ondine's Curse, the
profound hypoventilation occurs in Quiet sleep, whereas in Paradoxical sleep
respiration, although erratic, is reasonably well maintained (Fig 1).

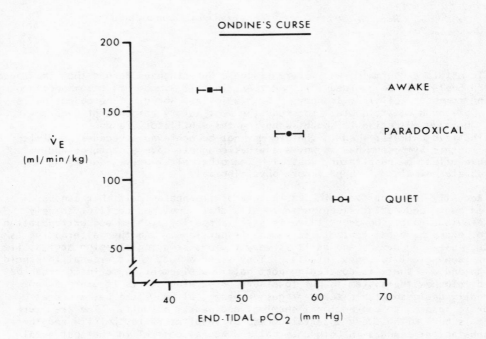

Fig. 1. Ventilation and $P_{A_{CO_2}}$ awake, in Paradoxical and Quiet
sleep, in an infant with Ondine's Curse.

The same conclusion was reached by Sullivan et al (2) by stepwise removal of
respiratory drives in sleeping dogs. After vagal block, hyperoxia and a
metabolic alkalosis, respiration was reduced to less than one breath/min in
Quiet sleep. In Paradoxical sleep the same procedure has a much smaller effect
on respiration.

<u>AROUSAL</u>

In many respects the ventilatory responses to chemical or mechanical loads
are irrelevant. Such challenges are normally dealt with by mobilizing the
behavioral system. If a sleeper obstructs his airway in a pillow the crucial
response is arousal and a positional change. Miller et al (3) showed that in

premature infants hypoxia not only depressed ventilation; the infants didn't
wake up. When re-tested a few weeks later hypoxia stimulated ventilation, but
of more importance, there was arousal and struggling within a minute or two.
Phillipson et al have shown that arousal occurs much later in response to
hypoxia (4) and hypercarbia (5) in Paradoxical sleep than in Quiet sleep (again
suggesting that metabolic drives are less relevant in Paradoxical sleep). The
arousal threshold not only varies with sleep state, sleep quality is important.
Patients with obstructive sleep apnea have frequent arousals but the astonishing
thing is that they can be completely obstructed for long periods before they
wake up. This suggests that continual sleep disruption has progressively
raised their arousal threshold. This may be important in the etiology of the
Sudden Infant Death Syndrome. Anderson and Rosenblith (6) showed that
obstructing the airway of normal infants produced prompt arousal whereas, in
infants who subsequently became SIDS victims, there was little response. It
is worth recalling that SIDS is very common after a minor cold, which frequently
causes sleep fragmentation which could further elevate the arousal threshold.

DIAPHRAGMATIC FUNCTION

1.   Tonic Activity

It is claimed that the diaphragm has no tonic activity (7), a paucity of
muscle spindles and a weak or absent stretch reflex (8).   However, Prechtl
et al (9) have recently shown that there is substantial end expiratory tonic
activity in the infants diaphragm.   It is difficult to distinguish tonic
activity from noise and the 'noise' is often filtered out.   Prechtl was able
to establish that this signal was tonic activity as it was abolished in State 2
or Paradoxical sleep.   Our results are in complete agreement; in both infants
and adults there is tonic diaphragmatic activity in the supine position which
is abolished in Paradoxical sleep.   Further, in man, the tonic activity of the
diaphragm can be increased by abdominal loading.   This implies the presence
of spindles in the diaphragm but these are scanty in the adult and confined to
the edge of the central tendon (10).   We also found that spindles were very
hard to find in the adult.   In contrast in the infant diaphragm they were very
abundant, appearing in almost every section in the central tendon area, with
up to ten spindles per section.   The difficulty in finding them in adults is
presumably due to 'dilution', by muscle fibre growth.

The importance of this stretch reflex is that it helps keep the abdominal
contents out of the thoracic cage.   When tonic activity is lost during
Paradoxical sleep, Henderson Smart and Read showed that there was a 30% fall
in infants' thoracic gas volume (11).

The difference between these results and those in animals may reflect the
greater gravitational stresses imposed on a large biped compared to those in a
small quadruped.   Afferent proprioceptive information in the phrenic is
certainly more important in humans than in animals.   Phrenic dorsal root
section produces diaphragmatic paralysis for several weeks in humans (12) but
has no effect on respiration in cats (13).

2.   Phasic Activity

Shortening of the diaphragm in infants, particularly during Paradoxical
sleep, often causes paradoxical inward motion of the rib cage. This is a
consequence of the anatomical arrangement of the ribs in the infant. The
relative antero - posterior diameter of the rib cage is larger than in the
adult because the ribs are vertically rather than caudally inclined (Fig 2).

The pump and bucket handles are thus already raised and the vector of the diaphragmatic contraction will decrease rib cage volume, unless vigorously opposed by intercostal activity, which is absent in this sleep state.

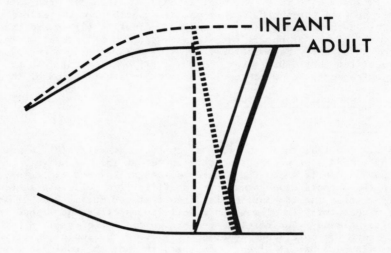

Fig. 2.   Schematic of the configuration of the ribs and
diaphragm comparing an infant and an adult.

As the diaphragm is now sucking in ribs rather than fresh air, to maintain the same tidal volume the work of breathing must increase.   However, the newborn diaphragm is poorly equipped to sustain high work loads as it has a low oxidative capacity (14).   To examine whether the infant diaphragm fatigues we used spectral frequency analysis of the surface diaphragmatic EMG as described by Kadefors et al (15).   During Quiet sleep the EMG spectrum was very similar to that of unfatigued adult skeletal muscle.   During Paradoxical sleep with marked rib cage distortion there were characteristic changes of fatigue: an increase in the low and a decrease in the high frequency power.   Similar fatigue patterns can also be demonstrated in infants who are being unsuccessfully weaned off ventilators.

The occurrence of diaphragmatic fatigue modified ventilatory control in a number of ways.   The commonest response is a gross body movement, followed by activation of the intercostals, with a fairly rapid loss of the diaphragmatic EMG fatigue pattern.   In infants with lung lesions this response is often inadequate and hypoventilation with CO_2 retention ensues.   Fatigue patterns frequently precede apnea.   In infants with normal lungs there is an increase in the total EMG power as the diaphragm fatigues.   This is accompanied by increased distortion of the rib cage and it is conceivable that the apnea is precipitated by an intercostal-phrenic inhibitory reflex.   In infants with lung problems the diaphragmatic EMG often gradually fades away and then stops, which is unlikely to be due to a distortion based reflex.

3.   Apnea

The major difference between respiration in the infant, particularly the premature infant, is the occurrence of life threatening central apnea.   This is very rare in older children and adults in the absence of a CNS lesion (although short respiratory pauses are common in Paradoxical sleep).   The basis for this is probably structural.   Sears (16) has emphasised the very large synaptic input required to depolarise a respiratory neurone.   This must be hard to achieve in the premature nervous system with its poorly developed dendritic arborisation, incomplete myelination and small neuro-transmitter stores.   The predominance of apnea in paradoxical sleep is probably due to a further reduction of inputs by inactivation of the gamma loop in the intercostals and diaphragm.

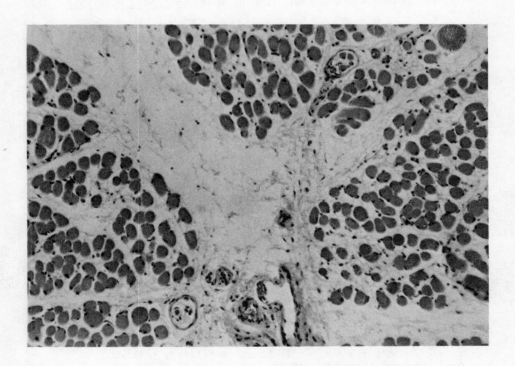

Fig. 3.   Microphotograph showing the presence of muscle
spindles in the infant diaphragm.

References

1.   Severinghaus, J., Ozanne G, and Massuda, Y. Measurement of the ventilatory
     response to hypoxia. Chest 70,121, (1976).

2.   Sullivan, C.E., Kozar, L.F., Murphy, E., and Phillipson, E.A. Primary role
     of respiratory afferents in sustaining breathing rhythm. J. Appl. Physiol.
     45:11,(1978).

3.   Miller, H.C. and Behrle, F. The effects of hypoxia on respiration of new-
     born infants. Paediatrics 14:93, (1954).

4.   Phillipson, E.A., Sullivan, C.E., Read, D.J.C., Murphy, E. and Kozar, L.F.
     Ventilatory and waking responses to hypoxia in sleeping dogs. J. Appl.
     Physiol 44:512,(1978).

5.   Phillipson, E.A., Kozar, L.F., Rebuck, A.S. and Murphy, E. Ventilatory
     and waking responses to CO_2 in sleeping dogs. Am. Rev. Resp. Dis.
     115:251,(1977).

6.   Anderson, R.B. and Rosenblith, J.F. Sudden Infant Death Syndrome: Early
     indicators. Biol. Neonate 18:395, (1971).

7.   Agostoni, E., and Sant'Ambrogio, G.   IN: The Respiratory Muscles. Eds.
     Campbell, E.J.M., Agostoni, E. and J. Newsom Davis. Pub. Lloyd Luke
     (London) 1970.

8.   Corda, M., Euler, C.von, and Lennerstrand, D.   Proprioceptive innervation
     of the diaphragm. J. Physiol (Lond) 178:161, (1965).

9.   Prechtl, H.F.R., Eykern, L.A. van and O'Brien, M.J.O. Early Human
     Develop. 1:265, (1977).

10. Winkler, P.G. and B. Delaloye. A propos de la presence de fuseaux
     neuro-musculaires dans le diaphragme   humain. Acta Anat 29:111, (1957).

11. Henderson Smart, D.J. and Read, D.J.C.   IN: Sleep Apnea Syndromes.
     Ed. Guilleminault C and W.C. Dement. Pub. A.R.Liss, New York, (1978).

12. Nathan, P.W., and Sears, T.A.   Effects of posterior root section on the
     activity of some muscles in man. J. Neurol. Neurosurg. Psychiat: 23,10,(1960)

13. Duron, B.   Postural and ventilatory functions of intercostal muscles.
     Acta Neurobiol. Exp: 33, 355, (1973).

14. Keens, T.G., Bryan, A.C., Levison, H. and Ianuzzo, C.D. Developmental
     pattern of muscle fiber types in human ventilatory muscles.
     J. Appl. Physiol. 44,909, (1978).

15. Kadefors, R., Kaiser, E. and Petersen, I.   Dynamic spectrum analysis of
     myo-potentials with special reference to muscle fatigue. Electromyography
     8:39, (1968).

16. Sears, T.A. The respiratory motor neurone and apneusis. Fed. Proc. 36:
     2412 (1977).

DISCUSSION

of the papers by Precthl et al. and Bryan and Bryan

The demonstration by Precthl et al. and by the Bryans that in the
newborn infants the relative contributions by the diaphragm and the
intercostals to the work of breathing is changing from one moment to
another gave rise to comments by Euler in support of the suggestion
that there may exist central nervous mechanisms whereby the participation in and proportional contribution to breathing of the different sets of respiratory muscles could be separately controlled in
relation e.g. to movements and posture of the trunk and to the sleep
states. It would seem likely that cerebellum is involved in such a
control. Whether or not the double representation of the motor output
from the bulbar respiratory control mechanisms i.e. from the NTS and
NRA groups in medulla may serve such a purpose remains an open question. The question was raised whether also in REM sleep the descending
pathways for automatic breathing were employed or whether in this
state the diaphragm is driven by the pathways employed by the 'behavioural' command signals.

Euler remarked that although the presence of muscle spindles in the
diaphragm have been conclusively shown e.g. for the cat both by
anatomical and functional evidence, including the demonstration of
fusimotor activation of these spindles (Corda et al., J.Physiol. 178,
161, 1965), nobody, so far, has ever been successful in provoking an
autogenetic excitation of phrenic motoneurons or a diaphragmatic
stretch reflex in spite of many efforts in that direction starting
with the classical work of Paul Hoffman and continuing with the
intracellular studies of Gill and Kuno (J.Physiol. 168, 274, 1963).
Widdicombe pointed out that many other afferents than those from
diaphragmatic muscle spindles would be of importance in controlling
the 'breaking' or 'tonic' activity in the diaphragm of the newborn.
Thus, tonic inspiration-facilitatory vagal reflexes e.g. to deflation
or compression of the lungs have been shown to occur both in the
adult and neonatal states.

The difference between fatigue and active inhibition or depression is
a key question and it would be of considerable importance to be able
to distinguish between the types of mechanical distorsions produced
by diaphragmatic fatigue and a non-fatigue decrease in diaphragmatic
activity.

There is considerable evidence for the occurrence of autogenetic
inhibition of the diaphragm. Inhibitory reflexes may also result from
Gr. III and IV muscle receptors in the diaphragm, which presumably
are responsible for the unpleasant sensations accompanying fatigue of
the diaphragm. Widdicombe made the point that if such inhibitory
reflexes were enhanced by fatigue in the diaphragm, this might
possibly contribute to the cause of apnoea. On the basis of the hypothesis of diaphragmatic fatigue and of the presence of tonic diaphragmatic activity one might expect a progressive fall in FRC with fatigue.
Whether or not such changes in FRC do occur had not been established
yet.

Harding asked if the recordings of tonic diaphragm activity really

originated from the diaphragm only or whether there might have been
a contribution from postural (intercostal) muscles as well. In the
lamb tonic diaphragmatic activity is never obtained from electrodes
in the central portion of the diaphragm. Prechtl replied that they
were absolutely sure that they were measuring activity from the diaphragm since the intercostal muscles behave so differently.

RESPIRATORY MUSCLE FATIGUE AND ITS EFFECTS ON THE BREATHING CYCLE

A. GRASSINO and F. BELLEMARE

Department of Physiology, McGill University and Department of Medicine, University of Montreal, Montreal, Canada

Studies of the breathing pattern in normal subjects at rest indicate that the minute ventilation ($\dot{V}_E$) tends to be held constant from breath to breath mainly because the mean inspiratory flow (V_T/T_I) remains constant. Departures from the mean V_E value were found to be dependent on variations in the expiratory time (T_E) (Refs. 1, 2) Cunningham and Gardner(3) further observed that increasing steady state levels of ventilation induced by CO_2 inhalation was accomplished by an increase in tidal volume (V_T) with the inspiratory time (T_I) remaining constant. They proposed that the general strategy for the respiratory control system was to increase V_E by increasing V_T/T_I. It was also pointed out that non chemical stimuli such as cortical influence (Ref. 2) external resistive loads (Refs. 4,5) or disease (Ref. 6) can deeply modify the subjacent chemical reflex. It is interesting to note that in most instances an increase in ventilation is mainly achieved by changes in V_T/T_I rather than by changes in T_I/T_{TOT}.

In the present study we have tested the possible interaction between <u>fatigue of</u> the respiratory muscles and the breathing cycle. The study consists of two parts: In the first part we examined the effect of the T_I/T_{TOT} on the time of appearance of a fatiguing pattern of contraction in the diaphragm; in the second part we performed a breath to breath analysis including the time and volume components the respiratory cycle, gastric pressure (Pg), mouth pressure (Pm) and EMG frequency analysis of the respiratory muscles in normal subjects breathing room air through high inspiratory resistance.

Effects of Changes in T_I/T_{TOT} on the Time of Appearance of a Fatiguing Pattern of Contraction in the Diaphragm.

Sustained or intermittent forceful muscle contraction of the fingers cause metabolic changes in the muscle leading to the appearance of a localized sensation of discomfort which may progress to intolerable pain (Ref. 7). The force of contraction falls gradually and a predetermined load can no longer be sustained. A similar phenomenon has been observed for the human respiratory muscles (Ref. 8). Lindström et al (9) have proposed that the slowly progressing metabolic changes in the fatiguing muscle are responsible for a decrease in the action potential velocity conduction which can be measured by surface EMG as a shift of the myoelectric power spectrum towards lower frequencies. Gross et al (10) have recently applied this technique to respiratory muscles and found that transdiaphragmatic pressure swings of about 50% of Pdi maximum resulted in a progressive decrease in the high frequency (H) component and an increase in the low frequency component (L) of the

EMG spectrum. The H/L ratio fall was interpreted as evidence of muscle changes
leading to fatigue. Pdi swings of 75% of Pdi max produced higher rates of decrease
with time in the H/L ratio of the EMG of the diaphragm than Pdi swings of 50%.

Methods

Four normal, healthy subjects with extensive experience as subjects for respiratory mechanics tests were studied.

The subjects breathe through a mouth piece, Fleisch pneumotachograph and a two-way
valve which separated the inspiratory from the expiratory line. The EMG of the
diaphragm was measured with an esophageal electrode and conditioned by a Hewlett
Packard bioelectric amplifier. In addition, Pg and Pm were measured in all subjects. All parameters were recorded on an eight channel tape recorder. The Pdi
swings were calculated by adding the value of elastic recoil of the lungs to the
sum of Pm and Pg. During the course of the test the subjects were asked to breathe

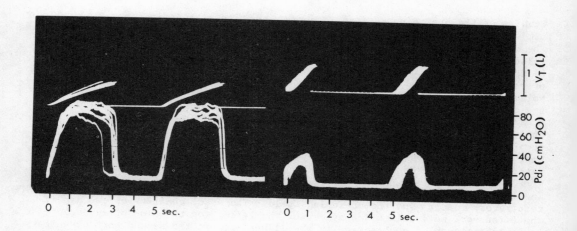

Fig.1. Respiratory cycle with T_I/T_{TOT} of .6 (left) and .3
(right). Each T_I/T_{TOT} was sustained at Pdi of 40,70 and 110 cm.
H_2O in separate runs. Tidal volume (V_T) and cycle duration
(T_{TOT}) were the same in all runs.

with a fixed T_I/T_{TOT} and Pdi for 10 minutes or less. To help accomplish this, they
were monitored from a storage oscilloscope their V_T (as measured by integration of
flow) and the time course of the breathing cycle, as shown in Fig. 1. Breathing
at T_I/T_{TOT} of .30 or .60 a variable resistance was added to the inspiratory line
of the valve and adjusted such as to enable the subject to generate with each
breath Pdi swings of about 40, 70 or 110 cm of H_2O. Each run lasted from 2 to 10
mins. A 30 min interval of rest was allowed between runs. Frequency of breathing
was constant at 12 breaths per minute, and V_T was selected in each individual
such as to provide a minute ventilation slightly higher than his resting ventilation. Pdi was displayed on the screen of the oscilloscope as well, and kept as
constant as possible.

Results

Fig. 2 shows on the left panel, the breath by breath H/L ratio of the diaphragm in one subject who is representative of the group. A significant fall in the H/L ratio can be seen starting at the 12th breath. The point of deflection (N) was

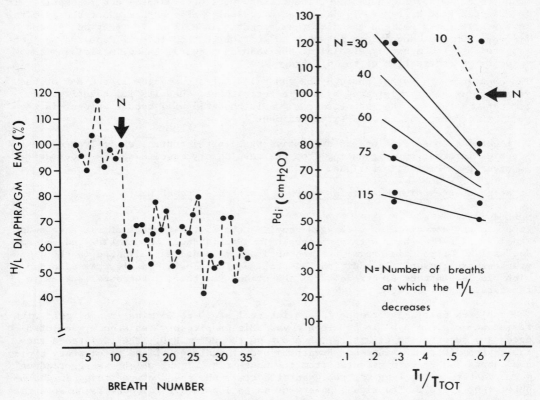

Fig. 2. Left: Time course of the high frequency/low frequency components (H/L) of the EMG of the diaphragm in a run sustained with T_I/T_{TOT} of .6 and P_{di} of 100 cm H_2O. N indicates the breath at which H/L decreased significantly. The 100% H/L was obtained by averaging the first 3 breaths. Right: Breath numbers (N) at which the H/L decreased as a function of the transdiaphragmatic pressure (P_{di}) and T_I/T_{TOT}. (o) indicates experimental results from runs obtained in two separate occasions in one subject. Lines with a negative slope are isobreath.

taken as an indication of the beginning of metabolic changes in the muscle leading to fatigue. On the right panel is shown the $T_I/T_{TOT}/P_{di}$ relationship. Each point represents the breath number at which the H/L ratio significantly decreased on each run. Isobreath isopleths were calculated by interpolation. At P_{di} below 50 cm of H_2O and up to 120 breaths there were no significant falls in the H/L ratio. Above that level an inverse relationship between the time of appearance of fatigue, and both T_I/T_{TOT} and P_{di} was observed. At P_{di} of 120 cm H_2O a fall in the H/L appeared from the 3rd breath and the run was sustained for only 2 mins. These results coincide with findings in other skeletal muscles (Ref. 7).

The application of this grid as a tool to quantify the actual course of a given pattern of breathing (example: breathing against loads) is somehow limited. In the first place it includes only the diaphragm and was calculated at a given T_{TOT} (5 sec). Furthermore each T_I/T_{TOT} was measured at a slightly different V_T/T_I in order to allow for a constant V_T, inspiratory work of breathing and isocapnia. It is expected that higher V_T/T_I, an index of velocity of contraction of the inspiratory muscles, may fatigue the diaphragm sooner than a lower V_T/T_I at any given T_I/T_{TOT}. On that account it is worth to mention that during all runs the subjects inspired by predominantly displacing the abdomen outward, hence, maximizing the velocity of contraction of the diaphragm.

The constancy of the P_{di} through the run rules out the changes in the H/L of the diaphragm as being originated by muscle recruitment. Despite its quantitative limitations the qualitative message shown in the grid will become evident in the analysis carried out in the next experiment.

We interpret these findings as suggestive that in the control of T_I/T_{TOT} some feedback information originating from the respiratory muscles may be necessary in order to avoid their fatigue.

Strategy of Breathing During Inspiratory Resistance Breathing

Methods

Five healthy normal males with ages ranging from 25 to 40 years of age have been studied while breathing with high inspiratory resistance. Mouth flow and V_T, Pm, Pg, and EMG of the diaphragm were measured and recorded as indicated in the previous experiment. In addition EMG from the intercostal muscles was recorded with bipolar surface electrodes from the second and third intercostal spaces in the paraesternal area.

The subjects initially breathe for an interval of 10 to 15 mins in a circuit with resistance of 1 cm H_2O l/sec. Then a variable inspiratory resistance was introduced and adjusted to elicit P_{di} of about 60 to 100 cm H_2O. The resistance runs lasted from 10 to 50 minutes. Breath by breath analyses of the respiratory cycle components and V_T were measured from the mouth flow signal which was recorded on magnetic tape. The tape was replayed at 8 times the speed of recording in a computer (PDP 11/70). The signal underwent an analog to digital conversion at a rate of 1000 samples per second giving 20 msec sample spacing in real time.

Further analysis was carried on from the digital data with a program written in basic and following an algorhythm similar to that described by Newsom Davis et al (2). The H/L ratio of the EMG and pressures were calculated with a digitizer from the strip chart record.

Results

Three subjects completed runs of 30 to 55 mins (subjects A, B and C). The other subjects (D and E) interrupted their run in the first 10 minutes because they felt incapable of continuing. They had a decrease in the H/L ratio of both muscles from the first few breaths and never completely recovered during the course of the run. The T_I/T_{TOT} was higher than .7 and a progressive fall in V_T/T_I (reaching values of .090 l/sec) and V_E was observed. There was a concomitant increase in end tidal CO_2. Repeated runs with the same resistance resulted in similar performances.

Figure 3 shows the initial 10 mins of the run in subject A. Following the ventilation tracing it can be noticed an initial decrease in V_E to 40% of the control values followed immediately by an increase in V_E. This increase is accomplished by an increase in T_I/T_{TOT} which rose to values of .8 (Fig. 3,(A)). V_T/T_I oscillates around a very low and constant value. In the intercostal muscles the H/L ratio remains

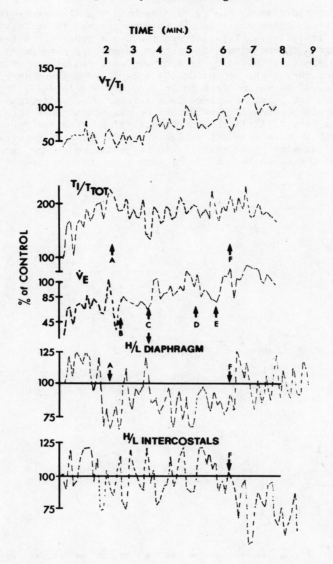

Fig.3. Breath by breath analyses in subject B breathing with
inspiratory resistance. Ordinate: T_I/T_{TOT}, V_E, V_T/T_I, and H/L
of the diaphragm and intercostal muscles. Abscissa: Time from
the introduction of the resistance. The dashed lines connect
individual breath   values. All parameters except Pg and Pm
are expressed 25% of their preresistance values.

constant up to the 6th.min (F).

The diaphragmatic H/L however, shows a fall in the last portion of the ascent of
T_I/T_{TOT} (A). Beyond point A, the T_I/T_{TOT} descends and the H/L of the diaphragm
returns to control values (B).

A new attempt to increase V_E starts, approaching the 4th minute (C). In this occasion the strategy changes. There is an upward trend in V_T/T_I with a smaller in phase increase in T_I/T_{TOT}. This pattern induces a progressive fall in the H/L ratio of the diaphragm. Beyond minute 5 (D) this attempt is terminated and a fall in V_E follows. Both ventilation and V_T/T_I approached pre-resistance values: T_I/T_{TOT} however, remains very high. At point (E) a new upward trend in V_E starts. In this case it is achieved by an increase in T_I/T_{TOT} (F) and in V_T/T_I; the diaphragmatic H/L remains low. At point (F) there is a switch; V_T/T_I increases and T_I/T_{TOT} decrease. In coincidence with the return of diaphragmatic H/L to control values is observed the first fall in the intercostal H/L. From the 7th min on V_T/T_I and V_E are successfully maintained at values close to those of non-resistive breathing. This run lasted 45 mins. The analyses of the pressure swings were omitted due to difficulties in the recording of the Pg signal in this portion of the run.

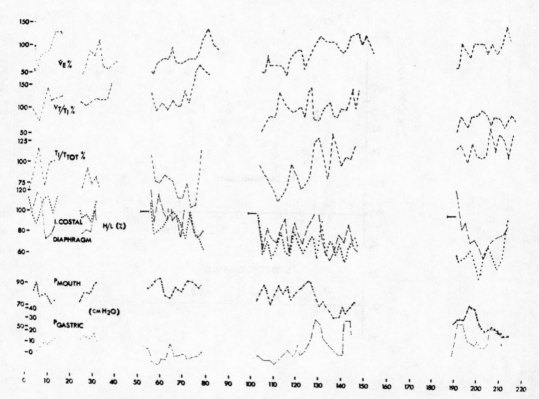

Fig.4. Breath by breath analysis in subject B breathing with inspiratory resistance. <u>Ordinate</u>: V_E, V_T/T_I, T_I/T_{TOT}, H/L of diaphragm and intercostal muscles, Pm and Pg. <u>Abscissa</u>: Breath number from the introduction of the resistance. Shown only the portions containing trends of increasing V_E.

Figure 4 shows a portion of the 50 min run obtained from subject B. It consists of a selection of parameters recorded breath by breath which are identified on the left side of each tracing. On the abscissa it is plotted the number of breaths from the beginning of the run.

In order to facilitate the visual inspection only those portions of the run in which

there was an upward trend in V_E are shown. Overall, the time course of V_E shows
cycles in which V_E oscillates from about 50% to 140% of the control(pre-resistance)
values in cycles of 10 to 40 breaths. Upon application of the inspiratory resistance there was a brief period of decrease in V_E, followed by the first upward
trend. The increases in V_E are achieved by predominantly increasing T_I/T_{TOT}
(cycles 4 and 5) or a combination of changes in the V_T/T_I and T_I/T_{TOT}. All cycles
started when either the diaphragm or intercostals EMG showed a H/L ratio close to
100% (non-fatigue) and was followed by a decrease in the H/L ratio.

P-mouth pressure and Pg indicates that each increase in V_E was in phase with an
upward trend in Pm, (cycle 2) Pg (cycle 1) or a combination of both. In most
cycles it can be seen out of phase trends between Pm and Pg which may be indica-
tive of trends in predominant intercostals or diaphragmatic contribution.

These analyses show several common trends which are repeated in the other subject,
as well, such as; a) the upward trends in V_E start when the diaphragm or intercostals H/L ratio is about 100%; b) the upward trends in ventilation are terminated
when in one of the muscles there is a fall in the H/L ratio; c) trends in increasing V_E are accomplished by a variety of V_T/T_I and T_I/T_{TOT} combinations; e) an
alternance between fatigue of the intercostals and diaphragm seems likely.

The presence of waves in V_E having periods of the order of 1 to 4 mins was suggested
previously in steady state breathing (Refs. 1, 11). Those studies include too
short periods of recording to allow definite conclusions about its characteristics
or mechanisms. The results of this study seems to show a similar tendency during
resistive breathing, with much wider oscillations in V_E. Definite conclusions,
however, cannot be drawn regarding the characteristics of the cycles,since the
present experimental protocol left some variables uncontrolled.

It is remarkable however, that in many cycles the termination of the upward trend
in ventilation coincides with a decrease in the H/L ratio of the EMG of the respiratory muscles.

If velocity of conduction of the membrane potentials is affected by accumulation of a
metabolite (Refs. 7,9) and the increasing trends in V_E are stopped when those changes
are evident, it is tempting to speculate that the fatiguing muscle may orginate
neural information which is centrally processed and originates, as a feed back an
unloading of the muscles by decreasing the V_T/T_I and/or T_I/T_{TOT}.

Summary

The time of appearance of a decrease in the H/L ratio of the EMG of the diaphragm
as a function of the T_I/T_{TOT} and P_{di} was studied in normal subjects. It was found
that the number of breaths performed before a significant decrease in the H/L ratio
occurred   inversely related to both Pdi and T_I/T_{TOT}. For a given Pdi, the H/L
ratio decreased earlier if breathing occurred at T_I/T_{TOT} of .60 as compared to .30.
We interpret these findings as an indication that the development of fatigue of the
diaphragm during loaded breathing may depend on the prevailing breathing pattern.

The analysis of the time course of the volume and time components of the respiratory
cycle, and the EMG frequency analyses during resistive inspiration suggests the
presence of mechanisms that seem to operate by trial and error in search for an
optimal pattern of breathing. These attempts are manifested by cycles of increasing
and decreasing V_E with time, each cycle carried out with a variety of combinations
of V_T/T_I and T_I/T_{TOT}, perhaps reflecting an interaction between the neural drive
and the prevailing metabolic state of the inspiratory muscles.

Acknowledgement

This research was supported by Conseil de la Recherche en Santé du Quebec and
Foundation Notre Dame. The authors wish to thank Mr. C. Pouliot for technical
assistance; Mrs. P. Bynoe for secretarial help; Mr. R. Thomson for the illustrations
Dr.J. Almirall and the Biomedical Engineering Unit for computer assistance.

References

1) I.P. Priban, An analysis of some short-term patterns of breathing in man
    at rest, J. Physiol. 166, 425 (1963).

2) J. Newsom Davis and D. Stagg, Interrelationships of the volume and time
    components of individual breaths in resting man, J. Physiol. 245, 481 (1975).

3) D.J.C. Cunningham and W.N. Gardner, The relation between tidal volume and
    inspiratory and expiratory times during steady state CO_2 inhalation in man,
    J. Physiol. 227, 50 (1972).

4) F. Zechman, F.G. Hall and W.E. Hull, Effects of graded resistances to tracheal
    air flow in man, J. Appl. Physiol. 10, 356 (1957).

5) M.D. Altose, S.G. Kelsen, N. N. Stanley, R.S. Levinson, N.S. Cherniack and
    A. Fishman, Effects of hypercapnia on mouth pressure during airway occlusion
    in conscious man, J. Appl. Physiol. 40, 338 (1976).

6) J. Sorli, A. Grassino, G. Lorange and J. Milic-Emili, Control of breathing in
    patients with chronic obstructive lung disease, Clin. Sci. Mol. Med. 54, 295
    (1978).

7) S. Rodbard and E. Bakay Pragay, Contraction frequency, blood supply, and muscle
    pain, J. Appl. Physiol. 24, 142 (1968).

8) C. Roussos and P. T. Macklem, Diaphragmatic fatigue in man, J. Appl. Physiol.
    43, 184 (1977).

9) L. Lindström, R. Kadefors and I.Petersen, An electromyographic index for
    localized muscle fatigue, J. Appl. Physiol. 43, 750 (1977).

10) D. Gross, A. Grassino, W. Ross and P. T. Macklem, The EMG pattern of diaphrag-
    matic fatigue, J. Appl. Physiol.(in press).

11) P. Dejours, R. Puccinelli, J. Armand and M. Dicharry, Breath to breath varia-
    tions of pulmonary gas exchange in resting man, Resp. Physiol. 1, 265 (1966).

INTERACTION OF NEURAL AND MECHANICAL FACTORS IN OBSTRUCTIVE SLEEP APNEA

J. E. REMMERS, W. J. deGROOT, E. K. SAUERLAND
and A. M. ANCH

Departments of Internal Medicine and Anatomy,
The University of Texas Medical Branch, Galveston, Texas, U.S.A.

INTRODUCTION

Respiratory disturbances during sleep are now recognized as a clinical disorder. The Pickwickian Syndrome probably represents a relatively common entity in which impairments of breathing during sleep produce a severe pathophysiology disturbance (1). This syndrome, occurring primarily in males, consists of hypersomnolence and cardiorespiratory failure in an obese patient. The pioneering work of Gastaut et. al. (2) established the association of this disease complex with periodic sleep apnea secondary to upper airway obstruction. The primacy of periodic sleep apnea during sleep in generating the disease complex has been demonstrated by the resolution of hypersomnolence and cardiorespiratory failure after tracheostomy (3). Phenomenologically, periodic airway obstruction usually consists of two repetitively alternating phases, one of airway patency and the other of airway occlusion (A.O.). The latter involves total inspiratory obstruction and partial expiratory obstruction; contraction of expiratory muscles can generate a very low flow through the obstructed upper airway.

Periodic AO during sleep results from occlusion of the oropharynx. This conclusion rests on three types of evidence: (1) pharyngeal intubation relieves AO (4); (2) supraglottic pressures equal esophageal pressures during inspiratory efforts against the occluded airway (4); and (3) radiographic and bronchoscopic visualizations reveal closure of the oropharyngeal airway (5,6,7,8). Although the site of occlusion during AO has now been established, the factors that lead to closure of the oropharynx remain in doubt. Two salient observations suggest alternate pathogenic mechanisms, one mechanical and one neural. On the one hand, weight loss or decrease in pharyngeal resistance usually leads amelioration of the syndrome (9), suggesting that structural alteration caused by adipose deposition produces important local mechanical alterations within the oropharynx. On the other hand, a sleep related deficit in motor activation of the upper airway musculature may contribute to AO. The oropharyngeal musculature, particularly the genioglossus muscle of the tongue, receives a respiratory modulation (10). Thach and Brouillette, in this volume, show that it acts to maintain a patent airway in rabbits (11). Posterior movement of the tongue causes oropharyngeal occlusion during anesthesia, probably because of diminished genioglossal activity (12), and the activity of this muscle declines during sleep (13).

The present communication summarizes the results of our research assessing the relative importance of passive mechanical factors versus active neural processes in the generation of oropharyngeal occlusion during sleep.

MOTOR CONTROL OF THE OROPHARYNGEAL AIRWAY DURING SLEEP

The various muscles of the upper airway are activated in synchrony with respiration. Specifically, the laryngeal abductors (14,15), the genioglossus (10), the medial pterygoids (16,17), the tensor veli palatini (16,17) and the alae nasi (18) all display inspiratory bursting, whereas the pharyngeal constrictors and laryngeal abductors exhibit expiratory activity, particularly in hypercapnic conditions (17,19). Perhaps the clearest parallel, both neurally and mechanically, exists between the laryngeal abductors and the genioglossus. Like the larynx, the oropharynx appears to be actively dilated during inspiration by contraction of the genioglossus muscle. In the supine posture this muscle displays a tonic expiratory activity as well (see Fig. 1). We have speculated that this normal behavior

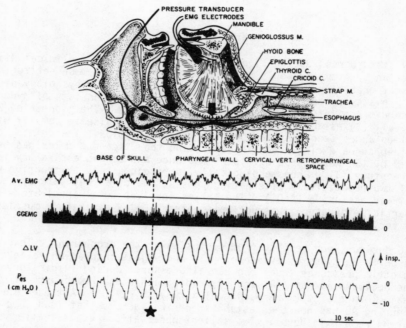

Fig. 1. Upper panel: A sagittal section of the human upper respiratory tract. VC: vocal cords. Pressure transducer shows the site of recording of pharyngeal (supraglottic) pressure. EMG electrode shows the position of intramuscular leads used in recording genioglossal EMG. The arrow marks the proposed site for interaction of genioglossal force and pharyngeal pressure. Lower panel: A recording showing the normal respiratory modulation of genioglossal activity during sleep. Top trace - average genioglossal EMG; second trace - raw EMG; third trace - changes in lung volume; bottom trace - esophageal pressure. Note that a genioglossal burst accompanies each inspiration (dashed line gives onset of inspiration) and tonic discharge persists during expiration. (Reprinted from J. Appl. Physiol., ref. 4)

insures a patent oropharynx by offsetting local mechanical factors that tend to close the airway, such as, subatmospheric pharyngeal pressure during inspiration or the action of gravity on the tongue in the supine posture. Thach and Brouillette, in this volume, provide convincing evidence in support of the former; the oropharyngeal airway of the anesthetized rabbit is much more resistant to the collapsing action of subatmospheric airway pressure when the genioglossus is innervated (11).

The activity of all the upper respiratory muscles, including genioglossus, diminishes during sleep, most strikingly during the REM phase (13,16,17,18,20). These normal alterations presumably mean that active maintenance of a patent upper airway is somewhat compromised during sleep (13,17,18,20). The diminution of laryngeal abduction increases upper airway resistance (21); the diminution of genioglossal contraction may lead to narrowing or collapse of the oropharynx if the airway pressures are quite negative or if the normal anatomical relations have been distorted (e.g., structural encroachment on the oropharyngeal lumen or opening the mouth).

PERIODIC PHENOMENA ASSOCIATED WITH A.O. DURING SLEEP

Periodic AO during sleep was documented in 12 obese hypersomnolent patients (4). In all patients, tidal breathing ceases intermittently despite persistence of rhythmic fluctuations in esophageal pressure, as shown in Fig. 2. During inspira-

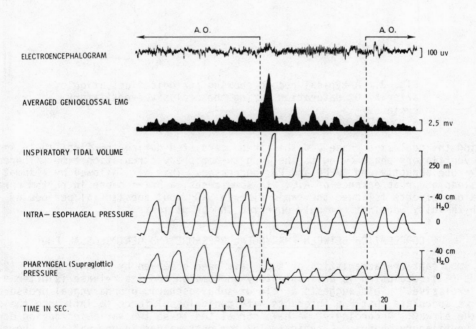

Fig. 2. Typical record obtained during periodic A.O. EEG evidence of arousal (alpha activity) occurs just prior to termination of occlusive phase, and sleep onset occurs coincident with onset of A.O. Note that the peak EMG coincides with termination of the occlusive phase. (Reprinted from J. Appl. Physiol., ref. 4)

tory efforts against the occluded airway (AO), pharyngeal (supraglottic) pressure
(Pph) and esophageal pressure (Pes) were nearly equal and increased steadily,
typically reaching values of 50-70 cmH2O after 30-45 sec. Genioglossal activity
occurred in rhythmic inspiratory bursts, waxing and waning in relation to the
periodic breathing cycle. The discharge was relatively low at the beginning of the
occlusive phase and was consistently the highest at the end of that phase.
Throughout the occlusive phase, genioglossal EMG (GGEMG), Pph and Pes increased
steadily as the patient became progressively more hypoxic. During the ventilatory
phase, GGEMG and Pes declined whereas Pph tended to be relatively low and constant.

These periodicities in Pes, Pph and GGEMG are associated with large fluctuations in
respiratory drive consequent to cyclic changes in chemical stimuli. Arterial oxygen saturation (SaO2) provides a valid index of the time course of hypoxic stimulation of the peripheral chemoreceptors as shown in Fig. 3. SaO2 decreased

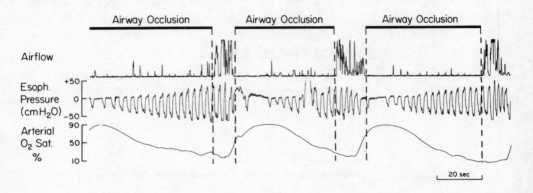

Fig. 3. A typical record showing periodic fluctuation of
arterial O2 saturation during the occlusive/ventilatory
cycle.

during the occlusive phase and this trend persisted during the first 10-15 sec. of
the ventilatory phase owing to the lung-to-periphery circulation time. Thereafter,
SaO2 rose abruptly and GGEMG and Pes decreased. This was followed by resumption
of sleep and reappearance of A.O. In some cases, a brief pause in rhythmic respiratory efforts followed the rapid rise in SaO2, but substantial periods of
arrhythmicity were not commonly observed in our patients.

CORRELATION BETWEEN PHARYNGEAL PRESSURE AND GENIOGLOSSAL EMG

Two important characteristics of A.O. have been observed by Gastaut et al. (2) and
by us (4): occlusion is an inspiratory phenomenon and its release is often sudden
or "explosive." This suggests a role of subatmospheric oropharyngeal pressure,
and we speculate that Pph interacts with genioglossal force to influence the state
of the airway. Accordingly, we have correlated these two variables during occluded
and ventilatory phases. A typical plot for peak values in one patient, shown in
Fig. 4, reveals two separate correlations, one for unoccluded breaths and one for
occluded efforts. Neither variable alone predicts the state of the airway, but
their combination uniquely describes whether or not the oropharynx is occluded.
The dashed line separates all unoccluded from occluded efforts and can be viewed
as indicating the values where a critical balance exists between the constricting
action of Pph and the dilating action of genioglossal force.

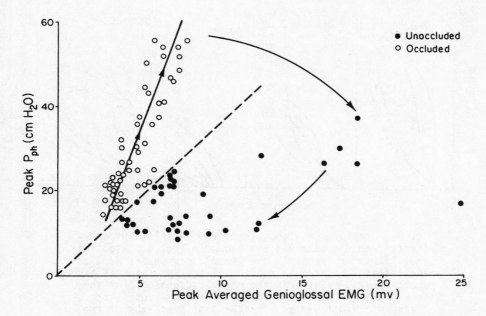

Fig. 4. Relation between peak pharyngeal pressure and peak
averaged genioglossal EMG for all inspiratory efforts during
a series of occlusive/ventilatory cycles. Note that the regression for unoccluded breaths is separated from that for
occluded efforts. The dashed line segregates the two. The
ventilatory phase begins with points lying at the extreme
right and ends with points lying just to the right of the
segregating line. During the occlusive phase points scatter
upward along the solid line, and termination of occlusion
is associated with rightward and downward movement of points
(upper arrow). (Reprinted from J. Appl. Physiol., ref. 4)

CAUSAL RELATIONSHIPS IN PERIODIC A.O.

In order to identify various factors' contribution to the periodicities observed in
our patients, we have analyzed separately the factors influencing onset, maintenance and termination of occlusion.

1.   <u>Onset of Occlusion</u> - the dynamic relationship between Pph and GGEMG during
the ventilatory phase provides some insights, as shown in Fig. 5. The initial
breaths in this phase (right panel) describe widely open, counter clockwise loops,
i.e., GGEMG leads Pph. This suggests that strong contraction of the genioglossus
early in inspiration dilates the oropharynx, minimizing the rise in Pph, thereby
maintaining the balance of forces in favor of a patent lumen. In subsequent
breaths (middle panel), the loop narrows, i.e., GGEMG and Pph change in phase.
Pharyngeal resistance has increased, presumably because a lower genioglossal force
has allowed the oropharynx to narrow. This means that the balance of forces is
shifting and is approaching a critical value (dashed line). In fact, the airway
occludes on the next breath. Overall, therefore, the ventilatory phase witnesses
a progressive shift in the balance between dilatory and constrictive forces that

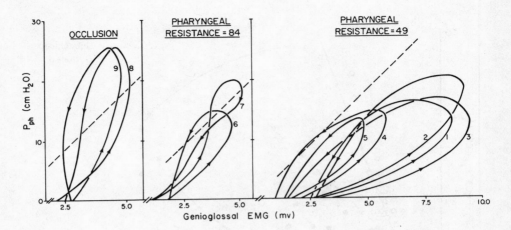

Fig. 5. Pressure/EMG loops for 9 sequential inspiratory
efforts from the same patient shown in Fig. 4. Right hand
panel: first 5 breaths in the ventilatory phase; Middle
panel: last 2 breaths in the ventilatory phase; Left hand
panel: first 2 breaths in the occlusive phase. For the
first 5 breaths the GGEMG leads Pph and the resistance
equals 49 cmH2O/1 per s. For the last 2 breaths of the
ventilatory phase the phase shift between the 2 variables
is less, and pharyngeal resistance equals 84 cmH2O/1 per s.
During the occlusive phase the loops are nearly vertical
and cross the segregating line (Reprinted from J. Appl.
Physiol., ref. 4)

ultimately leads to airway closure.

This proposed causal sequence for the institution of occlusion neglects the possible actions of other muscles that may tend to close the oropharynx. Bronchoscopic
and radiographic visualizations indicate that the site of initial closure may be
high in the oropharynx, at the level of the soft palate (7,22). Weitzman et al.
observed circumferential constriction here and postulate that contraction of con-
strictor muscles at the beginning of inspiration actively closes the pharynx at
the junction between the oropharynx and nasopharynx. What muscle groups may cause
this sphinteric action is uncertain. The normal behavior of the pharyngeal constrictors would not suggest a role for these muscles.

Another candidate is the soft palate. Relaxation of the tensor veli palatini might
narrow the airway at the level of the soft palate and increase pharyngeal resistance. This muscle displays an inspiratory bursting pattern entirely comparable
to the genioglossus, and it undergoes a similar diminution during sleep (17).
Anatomically, one can reasonably assume that tensor contraction maintains a patent
airway at the top of the oropharynx. Accordingly, one can advance an hypothesis
similar to that described for the genioglossus. The activity of the tensor might
decrease during the ventilatory phase causing an increase in pharyngeal resistance.
Greater sub-atmospheric values of Pph would tend to occlude the airway at this
site.

2. Maintenance of Occlusion - During the occlusive phase, Pph and GGEMG increase
together, describing a linear mutual relationship (Fig. 4). Peak Pph equals peak

Pes, and the latter value, in turn, reflects force developed by diaphragm and inspiratory intercostals during isometric contraction. Accordingly, the slope of
this regression represents the change in relative inspiratory motor output to the
two types of inspiratory muscles, those generating intrapleural pressure and those
acting to dilate the oropharynx. Therefore, the slope of this regression represents a fundamental characteristic of automatic respiratory motor control during
sleep when challenged by an asphyxiant stimulus. As depicted in Fig. 6, the slope

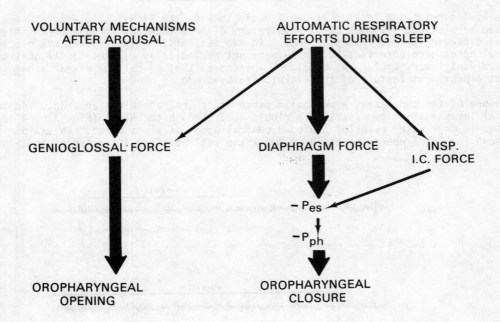

Fig. 6. Proposed schema depicting neural events during
periodic airway occlusion. During sleep the contraction
of the diaphragm is unchanged from wakefulness but the activities of the genioglossal and inspiratory intercostal
muscles is diminished. During airway occlusion, the recruitment of the genioglossus in relation to the diaphragm is
inadequate to open the airway. The occlusive phase is terminated by arousal and recruitment of non-automatic mechanisms which differentially activate genioglossal motoneurons.

indicates the relative recruitment of these two types of muscles when the sleeping
individual receives an hypoxic/hypercapnic stimulus. Assuming that the dashed line
in Fig. 4 represents the critical balance of forces acting on the oropharynx, we
conclude that the recruitment pattern in these patients favors maintenance of
occlusion, i.e., the slope is so steep that with increasing respiratory drive,
points move away from the dashed line.

Termination of Occlusion - Release of occlusion is characteristically associated
with a very pronounced GGEMG burst in which genioglossal discharge is elevated
from the beginning of the inspiratory effort. Another feature is antecedant EEG
evidence of arousal. These findings suggest the causal sequence depicted in

Fig. 6: hypoxic stimulation disrupts sleep which, in turn, engages non-automatic mechanisms projecting to genioglossal motoneurons, thereby increasing genioglossal force in relation to Pph so that the airway opens. On the Pph vs GGEMG plot, one observes a striking rightward and downward movement (upper arrow). In other words, the sudden activation of the genioglossus appears to reflect a neural discontinuity, and the fundamental characteristic governing recruitment of the two types of muscles during sleep no longer applies.

CENTRAL VERSUS OBSTRUCTIVE APNEA

We have carried out 24 studies on 12 patients with the Pickwickian Syndrome and have rarely observed absence of respiratory efforts (central apnea) for an interval exceeding 3 respiratory periods. In two patients, protracted periods of central apnea were observed, but these were not periodically related to the obstructive/ventilatory cycle. We conclude, therefore, that so-called "mixed" apnea is not a prominent feature of the Pickwickian Syndrome.

In one of the two cases, a metabolic cause of central apnea was apparent. An initial investigation demonstrated periodic A.O. through the night (Fig. 3). A second study 4 days later revealed profound central apnea at sleep onset. An example is shown in Fig. 7 where the observer awoke the patient after 2 minutes of apnea.

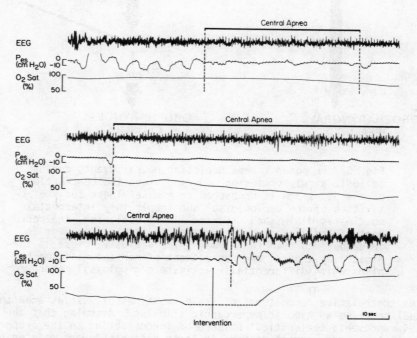

Fig. 7. A continuous trace recorded during a second study on the patient shown in Fig. 3. The record was obtained shortly after sleep onset and shows two prolonged periods of central apnea during which arterial O2 saturation drops to low levels. At the point marked intervention, the observer awoke the patient. The appearance of central apnea in this patient was associated with a severe metabolic alkalosis.

Arterial PO$_2$ at this time was 22 mmHg and the pH was 7.51. We relate this life-threatening episode to a severe metabolic alkalosis (plasma bicarbonate concentration = 33 mmHg) perhaps consequent to diuretic therapy. After repeated episodes of severe hypoxemia the metabolic alkalosis resolved somewhat, and a regular respiratory rhythm appeared. Ultimately, the acid-base balance returned to normal and periodic A.O., indistinguishable from that observed initially, was observed.

This case is reminiscent of the central apnea during sleep reported by Phillipson et al. (23) in dogs with a metabolic alkalosis, breathing oxygen and with vagal blockade. As in our case, the dogs displayed a normal respiratory rhythm while awake. This case emphasizes the dependence of the rhythm on chemical drive during sleep. Furthermore, it suggests that therapeutic agents that may cause metabolic alkalosis should be used with caution in such patients.

ACKNOWLEDGEMENTS

This research was supported by the National Heart, Lung and Blood Institute Research Grant HL-18007 and by Grant RR-73 from the General Clinical Research Centers Program of the Division of Research Resources, National Institutes of Health. J.E. Remmers is the recipient of National Institutes of Health Pulmonary Academic Award 5K07-HL-00131. A.M. Anch is a National Institutes of Health Postdoctoral Trainee (Grant HL-07217).

REFERENCES

(1) C. Guilleminault, A. Tilkian and W.C. Dement, The sleep apnea syndromes, Ann. Rev. Med. 27, 465-484 (1976).

(2) H. Gastaut, B. Duron, C.A. Tassinari, S. Lyagoubi and J. Saier, Mechanism of the respiratory pauses accompanying slumber in the Pickwickian Syndrome, Activitas Nervosa Super. 11, 209-215 (1969).

(3) G. Coccagna, M. Mantovani, F. Brignani, C. Parchi and E. Lugaresi, Tracheostomy in hypersomnia with periodic breathing, Bull. Physio-Pathol. Respirat. 8, 1217-1227 (1972).

(4) J.E. Remmers, W.J. deGroot, E.K. Sauerland and A.M. Anch, Pathogenesis of upper airway occlusion during sleep, J. Appl. Physiol. 44, 931-938 (1978).

(5) B.A. Schwartz and J.P. Escande, Respiration hypnique pickwickienne, In: The abnormalities of sleep in man, Eds. H. Gastaut, E. Lugaresi, G. Berti Ceroni and G. Coccagna, Bologna, Gaggi 209-214 (1968).

(6) R.E. Walsh, E.D. Michealson, L.E. Harkerload, A. Zighelboim and M.A. Sackner, Upper airway obstruction in obese patients with sleep disturbance and somnolence, Ann. Internal Med. 76, 185-192 (1972).

(7) S. Smirne and G. Comi, The obstructive mechanism in Pickwickian Syndrome: a serial x-ray study, Sleep Res. 4, 237 (1976).

(8) I. Karacan, C. Ware, C. Moore and B. Derrent, Disturbed sleep as a function of sleep apnea; too much sleep but not enough, Texas Med. 73, 49-56 (1977).

(9) C.A. Tassinari, B. DallaBernadina, F. Cirignotta and G. Ambrosetto, Apneic
     periods and the respiratory related arousal patterns during sleep in
     Pickwickian Syndrome. A polygraphic study, Bull. Physio-Pathol.
     Respirat. 8, 1087-1102 (1972).

(10) E.K. Sauerland and S.P. Mitchell, Electromyographic activity of intrinsic and
     extrinsic muscles of the human tongue, Texas Rept. Biol. Med. 33, 445-
     455 (1975).

(11) B.T. Thach and R.T. Brouillette, The respiratory function of pharyngeal mus-
     culature: relevance to clinical obstructive apnea, In this volume.

(12) P. Safar, L.A. Escarrago and F. Chang, Upper airway obstruction in the uncon-
     scious patient, J. Appl. Physiol. 14, 760-764 (1959).

(13) E.K. Sauerland and R.M. Harper, The human tongue during sleep: electromyogra-
     phic activity of the genioglossus muscle, Exptl. Neurol. 51, 160-170
     (1976).

(14) D. Bartlett, Jr., J.E. Remmers and H. Gautier, Laryngeal regulation of
     respiratory airflow, Respir. Physiol. 18, 194-204 (1973).

(15) J.E. Remmers and D. Bartlett, Jr., Reflex control of expiratory airflow and
     duration, J. Appl. Physiol. 42, 80-87 (1977).

(16) L.E. Hairston, E.K. Sauerland and W.C. Orr, The role of oropharyngeal muscles
     in respiration: An electromyographic study during wakefulness and sleep,
     Anat. Rec. 190, 411 (1978).

(17) L.E. Hairston, The role of oropharyngeal muscles during respiration: an elec-
     tromyographic study during wakefulness and sleep, Ph.D. Thesis, Univer-
     sity of Texas Medical Branch, Galveston, Texas (1978).

(18) J.H. Sherry and D. Megirian, State dependence of upper airway respiratory
     motoneurons: functions of the cricothyroid and nasolabial muscles of the
     unanesthetized rat, Electroenceph. Clin. Neurophysiol. 43, 218-228
     (1977).

(19) H. Gautier, J.E. Remmers and D. Bartlett, Jr., Control of the duration of ex-
     piration, Respir. Physiol. 18, 205-221 (1973).

(20) J. Orem, P. Norris and R. Lydic, Laryngeal abductor activity during sleep,
     Chest 73, 300-301 (1978).

(21) J. Orem, A. Netick and W.C. Dement, Increased upper airway resistance to
     breathing during sleep in the cat, Electroenceph. Clin. Neurophysiol.
     43, 14-22 (1977).

(22) E.D. Weitzman, C.P. Pollak, B. Borowiecki, B. Burack, R. Shprintzen and S.
     Rakoff, The hypersomnia-sleep apnea syndrome: site and mechanism of
     upper airway obstruction, In: Sleep Apnea Syndromes, eds. C. Guillemi-
     nault and W.C. Dement, Liss: New York 235-248 (1978).

(23) E.A. Phillipson, C.E. Sullivan, D.J.C. Read, E. Murphy and L.F. Kozar, Venti-
     latory and waking responses to hypoxia in sleeping dogs, J. Appl.
     Physiol. 44, 512-520 (1978).

Discussion after the paper by Lugaresi et al.

THE RESPIRATORY FUNCTION OF PHARYNGEAL MUSCULATURE: RELEVANCE TO CLINICAL OBSTRUCTIVE APNEA*

B. T. THACH and R. T. BROUILLETTE

Edward Malinckrodt Department of Pediatrics, Washington University School of Medicine, and the Division of Neonatology, St. Louis Children's Hospital, St. Louis, Missouri, U.S.A.

INTRODUCTION

Episodic upper airway obstruction ("obstructive apnea") is common during anesthesia in man (1). It also occurs during sleep in adults and children with idiopathic sleep apnea (2,3), in the Pickwickian syndrome (4,5,6), in children with adenoid hypertrophy (3,7), in the Pierre Robin syndrome (8,9), and in sudden infant death "near miss" infants (10,11,12). Some patients with obstructive apnea have documented anatomical abnormalities of the airway; some have abnormalities of central respiratory control, while others have no known abnormality. Use of monitoring techniques that detect obstructed breaths is enlarging this list of syndromes. Thus idiopathic apneic spells of preterm infants long assumed to be "central" or "diaphragmatic" in origin (13) have recently been shown to include obstructed respiratory efforts in many (10,14) or most (15) spells (Fig. 1).

In adult patients with sleep apnea, and in anesthetized subjects as well, there is strong evidence that the site of obstruction is in the oropharynx, behind the tongue (1,5). Other important questions regarding the mechanism of obstruction remain unanswered. How can the sudden onset and equally sudden recovery be explained? What has sleep in common with anesthesia that would explain why obstruction is associated with both? Why is there an association between sleep obstruction and partial airway obstruction (e.g., adenoid hypertrophy)? Why is a posture of cervical flexion associated with recurrent episodes of airway obstruction (15)?

Recently Remmers, de Groot, Sauerland, and Anch (5) formulated a comprehensive hypothesis for the mechanism of airway obstruction during sleep apnea which potentially explains these associations. This hypothesis, an amplification of one originally proposed by Gastaut, Tassinari and Duron (4), is based on observations of pharyngeal pressure and genioglossus muscle activity in "Pickwickian" patients with episodes of obstructive apnea. In Remmers' view, the genioglossus is a respiratory muscle whose activity is required to prevent pharyngeal closure due to

---

*These studies were supported in part by: The Life Seekers, N.I.H. grant 56545A, N.I.C.H.D. grant H.D. 10993-02, and by an American Lung Association Training Fellowship (Robert T. Brouillette). The authors are indebted to Lois Price and Sheila Prensky for assistance in preparing the manuscript and illustrations.

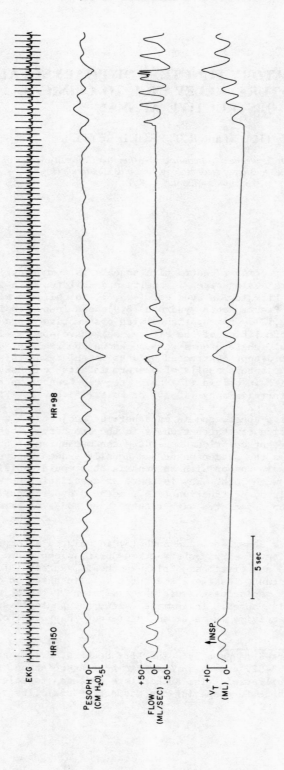

Fig. 1. Obstructive apnea. Two episodes of spontaneous airway obstruction in a preterm infant with the clinical diagnosis of "apnea of prematurity." Tracings, from top to bottom, are: electrocardiogram, esophageal pressure (15), nasal airflow and integrated tidal volume. Respiratory flow was recorded using nasal prongs and a screen flowmeter. The patient was sleeping, lying supine with the neck unflexed. Obstructed breaths are indicated by absent nasal airflow with esophageal pressure fluctuations. Bradycardia occurs during the first but not the second episode. Recovery from obstruction was spontaneous in each instance. Other spells recorded in this infant were "mixed apnea" - a period of diaphragmatic apnea preceding one or more obstructed inspiratory efforts prior to spontaneous recovery. Recordings made by the authors.

negative pressure during inspiration: "The oropharynx occludes whenever the constricting action of the transpharyngeal pressure exceeds the dilating action of genioglossus muscle force." Recent observations in an animal model provide a direct test of the Gastaut-Remmers hypothesis and extend this concept to include other pharyngeal muscles (16,17).

OBSERVATIONS OF THE RESPIRATORY FUNCTION OF PHARYNGEAL MUSCLES IN AN ANIMAL MODEL

We have examined upper airway patency in rabbits when transmural pressure is lowered. We insert an airway in one nostril, seal the mouth and other nostril, and place a non-obstructing canula in the thoracic trachea via a low tracheal incision. Pressures are recorded at the nose and trachea (Fig. 2). In dead animals, pressure is reduced in the airway by occluding the nasal opening and withdrawing air by syringe from the trachea. In spontaneously breathing animals, airway pressure is reduced by allowing the animal to inspire after the artificial nasal airway has been occluded.

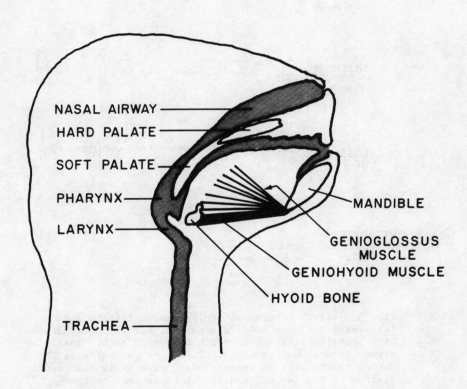

Fig. 2. Schematic of the extra-thoracic airway of the rabbit.

Our findings can be summarized as follows: 1) The pressure required to passively
collapse the upper airway ("closing pressure") in the post mortem animal is -5 to
-7 cm H$_2$O; the site of collapse appears to be the pharynx. 2) During nasal
occlusion maneuvers in living, lightly anesthetized animals, the airway remains
open at pressures down to -60 cm H$_2$O; the disparity between the pressures required
to produce airway closure in dead as opposed to living animals suggests that
muscular activity opposes closure in the latter case (Fig. 3). 3) Electromyographic EMG recordings from genioglossus and geniohyoid muscles reveal phasic
inspiratory activity. 4) Further observations indicate that these muscles
prevent airway closure during nasal loading maneuvers.

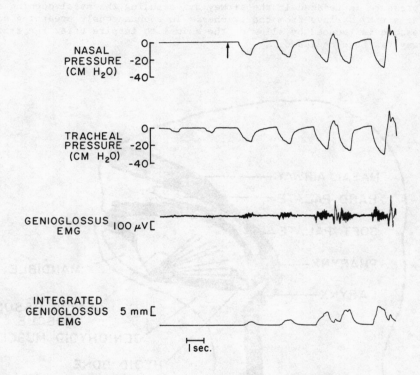

Fig. 3. Airway pressures, genioglossus activity and
integrated activity (34) in a rabbit, lightly anesthetized
with pentothol. Front of mouth is sealed shut. Nasal
airway is occluded at arrow. Increased genioglossus EMG
during inspiration of pre-occlusion breaths is just barely
visible in the raw EMG and is not registered by the
integrated EMG because of low amplification. Note recruitment of genioglossus activity in the first occluded breath
and progressive recruitment thereafter. Note identical
pressure traces at trachea and nose indicating upper airway
patency. In the fourth and fifth breaths, movement artifacts
in the EMG trace are associated with generalized somatic
movements and these probably indicate arousal.

Evidence that the genioglossus-geniohyoid muscles maintain airway patency is as
follows: 1) Closure during inspiration is observed when genioglossus-geniohyoid
activity is depressed by deep anesthesia or is abolished by denervation (section
of the hypoglossal nerves) (Fig. 4). 2) Following an occlusion maneuver in deeply
anesthetized animals, the airway closes during early inspiration; the transpharyngeal
pressure at which the airway closes is linearly related to peak integrated
genioglossus EMG. 3) Simulating the effect of genioglossus-geniohyoid contraction
in the dead animal by displacing the hyoid bone towards the muscular origin on the
mandible increases the amount of negative pressure required to produce closure -
in other words, anterior hyoid-tongue displacement "stiffens" the pharyngeal
airway.

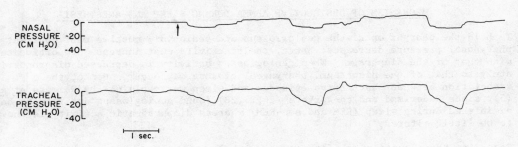

Fig. 4. Similar preparation as in Fig. 3 except that the
hypoglossal nerve (twelfth) has now been sectioned
bilaterally, paralyzing the genioglossus and geniohyoid
muscles. Artificial nasal airway is occluded at arrow.
Note that nasal pressure fails to decrease to levels as
low as tracheal pressure on these occluded inspirations
indicating airway closure. The lowest pressure reached
is termed airway "closing pressure." There is a slight
decrease in closing pressure from the first (C.P. = -8 cm
H_2O) to the third breath (C.P. = -11 cm H_2O).

It should be pointed out that our observations indicate that the genioglossus and
geniohyoid are the primary muscles that hold the airway open during inspiration;
however, these same observations indicate that they are not the sole muscles having
this effect. This conclusion is based on observations in bilaterally twelfth nerve
sectioned animals. During progressive asphyxia, there is a progressive decrease
in airway closing pressure (Fig. 4). We therefore conclude that additional muscles,
not innervated by the twelfth nerve and stimulated by asphyxia, influence closing
pressure to some degree. These muscles have yet to be identified.

Reflex Augmentation of Pharyngeal Muscular Activity During Respiratory Loading

When upstream resistance is increased, peak inspiratory airway pressures can be
expected to become more negative (18). In this situation, if pharyngeal pressure
falls below the critical closing pressure, closure will occur and tidal volume

will be compromised. One might predict reflex augmentation of genioglossus and geniohyoid activity in this circumstance. We have evidence for such reflexes in the rabbit. As can be seen in Fig. 3, when the nasal airway is suddenly occluded at end-expiration, genioglossus EMG activity of the first breath following occlusion is increased. This occurs before there could be an asphyxial change in blood gases, hence chemoreceptors can be ruled out as the mediators. By analogy to intercostal muscles and diaphragm, where similar responses to loading are observed (19), one might guess that Hering-Breuer stretch receptors and/or intrinsic muscle spindles are responsible. However, the latter can be ruled out, since the rabbit and other sub-primates have been found to lack genioglossus muscle spindles (20). Man, on the other hand, has numerous genioglossus spindles (21). Since the Hering-Breuer reflex is weak in man (22), it is tempting to speculate that genioglossus muscle spindles may be important in maintaining his pharyngeal airway in accommodation to varying naso-pharyngeal resistance.

MECHANISM OF OBSTRUCTIVE APNEA DURING SLEEP AND ANESTHESIA

To hold the pharynx open, the genioglossus and geniohyoid muscles must contract as pharyngeal pressure decreases; hence, their activity must increase proportionately with that of the diaphragm. When genioglossus activity is depressed disproportionately to that of the diaphragm, pharyngeal closure may occur. Hence, the association between obstructive episodes and sleep was explained by Remmers et al. (5), since Sauerland and co-workers (26,27,28) found genioglossus activity to be diminished during sleep (REM and non-REM) whereas diaphragmatic activity is known to be little altered.

Regarding the significance of the critical balance between genioglossus-geniohyoid and diaphragm activity, the rabbit offers a model for obstructive apnea during sleep since pentobarbital anesthesia depresses genioglossus muscle activity disproportionate to that of the diaphragm. In this laboratory model, the result of selective genioglossus-geniohyoid depression is an increased tendency for airway obstruction during nasal loading. In fact, these observations in the rabbit provide evidence for the mechanism of airway obstruction during general anesthesia in man. On the basis of indirect evidence, Safar et al. (1) concluded that obstruction during anesthesia was due to "flaccid pharyngeal walls" and a "relaxed tongue." It is interesting to note that Safar observed increased airway obstruction in obese anesthetized patients compared to non-obese controls. This may be on the basis of anatomical narrowing of the pharyngeal airway by adipose tissue as Remmers et al. (5) speculated. In any event, this observation links sleep obstructive apnea in obese "Pickwickian" subjects to pharyngeal obstruction induced by anesthesia. It is noteworthy that reduction of body weight in the "Pickwickian" patients can eliminate sleep apnea (6).

It should be pointed out that obstructing the nasal airway is required to demonstrate pharyngeal closure in the anesthetized rabbit, whereas closure is observed in sleeping or anesthetized man in the absence of any identifiable increased nasal resistance. This observation suggests that the rabbit pharynx may have a greater intrinsic rigidity (i.e., more negative post mortem closing pressure) than that of man. In other words, man may be more dependent on pharyngeal muscles for airway maintenance than other species.

MECHANISM OF PERIODICITY AND SPONTANEOUS RECOVERY FROM
RECURRENT OBSTRUCTIVE APNEA

Relevant to the phenomenon of spontaneous recovery from apnea are observations of the influence of progressive asphyxia on pharyngeal musculature of the rabbit. We have observed that asphyxia has an effect opposite to that of pentobarbital. Thus, genioglossus activity is preferentially increased over activity of inspiratory pressure generating muscles during progressive asphyxia. This can be seen in Fig. 5. Both integrated EMG and tracheal inspiratory pressure increase with successive occluded inspiratory efforts, presumably as a result of increasing chemoreceptor activity (29). This relation is not linear: There is greater increment in genioglossus EMG than in airway pressure. Since inspiratory pressure has been found to be proportionate to phrenic nerve activity (30), we conclude that as asphyxia increases, it becomes an increasingly more potent stimulus for the genioglossus muscle than for the diaphragm. This observation is of particular significance to the phenomenon of spontaneous recovery from obstructive apnea, since the ultimate effect of preferential genioglossus excitation would be relief of airway obstruction.

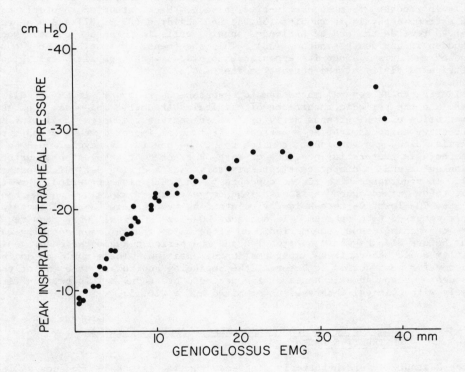

Fig. 5. Data obtained from rabbit prepared as in Fig. 3. Peak inspiratory tracheal pressures and peak integrated genioglossus EMG of inspiratory efforts following nasal occlusion maneuvers: Values to left are from breaths soon after onset of occlusions; values to right are from subsequent breaths. Progressive decrease in tracheal pressure and increase in genioglossus activity result from chemostimulation. Note the preferential augmentation of genioglossus activity compared to that of pressure generating muscles.

What is the origin of this differential effect of chemostimulation on two different respiratory muscles? Remmers et al. (5) have observed this phenomenon in patients during obstructive apnea episodes. Preferential recruitment of the genioglossus was associated with a generalized "arousal" pattern in the EEG. Remmers concluded that voluntary respiratory pathways of the forebrain were responsible for preferential excitation. We have observed behavioral arousal (increased somatic activity) during airway occlusion maneuvers in lightly anesthetized rabbits (Fig. 3), in which case preferential excitation of genioglossus is usually present. However, we also see preferential excitation when there is no evidence of behavioral arousal. Therefore, in rabbits at least, this phenomenon could primarily involve brain stem or "involuntary" respiratory pathways.

Studies of the relation of head-neck posture to upper airway patency suggest additional mechanisms for sponteneous recovery from obstructive apnea. Cervical extension has the effect of drawing the tongue forward thereby enlarging the pharyngeal airway (1,31,32). Involuntary cervical extension, therefore, could result in recovery from an obstructive episode. Neck extension regularly occurs with extreme asphyxia in rabbits (33,34) and children (35,36,37) and has been observed towards the end of prolonged apneic spells in infants who later succumbed to sudden infant death syndrome (38). This phenomenon is attributed to "cortical release" mechanisms since its appearance coincides with asphyxial depression of electrical activity of the cerebral cortex (34,37).

Considering these several mechanisms of spontaneous recovery, it is not difficult to explain the periodic recurrence of clinical obstructive episodes. The asphyxial augmentation of genioglossus activity (or neck extensor muscles) following an obstructive episode might be expected to last until improved ventilation corrected asphyxial blood gas tensions, at which point the obstructive cycle would be repeated. In preterm infants, one or more obstructed breaths often occur at the beginning or end of diaphragmatic respiratory pauses during periodic breathing (15). In accordance with recent concepts of the mechanism of periodic breathing (39), these "mixed apnea" episodes might conceivably be explained on the basis of a higher CO_2-lower O_2 threshold for maintaining hypocapneic "apnea" of genioglossus muscle compared to diaphragm. If a higher CO_2-lower O_2 level were required to drive the genioglossus, the periodic suppression of genioglossus activity would occur before diaphragmatic suppression and the periodic augmentation of genioglossus activity would occur after diaphragmatic augmentation. There would be an increased tendency for obstruction to occur at the beginning and towards the end of the episodes of diaphragmatic apnea during periodic breathing. This pattern fits closely with clinical observations of mixed apnea (10,15).

RELATION OF INCREASED NASAL RESISTANCE TO CLINICAL OBSTRUCTIVE APNEA

In the Gastaut-Remmers hypothesis, increased nasal resistance produces a "load" on the genioglossus muscle in the form of increased negative pharyngeal pressure swings during inspiration. Remmers et al. (5) view this as the basis for obstructive apneic episodes in children with adenoid and tonsil hypertrophy (3,7). The tendency for pharyngeal obstruction in such individuals is increased, since the "constricting action of the transpharyngeal pressure" potentially increases disproportionately to the "dilating action of genioglossus muscle force." The same mechanism could account for the increased incidence of apnea in sudden infant death "near miss" patients during episodes of otherwise uncomplicated naso-pharyngitis (23,24,25). Increased nasal resistance would be expected as a consequence of inflammatory edema of the nasal mucosa. As mentioned previously, prolonged apneic spells in these infants have been observed to be mixed or obstructive apnea (10,12).

MECHANISM OF PHARYNGEAL OBSTRUCTION ASSOCIATED WITH CERVICAL FLEXION AND WITH MICROGNATHIA

The frequency of mixed and obstructive apneic spells is increased in preterm infants when resting in a spontaneously assumed posture of cervical flexion (15). Some spells occur shortly after onset of flexion; however, others occur much later on. Therefore, the immediate mechanical effect of neck flexion by itself does not explain the association. Neck flexion displaces the base of the tongue backward towards the posterior pharyngeal wall (32,40); this maneuver invariably obstructs the airway of lightly anesthetized adults (1). In contrast, Shelton and Bosma (31) have shown that conscious subjects maintain or even increase their airway dimensions during voluntary neck flexion. Maintenance of the pharyngeal airway appeared to be the effect of "involuntary" activity of tongue muscles, since none of the subjects could voluntarily narrow his pharyngeal airway while maintaining a flexed posture. In the sleeping infant this postural regulation of genioglossus tone is presumably diminished often leading to complete airway obstruction when his neck is passively flexed (41). In this case, even when complete occlusion does not occur, if neck flexion displaces the tongue backward into the pharynx, increased shortening of the genioglossus muscle would be required to maintain normal airway dimensions. The genioglossus muscle in this instance is mechanically disadvantaged; increased neural input would be required to maintain airway patency. By similar logic, Remmers et al. (5) argued that structural encroachment on the pharyngeal lumen would require increased genioglossus activity to restore airway dimensions. In the absence of compensatory genioglossus activity, narrowing of the airway would impose a "load" on the genioglossus by increasing naso-pharyngeal resistance. Posterior displacement of the tongue is a well-known feature of congenital micrognathia (Pierre Robin syndrome) (8,31,42); therefore, the combination of increased pharyngeal resistance and a mechanically disadvantaged genioglossus muscle potentially explains the episodic obstructive apnea that characterizes this syndrome (8,9).

Why are obstructive and mixed apneic spells associated with neck flexion intermittent? Observations in healthy term infants suggest that the response of their pharyngeal muscles to asphyxia is similar to that of the rabbit (41). When the neck of a sleeping infant is passively flexed, one often sees complete obstruction of the first several respiratory efforts (Fig. 6). In subsequent respiratory efforts, the obstruction is frequently partially or completely relieved. Spontaneous restoration of airway patency can occur in the absence of behavioral arousal or change in the infant's neck posture.

Presumably, recovery of airway patency in these infants is due to asphyxial recruitment of genioglossus-geniohyoid muscles. Augmentation of diaphragmatic activity occurs during the first five post-occlusion breaths in infants (43,44). Since increased diaphragmatic activity would tend to maintain pharyngeal obstruction, restoration of the airway while in the flexed posture probably involves some degree of preferential activation of pharyngeal muscles. Periodic recurrence of obstructive episodes while the neck is maintained in a flexed posture would be on the same basis as periodic episodes in neutral neck postures. Following spontaneous recovery from an episode of obstruction, preferential recruitment of pharyngeal muscles would improve ventilation, relieve asphyxia and thereby create conditions which predispose to recurrence of obstruction.

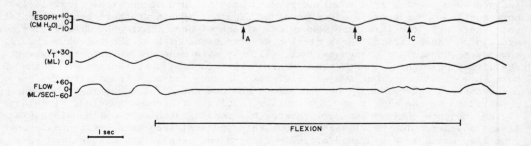

Fig. 6. Esophageal pressure, respiratory flow and integrated
flow (VT) recorded using a face mask in a sleeping term
infant. Note complete obstruction of the airway of first
inspiration after flexion (↑A). The second inspiratory
effort (↑B) produces slight flow (9 ml/sec.) and the third
(↑C) greater flow (28 ml/sec.). There is a progression
from infinite inspiratory resistance after onset of flexion
towards lower inspiratory resistance even though head-neck
posture did not change. The infant did not arouse during
the maneuver. Recordings by A.R. Stark and B.T. Thach (41).

SUMMARY

The genioglossus and geniohyoid muscles of the rabbit have phasic inspiratory
activity. These muscles normally function to hold the pharyngeal airway open at
low transmural pressure. Like other respiratory muscles, activity appears to be
servo-regulated by mechanoreceptors and chemoreceptors. These observations of
pharyngeal airway regulation in an animal model strongly support the Gastaut-
Remmers hypothesis for the mechanism of obstructive apnea in man. This hypothesis
can explain many heretofore unrelatable features of clinical obstructive apnea.
These include: 1) the prevalence of spells during sleep; 2) the relation of
episodes during sleep to those during anesthesia; 3) the mechanism of periodicity
in and spontaneous recovery from obstructive apnea; 4) obstructive apnea
associated with anatomical airway narrowing or increased nasal resistance;
5) increased episodes associated with cervical flexion; and 6) obstructive apnea
associated with micrognathia.

REFERENCES

(1) P. Safar, L.S. Escarraga and F. Chang, Upper airway obstruction in the
        unconscious patient, J. Appl. Physiol. 14, 760 (1959).
(2) C. Guilleminault, A. Tilkian, and W.C. Dement, The sleep apnea syndromes,
        Ann. Rev. Med. 27, 465 (1976).
(3) C. Guilleminault, F.L. Eldridge, F.B. Simmons, and W.C. Dement, Sleep apnea
        in eight children, Pediatrics 58, 23 (1976).

(4) H. Gastaut, C.A. Tassinari, and B. Duron, Polygraphic study of the episodic diurnal and nocturnal (hypnic and respiratory) manifestations of the Pickwick syndrome, Brain Research 2, 167 (1966).

(5) J.E. Remmers, W.J. de Groot, E.K. Sauerland, and A.M. Anch, Pathogenesis of upper airway occlusion during sleep, J. Appl. Physiol. 44, 931 (1978).

(6) M.D. Simpser, D.J. Strieder, M.E. Wohl, A. Rosenthal, and S. Rockenmacker, Sleep apnea in a child with the Pickwickian syndrome, Pediatrics 60, 290 (1977).

(7) R.E. Kravath, C.P. Pollak, and B. Borowieki, Hypoventilation during sleep in children who have lymphoid obstruction treated by nasopharyngeal tube and T and A, Pediatrics 59, 865 (1977).

(8) W.M. Dennison, The Pierre-Robin syndrome, Pediatrics 36, 336, (1965).

(9) L.M. Stern, E.W. Foukalsrud, P. Hassakis, and M.H. Jones, Management of Pierre-Robin syndrome in infancy by naso-esophageal intubation, Amer. J. Dis. Child. 124, 78 (1972).

(10) C. Guilleminault, R. Peraita, M. Souquet, and W.C. Dement, Apneas during sleep in infants: possible relationship with sudden infant death syndrome, Science 190, 677 (1975).

(11) C. Guilleminault, R. Ariagno, M. Souquet, and W.C. Dement, Abnormal polygraphic findings in near-miss sudden infant death, Lancet June, 1326 (1976).

(12) R.L. Ariagno, C. Guilleminault, and L.E. Nagel, Mixed and obstructive sleep apnea in 3-month-old control and near miss for sudden infant death syndrome infants, Pediat. Res. 12, 519 (1978).

(13) W.J.R. Daily, M. Klaus, and H.B. Meyer, Apnea in premature infants: monitoring-incidence, heart rate changes, and an effect of environmental temperature, Pediatrics 43, 510 (1969).

(14) A.F. Korner, C. Guilleminault, J. Van den Hoed, and R.B. Baldwin, Reduction of sleep apnea and bradycardia in preterm infants on oscillating waterbeds: a controlled polygraphic study, Pediatrics 61, 528 (1978).

(15) B.T. Thach and A.R. Stark, Spontaneous neck flexion and airway obstruction during apneic spells in preterm infants, J. Pediat., in press.

(16) R.T. Brouillette and B.T. Thach, Closing pressure of the extrathoracic airway, Fed. Proceedings 37, 554 (1978).

(17) R.T. Brouillette and B.T. Thach, A neuromuscular mechanism preventing airway obstruction, Pediat. Res. 12, 558 (1978).

(18) S.G. Kelson, M.D. Altose, M.N. Stanley, R.S. Levinson, N.S. Cherniack, and A.P. Fishman, Effect of hypoxia on the pressure developed by inspiratory muscles during airway occlusion, J. Appl. Physiol. 40, 372 (1976).

(19) G. Sant'Ambrogio and J.G. Widdicomb, Respiratory reflexes acting on the diaphragm and inspiratory intercostal muscles of the rabbit, J. Physiol. London 180, 766 (1965).

(20) A. Carleton, Observations on the problem of the proprioceptive innervation of the tongue, J. of Anat. 72, 502 (1938).

(21) J.P. Bowman (1971), The Muscle Spindle and Neural Control of the Tongue, Thomas, Springfield, IL.

(22) A. Guz, M.I. Noble, D. Trenchard, H.L. Cochrane, and A.R. Makey, Studies on the vagus nerves in man: their role in respiratory and circulatory control, Clin. Sci. 27, 293 (1964).

(23) A. Steinschneider, Prolonged apnea and the sudden infant death syndrome clinical and laboratory observations, Pediatrics 50, 646 (1972).

(24) A. Steinschneider, Nasopharyngitis and prolonged sleep apnea, Pediatrics 56, 967 (1975).

(25) A. Steinschneider, Nasopharyngitis and the sudden infant death syndrome, Pediatrics 60, 531 (1977).

(26) E.K. Sauerland and R.M. Harper, The human tongue during sleep: electromyographic activity of the genioglossus muscle, Exptl. Neurol. 51, 160 (1976).

(27) E.K. Sauerland and S. Mitchell, Electromyographic activity of intrinsic and

extrinsic muscles of the human tongue, <u>Texas Rep. Biol. Med</u>. 33, 445 (1975).

(28) E.K. Sauerland and S.P. Mitchell, Electromyographic activity of the human
     genioglossus muscle in response to respiration and to positional changes
     in the head, <u>Bull. Los Angeles Neurol. Soc</u>. 35, 69 (1970).

(29) M. Younes, W. Arkinstall, and J. Milic-Emili, Mechanism of rapid ventilatory
     compensation to added elastic loads in cats, <u>J. Appl. Physiol</u>. 35, 443,
     (1973).

(30) F.L. Eldridge, Relationship between respiratory nerve and muscle activity
     and muscle force output, <u>J. Appl. Physiol</u>. 39, 567 (1975).

(31) R.L. Shelton and J.F. Bosma, Maintenance of the pharyngeal airway, <u>J. Appl.
     Physiol</u>. 17, 209 (1962).

(32) S. Morikawa, P. Safar, and J. De Carlo, Influence of the head-jaw position
     upon upper airway patency, <u>Anesthesiol</u>. 22, 265, (1961).

(33) A.C.M. Campbell, K.W. Cross, G.S. Dawes, and A.I. Hyman, A comparison of air
     and O_2 in a hyperbaric chamber or by positive pressure ventilation in the
     resuscitation of newborn rabbits, <u>J. Pediat</u>. 68, 133 (1971).

(34) E.E. Lawson and B.T. Thach, Respiratory patterns during progressive asphyxia
     in newborn rabbits, <u>J. Appl. Physiol</u>. 43, 468 (1977).

(35) H. Gastaut and Y. Gastaut, Electroencephalography and clinical study of
     anoxic convulsions in children: their location within groups of infantile
     convulsions and their differentiation from epilepsy, <u>Electroencephalog.
     and Clin. Neurophysiol</u>. 10, 607 (1968).

(36) E.W. Gauk, L. Kidd, and J.S. Prichard, Mechanisms of seizures associated with
     breathholding spells, <u>New Eng. J. Med</u>. 268, 1436 (1963).

(37) C.T. Lombroso and P. Lerman, Breathholding spells (cyanotic and pallid
     infantile syncope), <u>Pediatrics</u> 39, 563 (1967).

(38) M.H. Stevens, Sudden unexplained death in infancy: observations on the natural
     mechanism of adoption of the face down position, <u>Amer. J. Dis. Child</u>. 110,
     243 (1965).

(39) N.S. Cherniack, C. von Euler, I. Homma, and I. Kao, Animal models of periodic
     breathing, (in this symposium volume).

(40) G.M. Ardran and F.H. Kemp, The mechanism of changes in form of the cervical
     airway in infancy, <u>Med. Radiogr. Photogr</u>. 44, 26 (1968).

(41) A.R. Stark and B.T. Thach, Mechanisms of airway obstruction leading to apnea
     in newborn infants, <u>J. Pediat</u>. 89, 982 (1976).

(42) P. Robin, Glossoptosis due to atresia and hypotrophy of the mandible, <u>Amer. J.
     Dis. Child</u>. 48, 541 (1934).

(43) H.W. Taeusch, S.C. Carson, I.D. Frantz, and J. Milic-Emili, Respiratory
     regulation after elastic loading and CO_2 rebreathing in normal term infants,
     <u>J. Pediat</u>. 88, 102 (1976).

(44) I.D. Frantz, S.M. Adler, I.F. Abroms, and B.T. Thach, Sleep state and
     maturation: respiratory response to airway occlusion in newborn infants,
     <u>J. Appl. Physiol</u>. 41, 634 (1976).

Discussion after the paper by Lugaresi et al.

POLYGRAPHIC AND CINERADIOGRAPHIC ASPECTS OF OBSTRUCTIVE APNEAS OCCURRING DURING SLEEP: PHYSIOPATHOLOGICAL IMPLICATIONS

E. LUGARESI, G. COCCAGNA and F. CIRIGNOTTA

Clinical Neurologica dell' Università di Bologna, Italy

Obstructive apneas appear during sleep intermittently in heavy snorers and almost continuously in patients suffering from "Hypersomnia with Periodic Apneas" (HPA). These apneas have negative consequences on alveolar ventilation and on circulation (1, 2). On the basis of personal polygraphic and cineradiographic observations, we would like to discuss briefly: 1) the reasons why in cases of heavy snoring, obstructive apneas occur in light slow sleep (stages 1-2) and in REM sleep, but not in deep slow sleep (stages 3-4); 2) the reasons why obstructive apneas are particularly prolonged during REM sleep; 3) the reasons why snoring and HPA are more frequent in men than in women; 4) the most likely mechanisms of the obstruction of the upper respiratory tracts, as suggested by the cineradiographic images.

1. Obstructive Apneas Appear During Snoring in Light Slow Sleep, but not in Deep Slow Sleep

Snoring is a prevalently inspiratory noise which is accompanied by a marked activity of intercostal muscles and by an abnormal increase in intrathoracic negative pressure: it is connected, therefore, with a stenosis of the upper airways.
This stenosis is particularly intense in deep slow sleep (stages 3-4): nevertheless, obstructive apneas appear in light sleep (stages 1-2) and in REM sleep (1). Figure 1 shows the polygraphic recording of a heavy snorer who had obstructive apneas during light sleep (stage 2), but never in deep slow sleep (stage 4), despite the fact that the inspiratory effort to overcome the obstruction of the upper airways was stronger in the latter stage (see intercostal EMG and intraesophageal pressure).

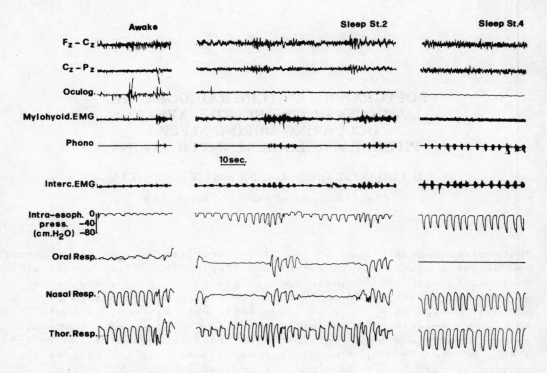

Fig. 1 – Polygraphic recording of a heavy snorer (for explanation see text)

Figure 2 shows the polygraphic recording of a mild form of HPA in which obstructive apneas appeared only in REM sleep, despite the fact in this stage of sleep the stenosis of the upper airways was much less intense than in deep slow sleep (see endoesophageal pressure).

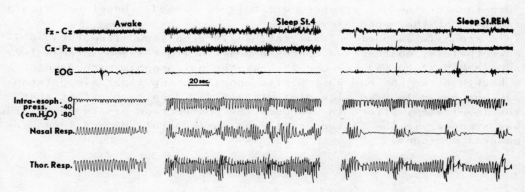

Fig. 2 – Polygraphic recording of a patient with a mild form of HPA

In heavy snorers and in mild forms of HPA, the appearance of obstructive apneas in sleep stages in which the stenosis of the upper
airways is less intense might be due to a phasic decrease in the
activity of respiratory centres resulting not only in a reduction
or arrest of the respiratory movements, but also in a decrease in the
tone of oro-pharingeal muscles. The latter phenomenon underlies the
complete obstruction of the upper airways.

2. Obstructive Apneas are Particularly Prolonged in the REM Stage

On the average, in severe cases of HPA, obstructive apneas had a
duration of 29 sec (range 11-140 sec) in Non-REM sleep and of 41 sec
(range 10-180 sec) in REM sleep (2).
The polygraphic aspects of apneas are also different in Non-REM sleep.
In Non-REM sleep, ineffective inspiratory efforts progressively
increase until breathing is resumed, whereas in REM sleep, they do
not show such a progressive intensification.
Figure 3 shows that during Non-REM sleep, in the course of a series
of obstructive apneas, the inspiratory efforts to overcome the
obstruction (see intraesophageal pressure) progressively increase,
reaching their maximum intensity just when oral and nasal respiration
is resumed.

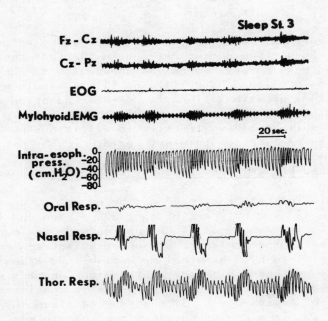

Fig. 3 - Polygraphic recording of an obstructive apnea
during Non-REM sleep

Figure 4 shows that in REM sleep, during a very protracted obstructive apnea, ineffective inspiratory efforts present an irregular pattern, and, above all, that their intensity do   not increase progressively during the suspension of oral and nasal airflow.

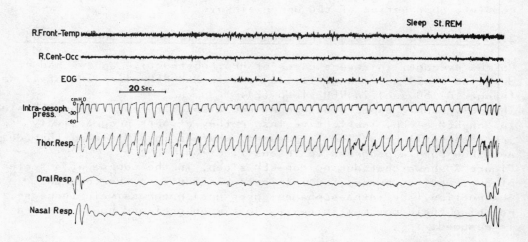

Fig. 4 - Polygraphic recording of a patient with HPA during REM sleep

The absence of an intensification in inspiratory efforts during apneas arising in REM sleep might be related to the fact that in this stage of sleep the respiratory centre, as shown with different techniques by Parmeggiani (3) and by Phillipson (4) is hardly excitable by different kinds of stimulation. The greater duration of apneas during REM sleep might be explained by the fact that in this stage of sleep chemical stimuli are less effective in eliciting the "arousal" necessary for respiration to start again.

3. Snoring and HPA are More Frequent in Men than in Women

An epidemiological study carried out by us on 3,000 persons has shown that, between 50 and 60 years of age, 30% of men and 18% of women snore habitually. Among our 35 HPA patients 33 are men and only 2 women. The marked predominance of men among snorers and HPA patients might be explained by a hormonal mechanism: the stimulating action of progesterone on the respiratory centre might protect women from these respiratory disturbances. This hypothesis is consistent with the observation of Newsom-Davis (5) that during sleep the respiratory response to CO_2 is more intense in women than in men.
Other important factors might be the different anatomical conformation of the upper airways.

4. Probable Mechanisms of the Obstruction of the Upper Airways
   (Presentation of a film)

The cineradiographic study of respiration during sleep and wakefulness
has allowed us to make the following observations:

1) In snorers, during inspiration, the hypnogenic stenosis of the
   upper airways causes an abnormal increase in negative intrathoracic
   pressure which, in its turn, promotes the donward stretching of
   the larynx and the further narrowing of the air-space between the
   tongue and the posterior wall of the pharynx.

2) In heavy snorers, and particularly in HPA patients, the phenomenon
   illustrated above may be so intense as to result in the complete
   occlusion of the oro-pharynx with a valve mechanism. The repeated,
   increasingly strong respiratory efforts than become ineffective,
   until the increase of the tone of the oro-pharyngeal muscles, on
   a sudden arousal, re-opens the upper airways.

3) In only one case the mechanism eliciting the apnea was the occlusior
   of the glottis. In this patient, the obstructive apnea came after
   a central (diaphragmatic) arrest of respiration. During this
   central arrest, the epiglottis slowly came down on the glottis.
   When breathing was resumed, during the first inspiratory act the
   occlusion of the glottis became total (this was demonstrated by
   the considerable increase in the air-space between the epiglottis
   and the posterior wall of the tongue) (Fig. 5).

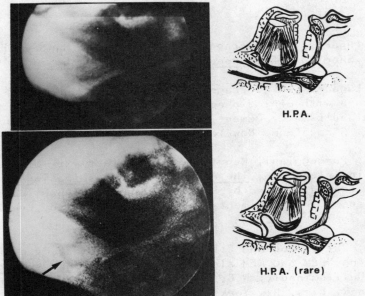

H.P.A.

H.P.A. (rare)

Fig. 5 - Obstructive apnea due to the collapse of the oro-
         pharyngeal wall (top) and to the valve-like drop
         of the epiglottis (arrow) on the glottis (bottom)

4) During obstructive apneas, the cardiac shadow enlarges and the pulmonary vessels are congested (Fig. 6).

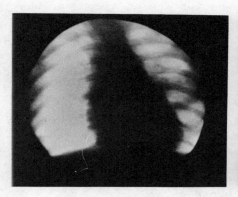 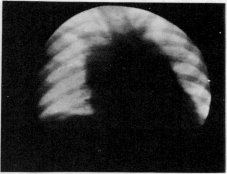

Fig. 6 - Cardiac shadow during quiet breathing (left) and obstructive apnea (right)

It would be important to investigate to which extent and with which mechanism this engorgement of the venous circulation is responsible for the pulmonary and systemic hypertension that appears during apneas.

REFERENCES

1. E. Lugaresi, G. Coccagna, P. Farneti, M. Mantovani and F. Cirignotta, Snoring - Electroenceph. clin. Neurophysiol. 39, 59 (1975)

2. E. Lugaresi, G. Coccagna, M. Mantovani, and F. Cirignotta, Hypersomnia with periodic apnea. - In: Narcolepsy. Edited by C. Guilleminault, W.C. Dement, P. Passouant - Advances in sleep research, vol. 3 Spectrum, New York 1976 p. 351.

3. P.L. Parmeggiani, Regulation of the activity of respiratory muscles during sleep. In: The regulation of respiration during sleep and anesthesia. Edited by R.S. Fitzgerald, H. Gautier, S. Lahiri Advances in experimental medicine and biology, vol. 99, Plenum, New York 1978 p. 47

4. E.A. Phillipson and C.E. Sullivan, Respiratory control mechanisms during NREM and REM sleep. - In: Sleep apnea syndromes. Edited by C. Guilleminault, W.C. Dement - Kroc Foundation Series, vol. 11 Alan R. Liss, New York 1978 p. 47

5. J. Newsom Davis, L. Loh, J. Nodal, and M. Charnock, Effects of sleep on the pattern of CO_2 stimulated breathing in males and females. - In: The regulation of respiration during sleep and anesthesia.

Edited by R.S. Fitzgerald, H. Gautier, S. Lahiri Advances in experimental medicine and biology, vol. 99 - Plenum, New York 1978 p. 79

DISCUSSION

on the papers by Remmers et al., Thach and Brouillette and
Lugaresi et al.

The cause of the obstructive apnoea in adults was discussed. Remmers reported that 80 to 90 per cent of the cases had abnormal airway anatomy such as micrognathia, enlarged tonsills or were very obese. But in the remaining 10 to 20 percent no anatomical explanation was found.

Snoring may be involved to a large extent in the initiation of airway occlusion. Thach remarked that even if people with normal airways usually do not get obstructed during sleep, obstructive apnoea is fairly common in lightly anaesthetized adults in prone or supine positions and that this condition appears in nearly every one when the neck is flexed.

Thach was asked by Widdicombe whether the genioglossus muscle is controlled like the diaphragm by the Hering-Breuer inflation reflex. Thach replied that this had been tested by vagotomy which abolished the response. Widdicombe remarked that the Hering-Breuer reflex is far weaker in man than in the rabbit and if this is true for the genioglossus muscle as for the diaphragm this might explain some of the differences between pharyngeal closure in man and rabbit.

SUBJECT INDEX

503

ABBREVIATIONS

CIA   central inspiratory activity

COPD chronic obstructive pulmo-
      nary disease

CPAP continuous positive airway
      pressure

CSF   cerebral spinal fluid

DRG   dorsal respiratory group
      (nuclear complex of tractus
      solitarius, NTS)

EMG   electromyography

EPSP excitatory postsynaptic
      potential

FBM   fetal breathing movements

FRC   functional residual capacity

IPSP inhibitory postsynaptic
      potential

ISF   interstitial fluid

kPa   kiloPascal (SI unit for
      pressure)
      1 kPa = 7.5 mm Hg
      (1 mm Hg = 0.133 kPa)

NPG   nucleus paragigantocellularis

NRA   nucleus retroambigualis

NTS   nucleus tractus solitarius
NST

Phr_T tidal phrenic activity

PSP   postsynaptic potential

REM   rapid eye movements

RMV   respiratory minute volume

SIDS sudden infant death syndrome

SWS   slow wave sleep

T_E duration of expiration

T_I duration of inspiration

T_{TOT} breath duration

$\dot{V}$ minute ventilation

VRG   ventral respiratory group
      (nucleus retroambigualis,
      NRA)

V_T tidal volume